Clinical Nutrition

Guest Editor

RAYMOND J. GEOR, BVSc, MVSc, PhD

VETERINARY CLINICS OF NORTH AMERICA: EQUINE PRACTICE

www.vetequine.theclinics.com

Consulting Editor
A. SIMON TURNER, BVSc, MS

April 2009 • Volume 25 • Number 1

SAUNDERS an imprint of ELSEVIER, Inc.

W.B. SAUNDERS COMPANY
A Division of Elsevier Inc.

1600 John F. Kennedy Boulevard • Suite 1800 • Philadelphia, Pennsylvania 19103

http://www.vetequine.theclinics.com

VETERINARY CLINICS OF NORTH AMERICA: EQUINE PRACTICE Volume 25, Number 1
April 2009 ISSN 0749-0739, ISBN-13: 978-1-4377-0556-0, ISBN-10: 1-4377-0556-1

Editor: John Vassallo; j.vassallo@elsevier.com
Developmental Editor: Donald Mumford

Veterinary Clinics of North America: Equine Practice (ISSN 0749-0739) is published in April, August, and December by Elsevier Inc., 360 Park Avenue South, New York, NY 10010-1710. Business and Editorial Offices: 1600 John F. Kennedy Blvd., Suite 1800, Philadelphia, PA 19103-2899. Customer Service office: 11830 Westline Industrial Drive, St. Louis, MO 63146. Subscription prices are $200.00 per year (domestic individuals), $332.00 per year (domestic institutions), $100.00 per year (domestic students/residents), $233.00 per year (Canadian individuals), $415.00 per year (Canadian institutions), $269.00 per year (international individuals), $415.00 per year (international institutions), and $136.00 per year (international and Canadian students/residents). To receive student/resident rate, orders must be accompanied by name of affiliated institution, date of term, and the signature of program/residency coordinator on institution letterhead. Orders will be billed at individual rate until proof of status is received. Foreign air speed delivery is included in all *Clinics* subscription prices. All prices are subject to change without notice. **POSTMASTER:** Send address changes to *Veterinary Clinics of North America: Equine Practice,* 11830 Westline Industrial Drive, St. Louis, MO 63146. Customer Service (orders, claims, online, change of address): Elsevier Periodicals Customer Service, 11830 Westline Industrial Drive, St. Louis, MO 63146. Tel: 1-800-654-2452 (U.S. and Canada); 314-453-7041 (outside U.S. and Canada). Fax: 314-523-5170. E-mail: journalscustomerservice-usa@elsevier.com (for print support); journalsonlinesupport-usa@elsevier (for online support).

Reprints. For copies of 100 or more of articles in this publication, please contact the Commercial Reprints Department, Elsevier Inc., 360 Park Avenue South, New York, NY 10010-1710. Tel.: 212-633-3812; Fax: 212-462-1935; E-mail: reprints@elsevier.com.

Veterinary Clinics of North America: Equine Practice is covered in *MEDLINE/PubMed (Index Medicus), Excerpta Medica, Current Contents/Agriculture, Biology and Environmental Sciences, and ISI.*

Printed and bound in the United Kingdom
Transferred to Digital Print 2011

Contributors

CONSULTING EDITOR

A. SIMON TURNER, BVSc, MS
Diplomate, American College of Veterinary Surgeons; Professor, Department of Clinical Sciences, College of Veterinary Medicine and Biomedical Sciences, Colorado State University, Fort Collins, Colorado

GUEST EDITOR

RAYMOND J. GEOR, BVSc, MVSc, PhD
Diplomate, American College of Veterinary Internal Medicine; Professor and Chairperson, Department of Large Animal Clinical Sciences, Veterinary Medical Center, College of Veterinary Medicine, Michigan State University, East Lansing, Michigan

AUTHORS

FRANK M. ANDREWS, DVM, MS
Diplomate, American College of Veterinary Internal Medicine; Director, Equine Health Studies Program; and LVMA Equine Committee Professor, Department of Veterinary Clinical Sciences, School of Veterinary Medicine, Louisiana State University, Baton Rouge, Louisiana

IVETA BECVAROVA, DVM, MS
Diplomate, American College of Veterinary Nutrition; Clinical Assistant Professor, Department of Large Animal Clinical Sciences, Virginia-Maryland Regional College of Veterinary Medicine, Virginia Tech, Blacksburg, Virginia

ELIZABETH A. CARR, DVM, PhD
Diplomate, American College of Veterinary Internal Medicine; Diplomate, American College of Veterinary Emergency and Critical Care; Associate Professor, Department of Large Animal Clinical Sciences, College of Veterinary Medicine, Michigan State University, East Lansing, Michigan

ANDY E. DURHAM, BSc, BVSc, CertEP, DEIM, MRCVS
Diplomate, European College of Equine Internal Medicine; The Liphook Equine Hospital, Liphook, Hampshire, United Kingdom

ANNA M. FIRSHMAN, BVSc, PhD
Diplomate, American College of Veterinary Internal Medicine; Department of Veterinary Population Medicine, University of Minnesota, Saint Paul, Minnesota

RAYMOND J. GEOR, BVSc, MVSc, PhD
Diplomate, American College of Veterinary Internal Medicine; Professor and Chairperson, Department of Large Animal Clinical Sciences, Veterinary Medical Center, College of Veterinary Medicine, Michigan State University, East Lansing, Michigan

PATRICIA HARRIS, MA, PhD, VetMB, MRCVS
Diplomate, European College of Veterinary Comparative Nutrition; WALTHAM Centre for Pet Nutrition, Leicestershire, United Kingdom

SUSAN J. HOLCOMBE, VMD, MS, PhD
Diplomate, American College of Veterinary Surgeons; Diplomate, American College of Veterinary Emergency and Critical Care; Associate Professor, Department of Large Animal Clinical Sciences, College of Veterinary Medicine, Michigan State University, East Lansing, Michigan

BECKY HOTHERSALL, PhD
Research Assistant, School of Veterinary Science, University of Bristol, Langford, United Kingdom

NICOLA G. JARVIS, BVetMed, MRCVS
Senior Veterinary Surgeon, Redwings Horse Sanctuary, Hapton, Norwich, Norfolk, England, United Kingdom

ERICA C. McKENZIE, BSc, BVMS, PhD
Diplomate, American College of Veterinary Internal Medicine; Department of Clinical Sciences, College of Veterinary Medicine, Oregon State University, Corvallis, Oregon

HAROLD C. McKENZIE III, DVM, MS
Diplomate, American College of Veterinary Internal Medicine; Assistant Professor of Equine Internal Medicine, Marion DuPont Equine Medical Center, Virginia-Maryland Regional College of Veterinary Medicine, Virginia Polytechnic and State University, Leesburg, Virginia

CHRISTINE NICOL, MA, DPhil
Professor of Animal Welfare, School of Veterinary Science, University of Bristol, Langford, United Kingdom

R. SCOTT PLEASANT, DVM, MS
Diplomate, American College of Veterinary Surgeons; Associate Professor, Department of Large Animal Clinical Sciences, Virginia-Maryland Regional College of Veterinary Medicine, Virginia Tech, Blacksburg, Virginia

RILLA E. REESE, BS
Graduate Student, Department of Animal Sciences and Large Animal Clinical Sciences, The University of Tennessee College of Veterinary Medicine, Knoxville, Tennessee

CRAIG D. THATCHER, DVM, MS, PhD
Diplomate, American College of Veterinary Nutrition; Professor, School of Applied Arts and Sciences, Arizona State University, Mesa, Arizona

Contents

Veterinarians are a primary source of nutritional information and advice for horse owners. This article reviews methods for clinical assessment of nutritional status and feeding programs that can be applied to an individual horse or group of horses. Physical examination, including measurement of body weight and evaluation of body condition score, estimation of nutrient requirements and the nutrient content of the horse's diet, and evaluation of the feeding method are important components of the assessment. Ongoing clinical assessment of health and body condition will gauge the need for reassessment of the feeding plan. Obvious indications for prompt reevaluation of diet and feeding include changes in health status (eg, body condition), life stage or physiologic state (eg, pregnancy), or performance status.

The feeding of "low carbohydrate" or "low glycemic" diets has been recommended for management of horses with metabolic and endocrine disorders in which insulin resistance is a component. A "low carbohydrate" diet is a misnomer, however, because horses require that a significant proportion of their daily ration comprises structural carbohydrates (fiber/forage) to maintain gut health and mental wellbeing. This article provides a detailed description of the different carbohydrates in equine feeds. It also reviews the terminology used to describe glucose and insulin responses to the ingestion of carbohydrates, in particular the concept of the glycemic index. Some of the factors that influence glycemic index in humans and the glycemic response to a meal in horses are also discussed.

Laminitis is a painful and debilitating condition of horses and ponies that has major economic and welfare implications. Anecdotal observations and the results of survey studies have indicated that most laminitis cases

to treatment. Effective pharmacologic agents are available to treat EGUS, but more comprehensive measures of environmental and dietary management are needed to decrease ulcer severity and recurrence. This article provides an understanding of dietary components and how feeds interact with stomach mucosal barrier function to cause EGUS. In addition, a secondary goal is to provide information on how diet and environmental management can reduce ulcer severity and prevent recurrence in horses with EGUS.

Nutrition of Critically Ill Horses 93

Elizabeth A. Carr and Susan J. Holcombe

Nutritional supplementation is becoming the standard of practice in equine medicine, although there are minimal data on nutritional support in critically ill horses and its association or effect on morbidity and mortality or length of hospital stay. Horses can be fed orally and when that is not possible, intravenously or parenterally. Enteral feeding is less expensive, more physiologic, improves immunity, and is easier and safer. This article reviews available information on the development of a nutritional plan for critically ill horses, and describes methods for and complications of enteral and parenteral feeding.

Feeding Management of Sick Neonatal Foals 109

Harold C. McKenzie III and Raymond J. Geor

Nutritional support of the foal can be challenging because of the constant changes in nutritional requirements and dietary composition during the transition from neonate to weanling. Additional complexity arises because of dilemmas regarding the means and route of delivery of nutrition to the foal, and the possibility that metabolic dysfunction may impair the ability of the foal to use nutrients appropriately. This article provides practical information on enteral and parenteral nutritional support of sick neonatal foals. The potential benefits of a conservative, hypocaloric feeding strategy, particularly in the very sick patient, are also discussed.

Optimal Diet of Horses with Chronic Exertional Myopathies 121

Erica C. McKenzie and Anna M. Firshman

Chronic exertional rhabdomyolysis represents a syndrome of recurrent exercise-associated muscle damage in horses that arises from a variety of etiologies. Major advances have been made in the understanding of the pathophysiology of this disease, and causative genetic defects have been recently identified for two conditions—polysaccharide storage myopathy of quarter horses, paints, warm bloods, and draft breeds. Dietary management in combination with a regular exercise regimen comprises the most effective means for control of clinical signs.

This article reviews the principles of feeding management for endurance horses. The amount and type of dietary energy (calories) are key considerations in dietary management, because (1) there is evidence that the body condition score, an indicator of overall energy balance, influences endurance exercise performance, and (2) the source of dietary energy (ie, carbohydrate versus fat calories) impacts health, metabolism, and athletic performance. Optimal performance is also dependent on provision of adequate feed, water, and electrolytes on race day.

This article reviews current thoughts on nutrition of the older horse in health and disease. Common causes of weight loss and poor body condition in old horses include dental or oral cavity abnormalities, pituitary pars intermedia dysfunction, and reduced feed intake attributable to competition from herd mates or pain associated with osteoarthritis. Feed intake and body condition may improve after institution of management changes. Thin but otherwise healthy old horses can benefit from a diet that provides 12% to 16% crude protein and includes highly digestible feedstuffs. In horses with severe irreversible dental problems, long-stem fiber (hay) should be replaced by soaked hay cubes, short chopped hay, or heavily soaked sugar beet pulp. Evidence of chronic endocrine, hepatic, or renal disease dictates dietary modifications.

This article reviews the effects of diet on equine feeding behavior and feeding patterns, before considering the evidence that diet affects reactivity in horses. A growing body of work suggests that fat- and fiber-based diets may result in calmer patterns of behavior, and possible mechanisms that may underpin these effects are discussed. In contrast, there is little evidence that herbal- or tryptophan-containing supplements influence equine behavior in any measurable way. The role of diet in the development of abnormal oral behaviors, particularly the oral stereotypy crib-biting, is also reviewed, and suggestions for future work are presented.

FORTHCOMING ISSUES

August 2009

New Perspectives in Equine Colic

Frank M. Andrews, DVM, MS, *Guest Editor*

December 2009

Practice Management

Reynolds Cowles, DVM, *Guest Editor*

April 2010

Laminitis, Part I

Christopher Pollitt, BVSc, PhD, *Guest Editor*

RECENT ISSUES

December 2008

Surgical Complications and Management Strategies

Laurie R. Goodrich, DVM, MS, PhD, *Guest Editor*

August 2008

Clinical Pathology

Bruce W. Parry, BVSc, PhD, *Guest Editor*

April 2008

Performance Horse Lameness and Orthopedics

Antonio M. Cruz, DVM, MVM, MSc, DrMedVet, *Guest Editor*

RELATED ISSUES

Veterinary Clinics of North America: Small Animal Practice (Vol. 36, No. 6)
Dietary Management and Nutrition
Claudia A. Kirk, DVM, PhD and Joseph W. Bartges, DVM, PhD, *Guest Editors*

Dedication

This issue is dedicated to the memory of Dr. David Kronfeld, eminent scientist, dedicated student mentor, and a pioneer of equine clinical nutrition and evidence-based medicine.

Vet Clin Equine 25 (2009) xi
doi:10.1016/j.cveq.2009.02.002 vetequine.theclinics.com
0749-0739/09/$ – see front matter

Preface

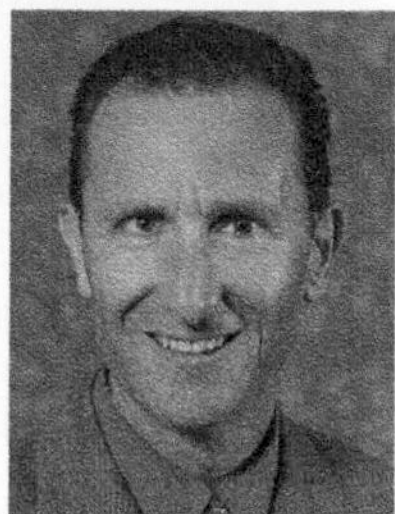

Raymond J. Geor, BVSc, MVSc, PhD
Guest Editor

A major focus of equine nutrition research has been to define nutrient requirements across different life stages and work functions (eg, sedentary versus athletic horses) and to examine the effect of different diets and feeding practices on aspects of health and productivity. The most recent edition (6th revised) of the National Research Council's *Nutrient Requirements of Horses* (published in 2007)[1] provides a very thorough review of current knowledge in the field of equine nutrition. Relatively few studies have examined the role of nutrition in various disease conditions or how disease may alter nutrient requirements. However, interest in clinical nutrition appears to be growing with the recognition that what (diet composition) and how (feeding methods) we feed horses and other equids can have profound effects on their health. Researchers have used epidemiologic approaches to evaluate associations between nutritional factors and disease events (eg, the effects of a recent change in diet on risk of colic).[2] Also, there have been controlled studies to evaluate the efficacy of different diets in horses with clinical conditions (eg, recurrent exertional rhabdomyolysis and polysaccharide storage myopathy). Please see the article by McKenzie and Firshman elsewhere in this issue for more information on this topic.

Equine veterinarians are a primary source of nutritional advice for horse owners and caregivers and, as such, must stay abreast of advances in equine nutrition to best serve the needs of their patients and clients. To that end, this issue of *Veterinary Clinics of North America: Equine Practice* provides up-to-date scientific findings and practical recommendations on a variety of nutritional topics that I hope will be a useful resource in your practice. The first article details approaches to the clinical assessment of nutritional status and feeding programs in an individual or group of horses. Several articles summarize research into how and why diet composition may alter the risk for conditions such as gastric ulcer syndrome, colic, laminitis, and chronic exertional myopathies. These articles also provide current recommendations for nutritional modifications in the management of disease. Two articles provide practical information for enteral and parenteral nutritional support of sick neonatal and mature horses. More studies in this area are needed to evaluate the impact of nutritional support in critically ill animals. Nonetheless, anecdotal observations suggest that providing nutrition to sick foals or horses is clinically beneficial. Undoubtedly, some of the feeding recommendations contained within will change as new scientific information comes to light.

Vet Clin Equine 25 (2009) xiii–xiv
doi:10.1016/j.cveq.2009.02.003 vetequine.theclinics.com

I offer my sincere thanks to the authors for their expertise and hard work. Thanks also to Simon Turner and John Vassallo for inviting me to serve as guest editor for this issue. Special thanks are due to John for his support and encouragement (and forbearance) as I strayed from deadlines!

Raymond J. Geor, BVSc, MVSc, PhD
Department of Large Animal Clinical Sciences
D-202 Veterinary Medical Center
College of Veterinary Medicine
Michigan State University
East Lansing, MI 48824, USA

E-mail address:
geor@cvm.msu.edu (R.J. Geor)

REFERENCES

1. Anonymous. Nutrient requirements of horses. In: National Research Council, editor. 6th revised edition. Washington (DC): National Academies Press; 2007.
2. Cohen ND, Peloso JG. Risk factors for history of colic and for chronic, intermittent colic in a population of horses. J Am Vet Med Assoc 1996;208:697–703.

Clinical Assessment of Nutritional Status and Feeding Programs in Horses

Iveta Becvarova, DVM, MS[a,*], R. Scott Pleasant, DVM, MS[a], Craig D. Thatcher, DVM, MS, PhD[b]

KEYWORDS

- Horse • Nutrition • Diet • Ration • Assessment
- Nutritional status • Feeding program
- Body condition score

Evaluation of nutritional status is an important part of clinical assessment since inadequate nutrition increases the risk of health and performance problems. As well, revealing relationships between abnormal physical signs and deficiencies or excesses of nutrients is critical for appropriate treatment. Performing nutritional assessment requires a basic knowledge of nutritional terminology (**Box 1**). Assessment of health history, diet history, physical examination, and laboratory tests identify existing malnutrition and individuals that are at risk of becoming malnourished. The clinical assessment of nutritional status and a feeding program consists of a sequence of logical steps. These steps consist of assessment of the horse or group of horses, and assessment of the current ration and feeding method. This assessment is followed by a new ration and feeding method recommendation if indicated. Periodic follow-ups are necessary to reevaluate the nutritional plan and determine whether alterations are indicated. Thus, assessment of nutritional status and feeding programs can be viewed as an iterative process.

ASSESSING AN INDIVIDUAL HORSE OR GROUP OF HORSES

Obtaining the History and Reviewing Records

A complete clinical history is necessary to determine factors that are important in tailoring a nutritional plan for a horse or group of horses. A signalment that includes breed, age, gender, reproductive status, level of exercise, and environment and

[a] Department of Large Animal Clinical Sciences, Virginia-Maryland Regional College of Veterinary Medicine, Phase II, Duckond Drive, Virginia Tech, Blacksburg, VA 24061, USA
[b] School of Applied Arts and Sciences, Arizona State University, 331R, Santa Catalina Hall, 7291 E. Sonoran Arroyo Mall, Mesa, AZ 85212, USA
* Corresponding author.
E-mail address: ivetak@vt.edu (I. Becvarova).

Vet Clin Equine 25 (2009) 1–21
doi:10.1016/j.cveq.2009.01.001
0749-0739/09/$ – see front matter. Published by Elsevier Inc.

Box 1
Nutritional terminology

Ad libitum. Free-choice access to feed.

Air dry. Approximately 90% dry matter. Feed that is dried by means of natural air movement.

Biologic value of a protein. The percentage of the protein of a feed or feed mixture that is usable as protein by the animal. A protein that has a high biologic value is said to be of a good quality.

Caloric. Pertaining to heat or energy.

Chelate. A cyclic compound that is formed between an organic molecule and a metallic ion.

Complete feed. A nutritionally adequate feed for animals other than humans; compounded to be fed as the sole ration and is capable of maintaining life and/or production without any additional substance being consumed except water.

Concentrate. A feed used with another to improve the nutritive balance of the total and intended to be further diluted and mixed to produce a supplement or complete feed.

Creep. An enclosure or feeder used for supplemental feeding of nursing young that excludes their dams.

Diet. Feed ingredients or mixture of ingredients including water, which is consumed by animals.

Dry forages. Feeds in the dry state that are bulky, low in weight per unit volume, and contain more than 18% crude fiber.

Easy keeper. An animal that grows or fattens rapidly on limited feed.

Electrolyte. A chemical compound that in solution dissociates by releasing ions.

Emaciated. An excessively thin condition of the body.

Energy. The capacity to perform work.

Energy feeds. Feeds that are high in energy and low in fiber (less than 18%), and that generally contain less than 20% protein.

Essential nutrients. Those nutrients that cannot be made in the body from other substances or that cannot be made in sufficient quantity to supply the animal's needs; hence they must be supplied in the ration.

Extruded. A process by which feed has been pressed, pushed, or protruded through orifices under pressure. The feed is subjected to increased pressure, friction, and attrition as it passes through a die opening. As the feed is released, it expands as steam is released because of the sudden drop in pressure.

Feed or feedstuff. Edible material that is consumed by animals and contributes energy and/or nutrients to the animal's diet.

Forage. The vegetative portion of plants in a fresh, dried, or ensiled state, which is fed to livestock (as pasture, hay, or silage).

Fructans. Polymers of fructose. Storage polysaccharides in plants. Not digested by mammalian enzyme but fermented by hind-gut microflora.

Grain. Seed from cereal plants.

Hard keeper. An animal that is unthrifty and grows or fattens slowly regardless of the quantity or quality of feed.

Hay. The aerial portion of grass or herbage especially cut and cured for animal feeding.

Hay belly. Horse's belly distended as a result of excessive feeding of bulky rations, such as hay, straw, or grass.

Hay quality. Physical and chemical characteristics of hay associated with palatability and abundance of feed nutrients.

Ingesta. Food or drink taken into the stomach.

Kjeldahl method. A method of determining the amount of nitrogen in an organic compound. Used as a part of Proximate analysis to determine crude protein (CP). CP = nitrogen (%) × 6.25.

Legume. A plant that has the ability to work symbiotically with bacteria to fix nitrogen from the air.

Macro minerals. The major minerals that are required in gram amounts per day—calcium, phosphorus, sodium, chlorine, potassium, magnesium, and sulfur.

Maintenance requirement. A ration that is adequate to prevent any loss or gain of tissue in the body when there is no production.

Malnutrition. Any disorder of nutrition. Used to indicate a state of inadequate (deficient or excessive) nutrition.

National Research Council (NRC). A division of the National Academy of Sciences established in 1916 to promote the effective use of scientific and technical resources. Periodically, this private, nonprofit organization of scientists publishes bulletins giving nutrient requirements and allowances of domestic animals.

Native pastures. Unseeded pastures native to the area.

Nitrogen. A chemical element essential to life. Animals get it from protein feeds; plants get it from the soil; and some bacteria get it directly from the air.

Nitrogen balance. The nitrogen in the feed intake minus the nitrogen in the feces, minus the nitrogen in the urine.

Nitrogen-free extract (NFE). Sugars, starches, pentoses, and non-nitrogenous organic acids. The percentage is calculated by subtracting the sum of the percentages of moisture, crude protein, crude fat, crude fiber, and ash from 100.

Nutrient allowances. Nutrient recommendations that allow for variations in feed composition; losses during storage and processing; periodic differences in needs of animals; age and size of animal; stage of gestation and lactation; activity level; the amount of stress; the system of management; the health, condition, and temperament; and the kind, quality, and amount of feed—all of which influence nutritive needs.

Nutrient requirements. Refers to meeting the animal's minimum needs, without margins of safety.

Nutrient. A feed constituent in a form and a level that will help support the life of an animal.

Palatability. Factors sensed by the animal in locating and consuming feed: appearance, odor, taste, texture, and temperature of the feed.

Parts per million (ppm). It equals milligrams per kilogram or milliliters per liter.

Pellets. Agglomerated feed formed by compacting and forcing through die openings by a mechanical process.

Premix. A uniform mixture of one or more microingredients with diluents and/or carrier.

Proximate analysis. A chemical analysis for evaluating feeds. Feeds are partitioned into the six fractions: 1. moisture, 2. crude protein, 3. ether extract (EE) or fat, 4. Ash, 5. crude fiber, 6. nitrogen-free extract (NFE).

Ration. The amount of total feed that is provided to one animal over a 24-hour period.

Supplement. A feed used with another to improve nutritive balance or performance of the total.

Sweet feed. A commercial horse feed that is characterized by its sweetness because of the addition of molasses.

TDN to Mcal. One pound of TDN = 2.0 Mcal or 2000 kcal.

Trace minerals (micro minerals). Mineral nutrients required by animals in micro amounts only—cobalt, copper, iodine, iron, manganese, selenium, and zinc.

housing should be obtained for each individual horse or for horses in the same category. Information on changes in body weight (BW), Body Condition Score (BCS), and growth rates should be obtained from medical and health records when possible. Health records should be carefully reviewed for medical diagnoses and/or surgical procedures performed, complications, the dates of problems, treatments, and hospitalizations. For example, if significant bowel resection has been performed, the current bowel anatomy should be noted. Laboratory tests and other diagnostic procedures that have been performed that could give information about the nutritional status of the horse should also be assessed. Obtaining a complete list of current and past medications is important, as some medications have important effects on metabolism and digestion. Medications that may alter physiologic status include drugs that modify metabolic rate (anabolic or catabolic drugs), glucose use, appetite, level of consciousness, gastrointestinal motility, digestive and absorptive capacity, fluid status, and immune status. Some medications are a significant source of nutrients, such as multivitamins, minerals, and trace elements, and should be accounted for in the ration. The use of alternative therapies should be investigated, such as administration of herbal products (plant-based drugs); nonplant-based products (enzymes, probiotics, hormones); or high doses of vitamins, minerals, and trace elements.

A detailed diet history is a critical component of the nutrition assessment process. This includes information on what is being fed and supplemented (type, amount, feeding frequency), and how the feed is offered (feeding management) (**Box 2**). Special attention should be given to feedstuff intolerances and hypersensitivities. Finally, changes in the horse's productivity (performance, growth, reproductive efficiency), appetite, feed intake, feeding behavior, activity, irritability, drinking pattern, bowel movement and urination pattern, bleeding tendencies, and rate of wound healing when applicable, should be recorded.

Nutrition-Focused Physical Examination

Physical examination assists in evaluation of nutritional status and in determining whether abnormalities have an underlying nutritional component. A complete physical examination should be performed with special attention given to those systems that are particularly responsive to nutrient deficiencies or excesses, and those that are necessary for delivery and assimilation of nutrients. Areas of emphasis include hydration status, mucous membranes, oral cavity, teeth, swallowing, hooves, rectum, cardiovascular and respiratory system, abdomen (shape, peristaltic movements), musculoskeletal system (muscle mass), and neurologic system.

BCS is a subjective method for estimating a horse's body fat stores and is an important tool for nutritional assessment. The BCS system that is used most commonly in horses was developed by researchers at Texas A & M University in the early 1980s.[1] The system scores horses on the amount of fat deposition at six body areas (neck, withers, behind the shoulders, over the ribs, along the topline, and around the tailhead) (**Fig. 1**). Each body area is assessed by visual appraisal and palpation and a score given based on descriptors (**Table 1**). The system ranks horses on a scale of 1 (emaciated) to 9 (extremely fat) (**Figs. 2–6**). Body condition scores of 4 to 6 are generally considered ideal. Although there is some variation in normal patterns of fat storage among different breeds, the system can be effectively used on all breeds and classes of horses. A history of reduced BCS may indicate a catabolic condition with or without the loss of lean muscle mass, whereas a history of BCS 7 to 9 is an indicator of overweight and obesity.

Both positive and negative energy balance also result in changes in BW. In the state of energy equilibrium, the energy intake equals the energy expenditure, and the horse's BW remains stable. Change in BW is a common early indicator of health problems. Knowing the horse's BW is also useful to determine the amount of feed and drugs required, to monitor the horse's health status, feeding management, and growth rate. Furthermore, mature adult BW is needed to determine nutrient requirements established by the National Research Council (NRC).[2] The horse's BW can be obtained with a walk-on scale or can be estimated. Body weight in horses is known to vary from 5% to 20% depending on the hydration status and on gastrointestinal fill.[3] Therefore, the time of feeding relative to weighing is critical. To minimize the error and at times when the walk-on scale is not available, the mature horse's body weight can be estimated from accurate body measurements, such as heart girth and body length measurement:[4]

$$lb \cdot body \cdot wt = [Heart \cdot girth(in)]^2 \times length(in)/330$$

$$kg \cdot body \cdot wt = [Heart \cdot girth(cm)]^2 \times length(cm)/11800$$

Heart girth is measured immediately behind the elbows following respiratory expiration. The weight tape is positioned according to the manufacturer's recommendation. Length is measured from the point of the shoulder to the tuber ischii.[5]

A slightly less accurate estimate of the horse's BW can be obtained from a heart girth measurement using a weight tape calibrated for horses. All measurements should be done in a consistent fashion and the horse should be standing on a flat, level surface. Significant error can be made by pulling the tape too tightly or in horses with heavy haircoats. An average of several measurements yields the most accurate body weight estimate.

Laboratory Tests and Diagnostics

Laboratory tests and other diagnostic procedures may be indicated in the nutritional assessment of some horses. Unfortunately, no one clinical nutrition marker or laboratory finding can completely determine a horse's nutritional status. In clinical practice, multiple tests need to be co-interpreted in relation to the history and health status for the most accurate assessment of a horse's condition.

The serum protein that is most commonly used to assess visceral protein status in horses is albumin. Albumin level accurately reflects visceral protein status and adequacy of protein intake in the absence of severe illness, inflammation, liver disease, fluid overload, or dehydration. If severe inflammation is present, serum albumin level is usually low because it is a negative acute-phase protein. Albumin is synthesized in the liver; therefore liver disease may result in slow rate of synthesis. Albumin level will be low as a result of overhydration and the dilutional effect of fluids, or abnormally elevated as a result of dehydration. In general, albumin level does not improve, despite adequate protein-energy intake, until the disease resolves. Albumin is a carrier for calcium, magnesium, and zinc. Therefore in hypoalbuminemia, the total plasma levels of these minerals will be lowered, whereas the unbound, physiologically active portion may be normal. Albumin in horses has a half-life of 19.4 days,[6] and therefore changes in albumin level will not immediately reflect protein-energy malnutrition. Serum albumin level may decrease with protein-losing enteropathy or nephropathy, severe parasitism, or blood loss. A direct relationship between vitamin A and lowered albumin has been observed in cows,[7] which was corrected by the administration of carotene. In horses, both hypo- and hypervitaminosis A have been associated with hypoalbuminemia.[8]

Box 2
Nutritional survey form used at the VA-MD Regional College of Veterinary Medicine

1. Are other species of animal kept on this farm? If yes, which ones?
2. How many employees work on the farm full time and part time?
3. How many and which employees are responsible for the feeding, watering, cleaning, grooming, breeding, and training?
4. What is the number of resident horses (horses that spend most of the year on the farm)?
5. How many visiting and resident animals do you have in each of the following groups during a typical year: foals, broodmares, stallions (breeding), and working horses (what type of work?).
6. What is the predominant source of grain (ie, home grown, home mixed, commercial bagged, commercial bulk)? List commercial brands.
7. How often do you feed grain and at what time?
8. What is the feeding sequence of grain and hay?
9. How often do you receive a new shipment of grain?
10. What type(s) of hay is/are fed to the horses?
11. Are there weeds present in the hay? List types of weeds found.
12. What is the predominant source of hay (ie, home grown, locally grown, out of state)?
13. How often do you get a new shipment of hay?
14. How often do you feed hay?
15. How is hay fed in the stable?
16. What cutting of hay is fed?
17. How is hay fed in the paddocks and/or pastures (ie, hay rack, hay net, on the ground)?
18. Where do you store the hay?
19. Do you routinely chemically analyze your hay? If yes, how often?
20. Do you feed salt? If yes, what kind of salt (ie, white salt, trace-mineralized salt)? List brand.
21. How do you feed the salt (ie, block, loose, mixed with grain)?
22. How often do you feed salt?
23. Do you feed supplements? If yes, which ones (ie, mineral, vitamin, electrolytes)? List brands.
24. How do you feed supplements (ie, block, loose, mixed with grain)?
25. Do the horses have access to supplements in the paddocks/pastures?
26. How often do you feed supplements?
27. What is the source of water in the stable (ie, well, city, pond/lake, stream)?
28. What is the source of water in the paddocks (ie, well, city, pond/lake, stream)?
29. What is the water delivery system in the stable (ie, automatic waterer, bucket)?
30. What is the water delivery system in the paddocks (ie, automatic waterer, bucket, tub)?
31. How often are the buckets in the stable checked for fullness?
32. How often are the buckets or tubs in the paddocks/pastures checked for fullness?
33. How often are buckets in the stable cleaned and what is the procedure?
34. What is the predominant type of forage in the paddocks/pastures?

35. What is your pasture management (fertilization, clipping, seeding, feces removal, vacuuming, dragging/harrowing, rotation)?
36. What is the length of time each day the horses are in the stall versus on the pasture? List for each group of horses or each horse.
37. List diseases and their frequency that have been a problem on the farm in the last year.
38. What kind of records do you keep (ie, health, breeding, training, feeding)?
39. How often and with what products do you deworm the horses on the farm?
40. Please, attach or draw a map of the farm with pastures and paddock.

Courtesy of Virginia-Maryland Regional College of Veterinary Medicine, Blacksburg, VA; with permission.

There are several other parameters that may assist in determining the horse's nutritional status on a basic chemistry and complete blood count panel. Nutritional causes of decreased blood urea nitrogen (BUN) include inadequate protein intake, starvation, and low protein turnover. Decreased creatinine signifies inadequate energy intake and decreased muscle mass. The nutritional causes of decreased hemoglobin and hematocrit include iron, copper and cobalt deficiency, folate deficiency, and inadequate protein intake. Synthesis of immunoglobulins and immune cells requires protein and selective amino acids. The consequences of dietary protein deficiency are impaired immune function and decreased antibody titer,[9] which can be reversed with protein repletion.[6] Total lymphocyte count is a measure of immune function and decreases with protein malnutrition.

Although not always diagnostic, concentrations of nutrients in the blood, serum, and plasma are helpful in determining the nutritional status and inadequate or excessive intakes of nutrients. The reason for the lack of diagnostic value is the effect of hydration status, excessive losses, and decreased excretion of nutrients. Nevertheless, abnormalities in serum electrolytes and acid-base balance may warrant treatment, either parenterally or enterally. A dietary excess of sodium, phosphorus, copper, molybdenum, iodine, selenium, fluoride, and vitamins A and D may cause an increase

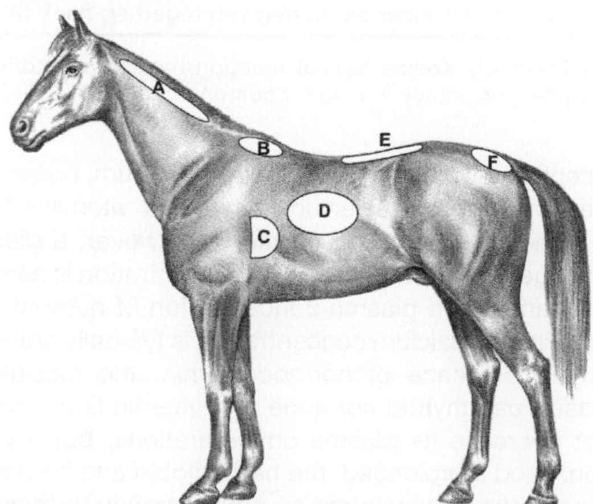

Fig. 1. The fat deposition at six body areas. A, neck; B, withers; C, behind the shoulder; D, ribs; E, topline; F, tailhead. (*Courtesy of* Virginia-Maryland Regional College of Veterinary Medicine and Virginia Cooperative Extension, Blacksburg, VA; with permission.)

Table 1
Description of Body Condition Scoring (BCS) system

Score	Description
1. Poor	Animal is extremely emaciated; spinous processes, ribs, tailhead, tuber coxae, and ischii project prominently; bone structure of withers, shoulders, and neck easily noticeable; no fatty tissue can be felt.
2. Very Thin	Animal is emaciated; slight fat covering over base of spinous processes; transverse processes of lumbar vertebrae feel rounded; spinous processes, ribs, tailhead, tuber coxae, and ischii are prominent; withers, shoulders, and neck structure faintly discernible.
3. Thin	Fat buildup about halfway on spinous processes; transverse processes cannot be felt; slight fat cover over ribs; spinous processes and ribs easily discernible; tailhead prominent, but individual vertebrae cannot be identified visually; tuber coxae appear rounded but easily discernible; tuber ischii not distinguishable; withers, shoulders, and neck accentuated.
4. Moderately Thin	Slight ridge along back; faint outline of ribs discernible; tailhead prominence depends on conformation, fat can be felt around it; tuber coxae not discernible; withers, shoulders, and neck not obviously thin.
5. Moderate	Back is flat (no crease or ridge); ribs not visually distinguishable but easily felt; fat around tailhead beginning to feel spongy; withers appear rounded over spinous processes; shoulders and neck blend smoothly into body.
6. Moderately Fleshy	May have slight crease down back; fat over ribs is spongy; fat around tailhead is soft; fat beginning to be deposited along the side of withers, behind shoulders, and along the sides of neck.
7. Fleshy	May have crease down back; individual ribs can be felt, but noticeable filling between ribs with fat; fat around tailhead is soft; fat deposited along withers, behind shoulders, and along neck.
8. Fat	Crease down back; difficult to feel ribs; fat around tailhead very soft; area along withers filled with fat; area behind shoulder filled with fat; noticeable thickening of neck; fat deposited along inner thighs.
9. Extremely Fat	Obvious crease down back; patchy fat appearing over ribs; bulging fat around tailhead, along withers, behind shoulders, and along neck; fat along with inner thighs may rub together; flank filled with fat.

Data from Henneke DR, Potter GD, Kreider JL, et al. Relationship between condition score, physical measurements and body fat percentage in mares. Equine Vet J 1983;15:371–2.

in their plasma concentration. A dietary deficiency of sodium, potassium, magnesium, phosphorus, copper, manganese, selenium, zinc, and vitamins A, E, and B_1 may cause a decrease in their plasma concentration.[8] However, a dietary deficiency or excess must be prolonged before the nutrient's concentration is altered in the plasma. Thus, the absence of an altered plasma concentration of nutrient does not exclude deficiency or excess. Plasma calcium concentration is typically not affected by dietary calcium intake. In the presence of normocalcemia, the calcium status can be measured as increased parathyroid hormone and vitamin D concentrations. An iron deficiency does not decrease its plasma concentrations, but it decreases plasma ferritin concentrations, and if prolonged, the hemoglobin and hematocrit. Iodine deficiency or iodine excess can be measured as concentration of triiodothyronine (T_3) in response to thyroid-stimulating hormone administration. The selenium status of horses can be evaluated by measuring serum, plasma, or whole blood selenium concentration. Whole blood selenium concentration is preferred to serum

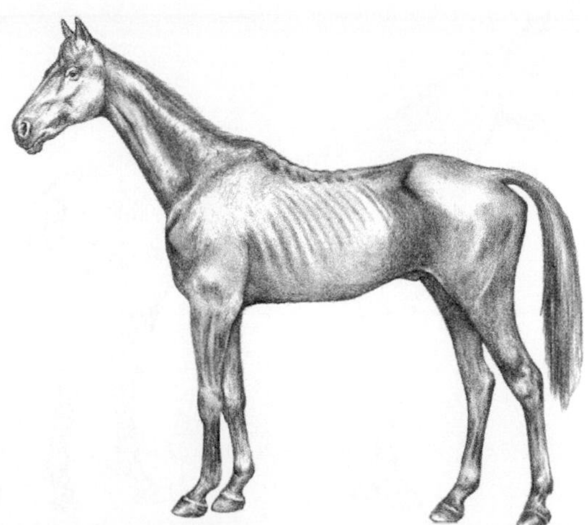

Fig. 2. Illustration demonstrating Body Condition Score of 1/9. (*Courtesy of* Virginia-Maryland Regional College of Veterinary Medicine and Virginia Cooperative Extension, Blacksburg, VA; with permission.)

concentration.[2] The common indicator of vitamin E status is serum α-tocopherol. Unfortunately, a single serum sample appears to be unsatisfactory because of the fluctuation of serum α-tocopherol within an individual horse over a 72-hour period from concentrations considered to be adequate through those considered marginal or deficient.[2] Therefore, obtaining single serum sample for α-tocopherol would be suitable to determine overall vitamin E status in a herd, whereas in one horse it is more appropriate to evaluate a minimum of three serum samples collected on consecutive days.[10]

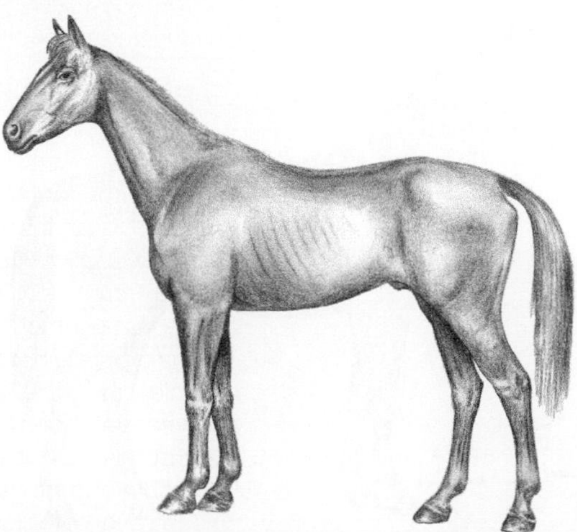

Fig. 3. Illustration demonstrating Body Condition Score of 3/9. (*Courtesy of* Virginia-Maryland Regional College of Veterinary Medicine and Virginia Cooperative Extension, Blacksburg, VA; with permission.)

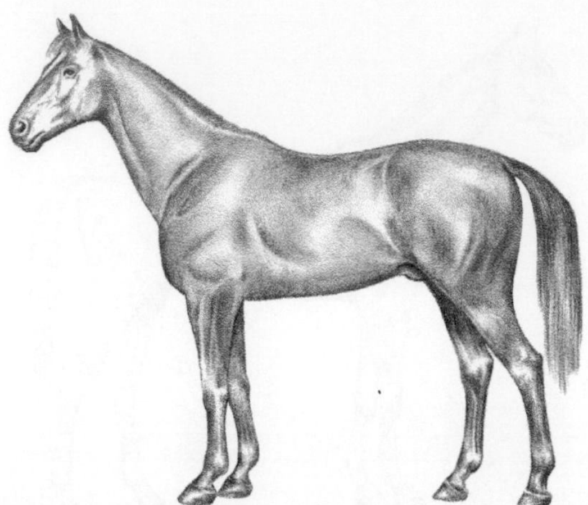

Fig. 4. Illustration demonstrating Body Condition Score of 5/9. (*Courtesy of* Virginia-Maryland Regional College of Veterinary Medicine and Virginia Cooperative Extension, Blacksburg, VA; with permission.)

The analysis of selenium, manganese, and zinc is most appropriate from whole blood (in EDTA or heparin as anticoagulant). Serum is an appropriate sample for measuring copper, iodine, iron, zinc, manganese, calcium, magnesium, phosphorus, vitamin A, β-carotene, and vitamin E. Plasma is appropriate for copper, zinc, manganese, vitamin A, β-carotene, and vitamin E. Samples for vitamin E, vitamin A, and β-carotene are sensitive to heat and light; therefore, tubes should be refrigerated, serum and plasma quickly separated from blood cells, with samples wrapped in tin foil, frozen, and delivered to the laboratory as soon as possible. To measure zinc concentration, it is recommended to use a vacuum tube that has been acid-washed

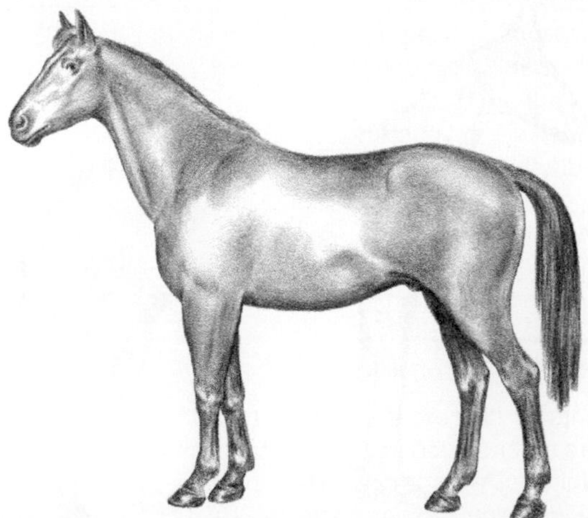

Fig. 5. Illustration demonstrating Body Condition Score of 7/9. (*Courtesy of* Virginia-Maryland Regional College of Veterinary Medicine and Virginia Cooperative Extension, Blacksburg, VA; with permission.)

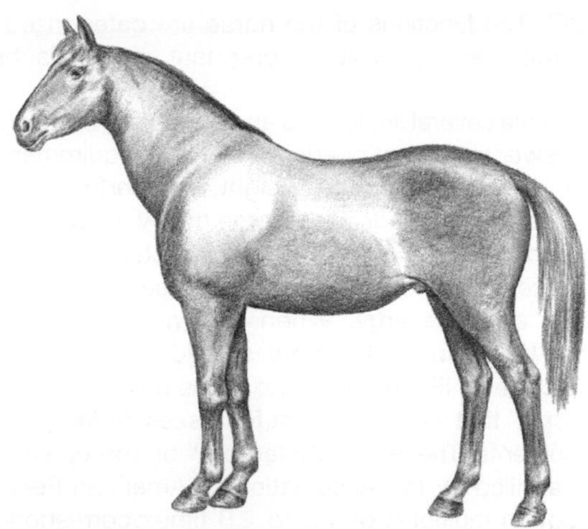

Fig. 6. Illustration demonstrating Body Condition Score of 9/9. (*Courtesy of* Virginia-Maryland Regional College of Veterinary Medicine and Virginia Cooperative Extension, Blacksburg, VA; with permission.)

and has a plastic (not rubber) stopper.[11] Measuring minerals other than zinc requires routine handling and refrigeration.

Nutrient contents of hoof, hair, and urine are considered an inadequate measurement of nutritional status because of their lack benefit in the diagnosis of nutrient imbalances.[8] If available, determining the concentration of a nutrient in certain body tissues, such as in a biopsy sample of liver tissue, may provide more diagnostic value. Reference intervals for the concentration of selected nutrients in horses have been established for blood, serum, plasma, and liver, and have been published elsewhere.[8]

When a group of horses or whole herd is evaluated for nutritional imbalances, it is important to sample a sufficient number of animals to obtain statistically representative results. Testing a minimum of seven animals within a group detects a difference of approximately 1 SD between the group tested and the reference population, with a 95% confidence interval.[11] The practical recommendation is to test 7 to 10 animals that are representative of the group from each population of concern. This applies for groups of 20 to more than 1000, assuming that animals in the group have all been managed the same. Horses on pasture, in stalls, growing horses, or horses in different stages of the reproductive cycle would represent separate groups.

In the summary, biomarkers of nutritional status are often difficult to interpret because they are affected by multiple factors. Therefore, clinicians should primarily rely on medical and dietary history, physical examination, BW and BCS changes, and routine blood work for assessment of nutritional status in horses.

Estimation of Nutrient Requirements

Nutrient requirements of horses and ponies have been estimated through feeding experiments, and are summarized in feeding standards. The most widely used feeding standards in the United States are those published by National Research Council (NRC)[2] and Kentucky Equine Research Inc. (KER). The nutrient requirements are expressed as amount of each nutrient needed per day for a specific life stage and function of a horse, and they are based on the mature BW. Nutrients are listed in weight units (g, mg, lb) and International Units (IU), and energy is expressed in Mcal of digestible energy (DE). The functions of the horse are categorized as adult maintenance, different exercise levels, stallions, pregnant mares, lactating mares, and growing horses.

Feeding standards have several limitations and should be primarily used as a guide, not as the ultimate answer to nutrient needs. First, NRC requirements are established for a population of horses of a given age, weight, and performance status. It is well known that the requirement of an individual horse may vary considerably even within a relatively small group. Second, published feeding standards were established in healthy horses, thus diseased horses may have increased or decreased requirements for selected nutrients and/or energy. When determining nutrient requirement of diseased horses, the key nutritional factors should be identified and their levels adjusted. Finally, the current NRC recommendations provide minimum requirements and lack a "safety factor" that would account for losses during digestion, absorption, and metabolism of nutrients. These "safety factors" on top of what is believed to be required have been applied by the Association of American Feed Control Officials (AAFCO)[12] on pet food in multiples of 1.3 to 2.0 times corresponding NRC values. Applying the same approach to a horse, the equine nutrient allowances would be about 1.2 times the NRC requirements for maintenance and up to 1.5 times for rapid growth.[13] In general, KER nutrient requirements are higher than NRC minimums, except for chloride, zinc, iodine, manganese, and vitamin E levels in some categories of horses. Feeding standards are useful and practical guides for clinicians and nutritionists to estimate nutrient and energy requirements.

ASSESSING THE DIET AND RATION

The diet and ration evaluation is used to identify nutritional imbalances that may relate to the health problems of an individual horse or group of horses.

Physical Evaluation of Feeds

The first step is to examine feedstuffs (grains, concentrates, hays, pastures) and supplements that are fed. The feeds in a feed room should be stored in closed and clean containers to prevent access to moisture, air, and pests. Vegetable oils should be stored protected from light and high temperatures to prevent rancidity. The feed turnover should be on a "first-in, first-out" basis. Hay should be protected from rain and moisture. All feeds should be physically evaluated using the senses for color, odor, presence of dust, weeds, foreign materials, feed components, and processing methods. Alfalfa hay that was cut after midsummer should be inspected for the presence of toxic blister beetles. Hay aroma should always be fresh and free of a musty or moldy odor, and should be free of dust.

The physical characteristics of hay quality include type of the hay (legume, grass), maturity at harvest, leaf-to-stem ratio, presence of seed heads, color, and moisture content. Signs of hay maturity include presence of seed heads, stems, coarseness, and low leaf-to-stem ratio. First cutting hays tend to be more mature, less digestible, consumed by horses in lower rates, and have lower nutritional value. When compared with second and third cutting hays, the first cutting hays often have higher yield because of higher cell wall contents (hemicellulose, cellulose, lignin), and a higher proportion of stems. They are often excellent choices for easy keepers and overweight/obese horses. In general, second and third cutting hays are leafier, more nutritious, and more digestible; contain a small number or have no seed heads; are soft on touch; and are consumed at higher rates than first cutting hays. Leaves, as compared with stems, provide increased photosynthetic capacity, are higher in nonstructural carbohydrates (sugars, starches, fructans) and protein, and lower in structural carbohydrates (pectin, hemicellulose, cellulose, and lignin). Thus leaves are more nutritious than stems.

Hay quality is greatly influenced by proper curing and storage. During curing, hay must be allowed to dry to less than 20% moisture. Hay that is baled too wet will mold, heat up, and presents a fire risk. Conversely, hay that is baled too dry will lose nutritious leaves from the mechanical process of raking and baling. This is particularly true for legumes. Nevertheless, even with the best management, the losses of nutrients between harvesting and feeding are between 10% and 20%. Hay yield and quality are further reduced if exposed to the rain during curing, through leaching of soluble components. Rain not only leaches nutrients (carotene, vitamin E, protein, water-soluble carbohydrates), but also increases leaf loss because of the extra mechanical operations during harvest.

The most desirable hay color is bright green. The green color indicates that the hay was properly cured, with no damage from rain, molds, or overheating during storage. Yellow or light brown color indicates that the hay has been rained on, sun-bleached, or was over-mature when cut. The amount of the green color present in forage gives an approximation of the amount of beta-carotene and alpha-tocopherol.[14] The green color indicates that the hay is rich in carotene, whereas yellow color or brown color signifies that the hay is low in carotene. Dark brown color and a tobaccolike odor may be the result of overheating during storage (caramelization) owing to excessive moisture content of the hay (>16%–18%) and metabolic activity of microbes (fungi).[15] Nevertheless, the hay color is the least important criterion on physical evaluation. Whereas sun-bleaching decreases carotene content and palatability, it typically occurs only on the side of the bale that was exposed to direct light, whereas the inside of the bale might be very green. Therefore, the sun-bleached hay should not be discriminated as seriously as rain-, heat-, or mold-damaged hay.

Measuring Feed Consumption

The second step is to measure the amount of feed consumed. It is important to understand that feeds should be fed by weight rather than volume because of the highly variable densities among feeds. Scales should be an essential inventory of every feed room (**Figs. 7** and **8**). Not only do grains and concentrates vary in weight per unit of volume, but hay bales and flakes also have different weights (even within the same harvest). The amounts of all supplements fed should be weighed as well. The amount of grain, concentrate, and supplements consumed is determined by subtracting the weight of leftovers from the amount fed. It is more difficult to determine the amount of hay consumed. This is especially true for horses that are fed from the ground and/or in groups. Feeding from the ground is associated with significant wastes that can be as high as 20%. For an accurate assessment, the amount of wasted hay should be weighed or, less ideally, estimated as a percentage. A particular challenge is the determination of voluntary pasture consumption, as DE and dry matter intake (DMI) can be highly variable in horses. For a mean daily energy intake of 16.4 Mcal DE, a 90% confidence interval (± 1.7 coefficient of variation) is 14.2 to 18.6 Mcal for mature horses and 11.9 to 20.9 for weanlings.[13] Voluntary DMI is based on BW, level of exercise, reproductive status, and growth stage. Estimates of voluntary DMI for grazing horses generally range from 1.5% to 3.1% of BW.[2] Daily DMI is highest for lactating mares, which on average consume 2.8% of BW, whereas the remaining categories

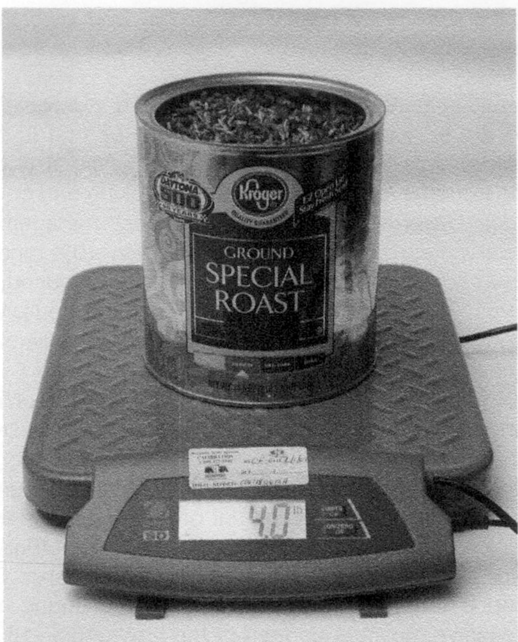

Fig. 7. Weighing the concentrate using a digital scale. (*Courtesy of* Virginia-Maryland Regional College of Veterinary Medicine and Virginia Cooperative Extension, Blacksburg, VA; with permission.)

of horses ingest approximately 2.0% of their BW.[2] Pasture intake can then be calculated, if the pasture dry matter (DM) is available from the chemical analysis, as follows:

1. Calculate lb of DMI

$$lb \cdot DMI = Body \cdot Weight(lb) \times (\%DMI \div 100),$$

where % DMI has a range of 1.5 to 3.1 for different categories of horses.[2]

2. Calculate lb of pasture consumed on an as-fed basis

$$lb \cdot pasture \cdot consumed = lb \cdot DMI \div (\%Pasture \cdot Drymatter \div 100)$$

Nutrient Content of Feeds

The third step is to obtain the nutrient content of feeds in the ration. This can be acquired from feed tags, nutrient databases, and chemical nutrient analyses. Commercially bagged feeds sold in the United States must have a tag attached to the bag or a label on the bag. Regulations for the feed tags in the United States are determined by the AAFCO[12] and include the product and brand name, inclusion statement of drugs, purpose and use statement, guarantees of limits to concentrations of certain nutrients, ingredient list, directions for use, warning or caution statement, quantity statement, and contact information for the manufacturer or person responsible for distributing the feed. During the farm visit, it is helpful to collect or make copies of all tags from the feeds and supplements for later evaluation. The guaranteed analysis on the tag has several limitations. First, it provides concentration of only a limited number of nutrients. Second, these concentrations guarantee only that

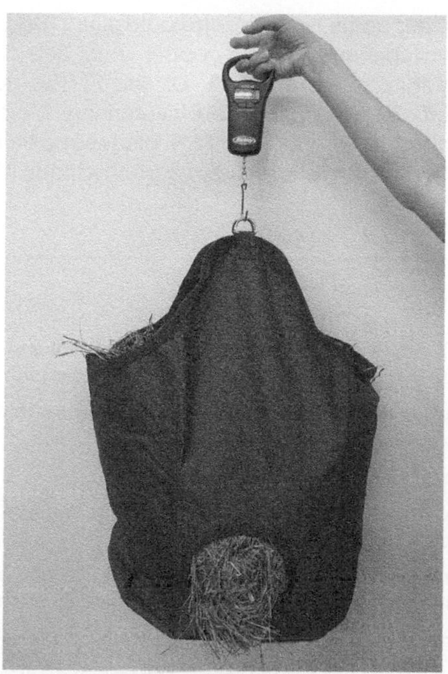

Fig. 8. Weighing the hay using a hanging scale. (*Courtesy of* Virginia-Maryland Regional College of Veterinary Medicine and Virginia Cooperative Extension, Blacksburg, VA; with permission.)

minimums were met and maximums were not exceeded. Therefore, for more accurate nutrient concentrations, chemical analysis should be obtained from the manufacturer or feeds should be chemically analyzed by an appropriate laboratory. Nutrient concentrations in feeds are determined by various wet chemistry procedures, which take several days, or by a quick but less reliable Near Infrared Reflectance (NIR) analysis.

The chemical analysis of the feed is only as good as the sampling method used. If the feed sample is not representative, the analysis has no value. The feed sample size sent to the laboratory should be approximately 1 lb or 450 g. At least two samples of each grain or concentrate should be taken, combined and thoroughly mixed. Hay samples should always be taken with a hay probe and drill. Ten percent of bales or at least 10 bales should be cored in the center of the small end between the strings. The samples should be combined in a clean bucket, thoroughly mixed, placed into a 1-qt size sealable plastic bag, and sent to the laboratory. Pastures should be sampled by walking the two diagonals and clipping a handful of forage at the grazing height (top 6 in or 15.2 cm) with shears. Weeds and ungrazed patches (defecation areas) should be avoided because they do not represent the pasture that is grazed. The forage sample must be clean, and devoid of soil and roots. The pasture should be clipped into 1- to 2-in (2.54–5.08-cm) strips into the plastic bucket, thoroughly mixed, placed into a 1-qt size sealable plastic bag and transported in a cooler on ice. Pasture samples should be frozen as soon as possible after the sampling and sent on ice overnight to the laboratory for analysis. Feed samples should always be properly labeled for identification and tracking purposes.

The basic nutrient profile of horse feeds includes DM, DE, crude protein (CP), acid detergent fiber (ADF), neutral detergent fiber (NDF), crude fat (EE, ether extract), calcium, magnesium, phosphorus, sodium, and potassium (**Box 3**). Trace element and vitamin analyses are available and include copper, zinc, selenium, iron, manganese, molybdenum, iodine, sulfur, and vitamins A, D, and E. The nutrient profile that we commonly use at VA-MD Regional College of Veterinary Medicine and is available from Equi-Analytical Laboratories, Ithaca, NY, includes moisture, DM, DE, CP, estimated lysine, ADF, NDF, starch, water-soluble carbohydrates (WSC), ethanol-soluble

Box 3
Interpreting chemical analysis

Acid detergent fiber (ADF): a measure of cellulose and lignin. Cellulose has variable digestibility and lignin is indigestible. Therefore, ADF is negatively correlated with overall digestibility.

As fed basis (as is; as sampled): nutrient concentration in the natural state of the sample, including moisture.

Ash: a measure of the total mineral content of the sample.

Crude fat: determined by ether extraction. Includes mainly fat, but also plant pigments, esters, aldehydes, and fat soluble vitamins.

Crude fiber (CF): an older method of fiber analysis that preceded NDF and ADF. Accounts for most of the cellulose and only portion of lignin. Poor method to quantify fiber in forages.

Crude protein (CP): the true protein and non-protein nitrogen in the sample.

Digestible energy (DE): the amount of energy that is apparently digested and absorbed by the animal. DE (Mcal) = Intake (gross) Energy – Energy in the feces.

Dry matter (DM): the percentage of all components of the feed sample except water (100% – moisture).

Dry matter basis (DMB): nutrient concentration in the sample with the water removed. DMB = (% nutrient As fed × % water in the sample) ÷ 100.

Ethanol soluble carbohydrates (ESC): carbohydrates solubilized and extracted in 80% ethanol. Includes primarily monosaccharides and disaccharides.

Lysine (Lys): an essential amino acid required for growth.

Moisture: the percent water in the feed sample.

Neutral detergent fiber (NDF): a measure of cellulose, hemicellulose, and lignin (plant cell wall contents) representing the bulk (fiber content) of the forage. NDF is negatively correlated with forage intake.

Non-fiber carbohydrates (NFC): a calculated value estimating non-cell wall (non-fiber) carbohydrates. Includes starch, sugar, pectin and fermentation acids. NFC (%) = 100 – (CP% + NDF% + Fat% + Ash%).

Relative feed value (RFV): an index for ranking quality of forages based on digestibility and intake potential. RFV is calculated from ADF and NDF. A RFV of 100 is considered the average score and represents an alfalfa hay containing 41% ADF and 53% NDF on a dry matter basis. The higher the RFV, the better the hay quality.

Relative forage quality (RFQ): an index for ranking forages. RFQ is calculated from CP, ADF, NDF, fat, ash, and NDF digestibility measured at 48 hours. RFQ is based on the same scoring as RFV with an average score of 100. The higher the RFQ, the better the quality.

Starch: a polysaccharide digestible with mammalian enzymes.

Total digestible nutrients (TDN): the percentage of the sum of the digestible protein, digestible nitrogen-free extract (NFE), digestible crude fiber, and 2.25 × the digestible fat.

Water soluble carbohydrates (WSC): carbohydrates solubilized and extracted in water. Includes monosaccharides, disaccharides, and some polysaccharides, mainly fructans.

carbohydrates (ESC), fat, calcium, phosphorus, magnesium, potassium, sodium, iron, zinc, copper, manganese, and molybdenum. Nonstructural carbohydrates (NSC) are subjected to a variety of interpretations and usually calculated as WSC + starch or ESC + starch (see *Primer on Dietary Carbohydrates and Utility of the Glycemic Index in Equine Nutrition* in this issue).

Ration Evaluation

The fourth step is to evaluate the ration. There are multiple methods used for ration evaluation, ranging from comparing a limited number of nutrients with the published standards to computer-based programs that allow the evaluation of multiple nutrients at once. Individuals who have limited experience and knowledge of horse nutritional physiology and use of feeds should contact an experienced nutritionist to perform ration evaluation and formulation of a balanced ration. The simple method to evaluate selected nutrients includes summarizing the amount of each nutrient consumed from feeds and comparing the summarized value with a feeding standard (NRC or KER). To do that, nutritional analysis of the feed and the amount of the feed consumed must be known. The horse's BW and the level of exercise are needed for determination of nutrient requirements from feeding standards.

The simple ration evaluation can be performed using nutrient content on an as-fed (AF) basis, which is available from the chemical analysis. The concentration of each variable (ie, nutrient, energy, DM) in the feed (ie, g/kg AF, mg/kg AF, IU/kg AF) is multiplied by the amount of feed consumed per day. The amount of each variable is then summarized and compared with a selected feeding standard (NRC or KER) (**Table 2**).

The calculations used to evaluate several parameters are time consuming and subjected to error. There are several specifically designed computer software programs available to calculate the total daily ration and compare the sets of values with nutritional standards, such as NRC or KER. Our nutrition group at the VA-MD Regional College of Veterinary Medicine uses Microsteed (Kentucky Equine Research Inc., Versailles, KY). This software program evaluates a ration by comparing estimated dietary intake (using stored data on the nutrient profiles of common feedstuffs) with either the KER or NRC nutrient requirements for the age and physiologic state of the horse.[16]

When evaluating and designing proper feeding programs for a group of horses, it is helpful to categorize the horses based on their body weight, BCS, reproductive and performance status, and age. A representative number of horses from each category are then evaluated. The ration is evaluated and formulated for each category, using averages of obtained variables.

ASSESSING THE FEEDING METHOD

Another essential component of nutritional assessment (and the iterative process) is to evaluate the appropriateness of the feeding route and how the feed is offered. The adequacy of the feeding route depends on the clinical status of the horse. Although most horses are able to feed themselves, nutritional support is indicated in all horses that have a history of anorexia/hyporexia for 3 days and more or have a recent history of weight loss of 10% and more (see *Nutrition of the Critically Ill Horse* in this issue). In a clinical setting, it is critical to evaluate the function of the gastrointestinal tract, the expected clinical course of disease, and the anticipated duration of the gastrointestinal tract malfunction. Based on these evaluations, enteral or parenteral nutritional support is selected. Assisted enteral feeding should be performed via a feeding tube. Parenteral nutrition should be initiated whenever the gastrointestinal tract is dysfunctional and the enteral route is unavailable. The indicators of the adequacy of

Table 2
Ration evaluation example

	Feed Ingredient Nutrient Composition From Chemical Analysis					
	DM %	DE (Mcal/ kg·AF)	CP (% AF)	Ca (% AF)		
Concentrate	89	3.4	11.0	0.8		
Grass hay	93	1.9	11.3	0.4		
Pasture	25	0.6	5.5	0.1		
Calculations						
Variable	Concentrate	Grass hay	Pasture (estimated)	Ration (total)	KER requirement	NRC requirement
DMI, kg/d[a]	0.89	5.58	3.53[b]	10 (~2% BW)	7.5	7.5–15.5 (1.5%–3.1% BW)
DE, Mcal/d	3.4	11.4	8.47[c]	23.3	16.4	16.7
CP, g/d[d]	110	678	777	1565	681	630
Ca, g/d[e]	8	24	14.1	46.1	29.9	20.0

Interpretation: The current ration is meeting and exceeding KER allowances and NRC minimum requirements in all selected parameters (DMI, DE, CP, and Ca).

Evaluate the nutrient profile of a ration for a 500-kg horse at average maintenance. The ration consists of 6 kg of grass hay, 1 kg of concentrate. The horse is turned out on a grass pasture 8 hours a day.

Abbreviations: DMI, dry matter intake; DM, dry matter basis; d, day; AF, as-fed basis; DE, digestible energy; BW, body weight; CP, crude protein; Ca, calcium; KER, Kentucky Equine Research Inc.; NRC, National Research Council.

[a] DMI, kg = (kg AF × DM percentage) ÷ 100. Example of calculation for concentrate: DMI, kg = (1 × 89) ÷ 100 = 0.89 kg.

[b] $DMI_{pasture}$, $kg/d = DMI_{total\ ration} - (DMI_{concentrate} + DMI_{hay}) = 10 - (0.89 + 5.58) = 3.53 kg/d$

[c] $DE_{pasture,Mcal/d} = Pasture \cdot intake, kg \cdot AF/d \times DE_{pasture,Mcal/kg \cdot AF} = [(DMI_{pasture,kg/d} \div DM \cdot percentage) \times 100] \times DE_{pasture,Mcal/kg \cdot AF} = [(3.53 \div 25) \times 100] \times 0.6 = 8.47$ *Mcal/d.*

[d] CP g/d = (% CP AF × 10) × kg feed/d. Example of calculation for concentrate: CP g/d = (11 × 10) × 1 = 110 g/d.

[e] Ca g/d = (% Ca AF × 10) × kg feed/d. Example of calculation for concentrate: Ca g/d = (0.8 × 10) × 1 = 8 g/d.

the feeding method are clinical status, and intake of energy and nutrients that meet the horse's requirements.

Water and forage are two essential components of the horse's ration, whereas grains and concentrates are optional and fed to make up the deficiencies in the forage. Horses should have adequate quantities of good-quality palatable water readily available at all times. Sources of drinking water should be checked ideally twice daily for fullness and cleanliness. The function of water heaters should be checked during freezing ambient temperatures. Water containers should be maintained clean and should be disinfected once a week. Drinking water before and after feeding does not affect feed digestibility but thirsty horses will reduce feed intake if water is not available before or during feeding.[17]

Proper forage feeding management minimizes forage losses (especially nutritious leaves), forage fecal contamination, and inhalation of dust. Hay should be fed from hay feeders (hay racks or nets, feed troughs, feed bunks) that keep the forage off the ground. The hay feeder should not be placed above horse's shoulder level, to avoid the dust getting into horse's eyes and airways. It is common to observe horses to pull hay from the feeder and then ingest it from the ground. This occurs because horses have the desire to see what is going on around them while eating. However, feeding forage from the ground increases hay waste, fecal contamination, and the risk of intestinal parasitism and dirt consumption. Dirt ingestion may be responsible for sand colic, enterolith formation, and intestinal impaction.[18] When feeding from the ground, the amount of waste should be estimated and added on the top of the calculated ration. If fed from the ground, the hay should be placed on a firm and dry area.

Grains should be fed in a feeder. Wooden, plastic, or rubber feeding pans are preferable for nonstabled horses. Free-choice trace-mineralized salt or vitamin-mineral supplement should be located close to the water source.

The natural feeding behavior of horses is to eat small meals frequently. If the feed is available to them, horses will eat hourly during the day and every 2 to 3 hours during the night.[19] Therefore, the feeds should be fed in equally divided amounts, as near the same time each day. The intervals between feedings should be as even as practical and the feeding frequency should be at least twice daily.[18]

Voluntary intake in horses is influenced by weather, palatability of feed, interactions with other horses (pecking order), and energy intake. If allowed free access to unlimited amounts of feeds (hay, pasture, grain, concentrate), horses may consume excessive amounts of nonstructural carbohydrates that may cause digestive upset, colic, or laminitis. Free access to forage is associated with obesity. Therefore, the best feeding management practice is to feed measured amounts of feed and control pasture intake to maintain optimal BCS.

FEEDING PLAN

There are two outcomes of the nutritional assessment. First, the current ration and/or feeding management are appropriate and there is no need for modification. Second, a more appropriate ration and feeding method are implemented. When changing the diet, all changes should be gradual over at least 10 to 14 days to avoid gastrointestinal upsets.

MONITORING NUTRITIONAL STATUS AND REASSESSMENT

Once the feeding plan is established, the next important step is to establish a monitoring plan that will allow adjustments to be made as needed. Obviously, adjustments in diet and feeding are justified only when the assessment reveals an inadequacy in the current plan. The frequency of monitoring nutritional and health status ranges from once daily in healthy horses to every hour in critically ill horses. Observations are made on feeding behavior, appetite, attitude, and amount of feed consumed. Frequency of defecation and fecal quality should be checked daily. Bodyweight and BCS should be evaluated and recorded monthly in healthy horses and daily in critically ill horses. Ideal BCS ranges from 4 to 6/9, depending on the horse's function and life stage. Physical examination and laboratory tests should be repeated whenever indicated.

In summary, the assessment of nutritional status and feeding programs consists of several steps that should be repeated whenever there is a change in the health, life stage, or performance status of a horse. The process starts with assessment of an individual or group of horses, and is followed by a nutrition-focused physical examination that includes obtaining BW and BCS. The next step is performing additional diagnostic laboratory tests and determining nutrient and energy requirements. Assessment of the diet and the feeding method follows. Introduction of a new feeding plan should be implemented if the existing feeding plan is not appropriate. The feeding plan should be reassessed and adjusted periodically.

ACKNOWLEDGMENT

We acknowledge Terry Lawrence, graphic designer and medical illustrator.

REFERENCES

1. Henneke DR, Potter GD, Kreider JL, et al. Relationship between condition score, physical measurements and body fat percentage in mares. Equine Vet J 1983;15: 371–2.
2. National Research Council. Nutrient requirements of horses. 6th edition. Washington, DC: The National Academies Press; 2007.
3. Webb AI, Weaver BM. Body composition of horses. Equine Vet J 1979;11:39–47.
4. Caroll C, Huntington P. Body condition scoring and weight estimation of horses. Equine Vet J 1988;20(1):41–5.
5. Ellis JM, Hollands T. Accuracy of different methods of estimating the weight of horses. Vet Rec 1998;143(12):335–6.
6. Kaneko JJ. Serum proteins and the dysproteinemias. In: Kaneko JJ, Harvey JW, Bruss ML, editors. Clinical biochemistry of domestic animals. 5th edition. San Diego (CA): Academic Press; 1997. p. 117–37.
7. Erwin ES, Varnell TR, Page HM. Relationship to vitamin A and carotene to bovine serum proteins. Proc Soc Exp Biol Med 1959;100(2):373–5.
8. Lewis LD. Diagnosis of equine nutritional imbalances. In: Lewis LD, editor. Equine clinical nutrition: feeding and care. Media (PA): Williams & Wilkins; 1995. p. 438–46.
9. Li P, Yin Y, Li D, et al. Amino acids and immune function. Br J Nutr 2007;98: 237–52.
10. Craig AM, Blythe LL, Lassen ED, et al. Variations of serum vitamin E, cholesterol, and total serum lipid concentrations in horses during a 72-hour period. Am J Vet Res 1989;50(9):1527–31.
11. Maas J. Diagnostic considerations for evaluating nutritional problems in cattle. Vet Clin North Am Food Anim Pract 2007;23:527–39.
12. Official Publication Association of American Feed Control Officials Incorporated 2008.

13. Kronfeld D. A practical method for ration evaluation and diet formulation: an introduction of sensitivity analysis. In: Pagan JD, Geor RJ, editors. Advances in equine nutrition II. Nottingham (UK): Nottingham University Press; 2001. p. 1–12.
14. Lewis LD. Vitamins for horses. In: Lewis LD, editor. Equine clinical nutrition: feeding and care. Media (PA): Williams & Wilkins; 1995. p. 64–86.
15. Baylor JE. Hay management in North America. In: Bolsen KK, editor. Field guide for hay and silage management in North America. West Des Moines (IA): NFIA; 1991. p. 13–32.
16. Pagan JD, Jackson S, Duren S. Computing horse nutrition: how to properly conduct an equine nutrition evaluation using microsteed™ equine ration evaluation software. World Equine Vet Rev 1996;1(2):10B11–7.
17. Lewis LD. Water, energy, protein, carbohydrates, and fats for horses. In: Lewis LD, editor. Equine clinical nutrition: feeding and care. Media (PA): Williams & Wilkins; 1995. p. 3–22.
18. Lewis LD. General horse feeding practices. In: Lewis LD, editor. Equine clinical nutrition: feeding and care. Media (PA): Williams & Wilkins; 1995. p. 185–93.
19. Houpt KA. Feeding problems. Vet Clin North Am Equine Pract 1982;4(7):17–20.

Primer on Dietary Carbohydrates and Utility of the Glycemic Index in Equine Nutrition

Patricia Harris, MA, PhD, VetMB, MRCVS[a,*], Raymond J. Geor, BVSc, MVSc, PhD[b]

KEYWORDS

- Horse • Carbohydrates • Nonstructural carbohydrates
- Fructans • Glucose • Insulin

The horse, a nonruminant herbivore, is well suited to a high-carbohydrate diet consisting predominantly of graminoids (eg, grasses, sedges, and rushes). Plant carbohydrates in equine feeds can be subdivided into the structural carbohydrates (SC), which largely make up the fibrous portion of the diet and originate from the plant cell wall, and the nonstructural carbohydrates (NSC), which originate from the cell content. Together, the NSC and SC constitute the main energy-yielding portions of the diet. Domestication and the requirement for high-energy intakes have resulted in the addition of alternative carbohydrate sources with high NSC content (eg, cereal grains) to the diet. In addition, many pastures contain forage species with far higher NSC contents (sugar, starch, and fructans) than the horse's evolutionary grasslands. Such pastures can result in marked changes of blood glucose and insulin similar to the changes that occur with the feeding of large cereal-based meals.[1] These fluctuations in turn have been linked to abnormalities in growth, development of insulin resistance, and an increased risk of laminitis and/or obesity.[2–4] This hypothesis that fluctuations in glucose and insulin have been linked with a number of diseases has stimulated research into the glycemic and insulinemic effects of different feeds and the influence of different dietary carbohydrates. In addition, it has driven commercial interest in the

---

Parts of this article, with kind permission, were adapted from Harris PA, Geor RJ. Relevance and standardisation of the terms glycemic index and glycemic response. In: Lindner A, editor. Applied Equine Nutrition and Training, Proceedings of Equine Nutrition Conference (ENUCO). Netherlands: Wageningen Academic Publishers; 2007. p. 57–78.

[a] WALTHAM Centre for Pet Nutrition, Freeby Lane, Waltham-on-the-Wolds, Melton Mowbray, Leicestershire LE14 4RT, UK
[b] Department of Large Animal Clinical Sciences, D-202 Veterinary Medical Center, College of Veterinary Medicine, Michigan State University, East Lansing, MI 48824, USA
* Corresponding author.
E-mail address: pat.harris@eu.effem.com (P. Harris).

Vet Clin Equine 25 (2009) 23–37
doi:10.1016/j.cveq.2009.01.006
vetequine.theclinics.com

development of low-starch feeds that result in a lowered glycemic response that may offer health benefits to the horse.

This article provides a detailed description of the different carbohydrates in equine feeds. It also reviews the terminology used to describe glucose and insulin responses to the ingestion of carbohydrates, in particular the concept of the glycemic index (GI). Some of the factors that influence the GI in humans and the glycemic response to a meal in horses are also discussed.

DIETARY CARBOHYDRATES

All carbohydrates contain similar amounts of gross energy. When used by the horse, however, they provide variable amounts of digestible energy, metabolizable energy, and/or net energy.[5] Carbohydrates digested and absorbed as monosaccharides in the small intestine yield (ie, more energy) than carbohydrates digested by microbial action (predominantly fermentation), and there tends to be a glycemic response to the ingestion of such carbohydrates. The type of linkage between the monosaccharide residues in the carbohydrate also affects the site of digestion, and thus the nutritional value, of these compounds. Hydrolysis of the α1-6 and the α1-4 linkages of starch and maltose, for example, can occur in the equine small intestine, but horses do not produce the enzymes necessary to digest the β1-4 linkages found in cellulose or the mixed linkages found in hemicellulose. Therefore, digestion of cellulose and hemicellulose must occur as a result of microbial fermentation, which does not result in a pronounced glycemic response. Stachyose, raffinose, β-glucans, fructooligosaccharides (or fructans), and pectin also are thought to be resistant to enzymatic hydrolysis. Thus, an understanding of the various carbohydrate components in plants (and the means of digestion) is needed to determine the potential for a feed to result in a glycemic response.

Terminology

Simple sugars

Through the process of photosynthesis in the green tissues of plants, whereby atmospheric carbon dioxide is "fixed" in the presence of light and water, simple sugars (mono- or disaccharides—glucose, fructose, and sucrose) are produced. These simple sugars can be used immediately by the plant to supply energy for metabolism, protein synthesis, and growth. Alternatively, they can be elaborated into more complex oligosaccharides (eg, raffinose and stachyose) or the structural polysaccharides of the plant cell wall (eg, cellulose, hemicellulose, and pectin). When sugar production exceeds immediate requirements for metabolism, the excess sugars are polymerized to form storage or reserve carbohydrates. These storage carbohydrates are predominantly in the form of starch or fructan, and these components together with the simple sugars and the oligosaccharides comprise the NSC fraction of the diet.

Free monosaccharides actually occur in low concentrations in plants. Levels of sucrose are rarely greater than 100 g/kg dry matter (DM), and the upper threshold level of sucrose in ryegrass leaves was reported to be approximately 60 to 75 g sucrose/kg DM, with fructan synthesis commencing above this level.[6]

Under certain circumstances, nonplant sources of simple sugars also are important in equine nutrition. For example, lactose, a disaccharide composed of glucose and galactose, is a primary nutrient source for the nursing foal.

Oligosaccharides

Members of the raffinose family of oligosaccharides are alpha-galactosyl derivatives of sucrose. The most common are the trisaccharide, raffinose (composed of galactose, fructose, and glucose) and the tetrasaccharide, stachyose. These oligosaccharides can be found in a variety of vegetables, sugar beet molasses, and whole grains. Soybean oligosaccharides comprise approximately 5% of DM in whole beans and up to 8% of DM in soybean meal. Together, raffinose and stachyose rank second only to sucrose in abundance as water-soluble carbohydrates (WSC). Unlike sucrose, however, they cannot be digested by mammalian enzymes, because the necessary enzyme, α-galactosidase, is not found in monogastric species. A few less commonly found oligosaccharides, such as maltotriose, can be digested by mammalian enzymes, however.

Structural polysaccharides

Structural polysaccharides include dietary fiber that is comprised of cellulose, pectin, and hemicelluloses, along with mannans, galactans, and xyloglucans. Total nonstarch polysaccharides are the sum of the water-soluble and water-insoluble nonstarch polysaccharides and include the sum of cellulosic and non-cellulosic polysaccharides. Pectic polymers tend to be the major component of the water-insoluble fraction. Although some of the nonstarch polysaccharides are water soluble, these are not digestible by mammalian enzymes, and digestion therefore can occur only through fermentation. This fermentation may occur proximal to the cecum.

Starch

Starch is the main storage polysaccharide in the majority of higher plants, including the forage legumes (clover, lucerne/alfalfa). Starch is stored in both the vegetative tissues (ie, nonreproductive tissues such as leaves, stem) and the reproductive tissues (eg, flowers, seeds). Although pasture grasses grown in temperate climates, such as those found in the United Kingdom and parts of the United States, store starch in their seeds, starch is only a minor constituent of the storage carbohydrates in their vegetative tissues.[7] The amount of starch present therefore depends on the plant, environmental conditions, and the time of year. This variation has been summarized as follows:[8] typically, the starch content of grass seed ranges from approximately 330 to 440 g starch/kg seed DM,[9] whereas that of oats, peas, barley, and maize generally constitutes approximately 410, 420, 550, and 690 g/kg seed DM, respectively.[10] The amount of starch stored in the leaves of legumes rarely exceeds 75 g starch/kg DM, however,[11] because in leaves starch is synthesized and stored in the plastids, and when the plastids are saturated with starch, starch synthesis ceases.

Starch consists of polymers of glucose, which occur in two forms: amylose and amylopectin. The former is a linear α-(1-4) linked molecule, whereas the latter is a larger, highly branched molecule containing both α-(1-4) and α-(1-6) linkages. The ratio of amylose to amylopectin depends largely on the botanic origin of the starch. For example, in wheat flour amylose is around 30% of the total starch, whereas maize can contain up to 70% amylose. Glucose availability in the small intestine tends to be higher for starches with high amylopectin content. The molecular weight of the starch is another factor that affects digestibility, with high-molecular-weight forms tending to be more resistant to hydrolysis by mammalian enzymes.

The extent to which starch is digested pre-cecally depends on many factors, including the availability of the starch to mammalian enzymes (eg, the extent to which any outer husk or hull has been broken down), the ratio of amylose to amylopectin within the starch granule, the nature of the starch granule itself, the effect of processing (thermal treatment, for example, improves the digestibility of corn and barley starch), and the rate of intestinal passage. Ingestion of excessive levels of starch may exceed the relatively limited amylolytic capacity of the equine foregut.[12] Any undigested starch (including resistant starch) that has not been fermented in the stomach and small intestine by resident microbes will pass into the large intestine, where it will be fermented, yielding less net energy than when it is absorbed as glucose. Resistant starch includes starch that is not accessible to digestive enzymes because of its structure or encapsulation in plant cell structures and starch that has been modified by certain types of processing.[13,14]

A system for characterizing the availability of the starch found in various horse feeds has not been developed but could be a useful tool in equine nutrition.

Fructan

Fructan is the major storage carbohydrate of the vegetative tissues of temperate grasses. "Fructan" is a collective term for oligo- and polyfructosyl sucrose. Depending on the number of fructose molecules, fructans can be described as oligosaccharides (< 10 monosaccharide units) or polysaccharides (> 10 units). Fructans also can be divided broadly into three groups characterized by their glycosidic linkages. Different fructan types are found in the different plants, and these differences may influence the rate and extent of their digestion in the horse, as does the molecular size of the fructan. Timothy and cocksfoot tend to have larger fructans (degree of polymerization [DP] of 100 or more), whereas ryegrass fructans typically have a DP of 30 to 40, and oat fructan is much smaller with an average DP of 5.[8]

High levels of fructan can accumulate in the vegetative tissues of pasture grasses as fructans are translocated away from the site of production to the vacuoles of the stem.[8] Fructan levels in excess of 400 g/kg DM have been reported for *Bromus* spp.[15] and in a 3-year Northern European study of the WSC components (sugar and fructan) in the vegetative structures of temperate grasses, fructan contents of up to 279 g/kg DM were recorded.[8] Fructan accumulation (unlike accumulation of starch) can occur below the temperature threshold for plant growth (approximately 6°C).[16,17] Therefore, cold, bright days that result in high rates of photosynthesis but negligible plant growth may lead to the production of large quantities of excess sucrose and, in turn, to significant fructan accumulation. In addition to grasses, various pasture weed species accumulate fructan. These species include common dandelion (*Taraxacum officinale*), sow-thistle (*Sonchus* spp.), and chicory (*Cichorium intybus*).

Collective Terms

Water-soluble carbohydrates

The WSC fraction includes the simple sugars (eg, glucose, sucrose, fructose) and the more complex sugars (oligosaccharides and fructans). Some nonstarch polysaccharides also are water soluble. Although not all these components can be digested by mammalian enzymes, the majority can be fermented rapidly by gram-positive bacteria, resulting in the production of lactic acid. It is important to note that starch, which also can be fermented in this way, is not included in this term.

In the aforementioned study of grasses in Northern Europe,[8] total WSC contents ranged from less than 100 to more than 385 g/kg DM, and fructan accounted for 55% to 75% of the total WSC fraction. The corresponding proportions of sucrose, fructose, and glucose were 16% to 22%, 6% to 12% and 3% to 10% DM, respectively.

Some commercial laboratories measure WSC (ie, free sugars plus oligosaccharides and fructans) but report it as "sugar," whereas others use the term "sugar" to describe the free sugar fraction only. A more accurate and consistent description of the measured (or calculated) fractions is needed.

Ethanol-soluble carbohydrates

The term "ethanol-soluble carbohydrates" (ESC) is relatively new and has been used in an attempt to characterize better the components of the WSC that are digestible by mammalian enzymes (eg, simple [mono- and disaccharide] sugars). Additionally, the difference between the WSC and ESC fractions has been used to approximate the amount of fructan in a particular feedstuff. This estimate may be inaccurate, however, in that some oligosaccharides (including some fructans) may be measured in the ESC fraction. Further work is needed to determine the utility of ESC in equine nutrition (ie, as a predictor of glycemic response to a feed).

Nonstructural carbohydrates

NSC often is taken to approximate the material within the feed or feedstuff that potentially can be fermented rapidly to lactic acid. NSC includes the mono- and disaccharides, oligosaccharides (including fructan), fructan polysaccharides, and starch. The concentrations of WSC, particularly the fructan component, in pasture grasses can vary greatly. This variation can be observed from season to season, from day to day, and from hour to hour.[8] There also is variation in the starch content of legume leaves, although those starch levels tend to be somewhat lower than the levels of the WSC/fructan fractions in grasses. There still is some debate about the optimal way to measure the NSC content of feeds, and some confusion has arisen from different methods being used in different publications. The most commonly used system of analysis for feeds was initially developed by Van Soest.[17] The system can analyze the feed for neutral detergent solubles and neutral detergent fiber (NDF). The NDF fraction contains cellulose, most of the hemicellulose, and lignin. Until recently the NSC content of a feed was determined from the feed analysis and was reported according to the following equation (ie, it estimated NSC "by difference"):

$$NSC = 100 - (crude\ protein\% + NDF\% + moisture\% + fat\% + ash\%)$$

This estimate was taken to represent the combined sugar, starch, and fructan content of the feed. However, unfortunately, it also includes pectins, gums, and mucilages that, unlike starch, sugar, and fructan, are not subject to very rapid fermentation and therefore do not induce the marked changes in lactic acid concentrations and pH within the hindgut that can occur with excess intake of sugars, starch, or fructan. Therefore, the NSC "by difference" fraction now is referred to as "nonfiber carbohydrate" (NFC). The quantitative difference between measured NSC and NFC is small for some feeds (eg, cereal grains) but can be quite large for other feeds (eg, feeds with substantial pectin such as sugar beet pulp). Also, with some analytical techniques the NDF fraction can include nitrogen-containing elements. When the equation given earlier is used to estimate the NFC, these nitrogen-containing elements will, in effect, be removed twice (via the crude protein and the NDF), resulting in a slightly reduced value.

Few commercial feed analysis laboratories completely fractionate the carbohydrates that make up the NSC, but in most feeds the amount of NSC can be approximated by summing the amount of starch and WSC. The extent to which the sum of starch and WSC accounts for all NSC depends on the analytical procedures used to measure these fractions. This determination probably more accurately reflects the potential for a feed to be fermented rapidly to produce lactic acid. The amount of starch, in particular, that is fermented rapidly rather than digested via mammalian enzymes depends on many factors, including how and where the starch is stored in the feed material, how the feed has been processed, how much is being fed, and possibly what it has been fed with (eg, oat starch tends to be digested efficiently in the small intestine regardless of processing). **Fig. 1** provides a simple chart highlighting the differences between WSC, NSC, and NFC. The reader is referred elsewhere for a more detailed schematic of the different feed carbohydrates.[18]

GLYCEMIC INDEX

In humans, obesity (and associated metabolic disorders) is one of the most important public health concerns, but the advice to reduce total dietary fat, in an attempt to reduce calorie intake, often leads to reciprocal increases in carbohydrate intake. This increased carbohydrate intake, in turn, may entail risk to health, because not all carbohydrates produce the same metabolic effects. In particular they differ in the extent to which they raise blood glucose and insulin concentrations.[19] The concept of the GI was developed approximately 25 years ago[20] as a means to classify carbohydrate-containing foods based on their potential for raising the blood glucose level. Since then numerous studies have looked at the role of GI and glycemic load (GL) in the prevention and management of type 2 diabetes, cardiovascular disease, obesity, and other chronic diseases such as cancer.[19,20] The true impact of changing from a high- to a low-GI diet remains controversial, however, with many conflicting studies, in part because study designs are confounded by the use of multiple dietary manipulations, rather than just a change to a low-GI diet.[19,21,22] In addition, although numerous international tables contain published data on the GI's of individual human foods,[23] these values do not take into account regional or individual differences in foods or food preparation.[21] Despite this obvious limitation, most human studies looking at the influence of GI on health and disease risk use estimated GI values based on such tables and food questionnaires rather than actual GI data for the foods used.[21]

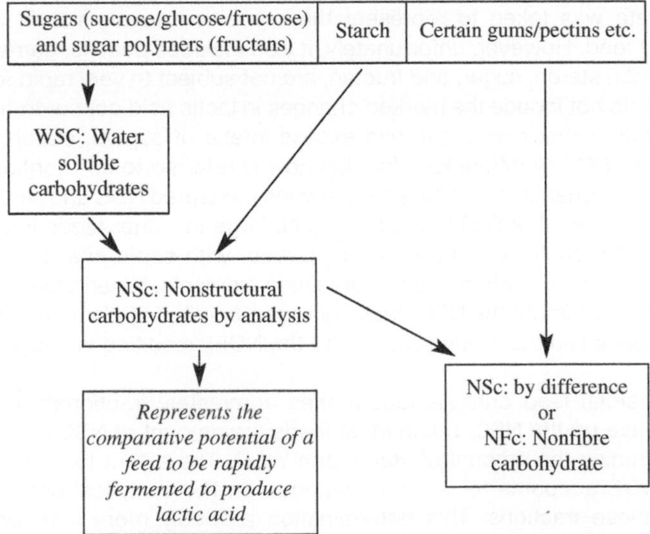

Fig. 1. Schematic guide to the nutrients included in the terms water-soluble carbohydrate (WSC), nonstructural carbohydrate (NSC), and nonfiber carbohydrate (NFC). (*Adapted from* Harris P, Geor R. Nutritional countermeasures to laminitis. In: Harris PA, Hill SJ, Elliot J, et al, editors. The latest findings in laminitis research. The 1st WALTHAM-Royal Veterinary College Laminitis Conference; 2007. p. 29–38; with permission.)

Terminology in Humans

Available carbohydrates

Available carbohydrates are simple sugars such as lactose, glucose, sucrose, fructose (maltodextrins, maltose), and available starch. These carbohydrates can be digested by mammalian enzymes, predominantly within the small intestine, to hexoses, which can be absorbed from the small intestine; if they escape digestion in the small intestine, they can be fermented rapidly (often to lactic acid as well as to other short-chain fatty acids) in the hindgut.

Glycemic response

The glycemic response is the incremental area under the plasma glucose versus time curve elicited by a meal. There are several ways of determining area under the curve (AUC); the most commonly used is the incremental method that includes the area over the baseline glucose concentration, ignoring the area of the curve that falls below baseline.

Glycemic index

The GI is the classification carbohydrate foods according to their potential for raising the blood glucose level.[24] The GI has been defined[25] as the ratio of the incremental area under the glycemic response curve elicited by the test food (F) providing a fixed amount of carbohydrate and the reference food providing the same amount of carbohydrate (R) when fed on separate occasions to the same subject:

$$GI = 100 \times AUC_F / AUC_R$$

Fundamentally, foods with a high GI produce a higher peak and greater overall blood glucose response than foods with a low GI (which release glucose into the blood at a slower rate). In humans, a low-GI food is one with a GI of 55 or less, whereas a high-GI food has a value of 70 or more. Ideally, the value of the AUC_R should be the average of two or three tests of the reference food. It has been stated that the GI value should reflect the response to 50 g of available carbohydrate in the test food in comparison with either 50 g of glucose or 50 g of available carbohydrate from white bread. A concern, however, is how to estimate the available carbohydrate load. One definition is the total carbohydrate minus dietary fiber analyzed by the Association of Analytical Communities method, but this method may overestimate the available glycemic carbohydrate load and therefore result in smaller portion sizes. An alternative approach is to use total starch minus resistant starch (see[24,26]). It is important to note that the GI is a biologic measurement; that is, it reflects the response in humans rather than being an analytical test in the laboratory. A number of criticisms have been raised, including the cost and difficulty of determining the GI of a food, the inherent variability of the results, and misunderstandings of the results and what they might mean.[25]

Relative glucose or insulin response or relative glycemic effect

The relative glucose response has been used to compare the glucose or insulin response elicited by a portion of food containing 50 g total carbohydrates relative to 50 or 75 g glucose.

Glycemic load

The GL has been defined as the GI times the amount of available carbohydrates in the portion of food (ie, the product of GI and the amount of glycemic carbohydrates in a serving of food).[27] Some authors use the term "relative GL," that is, GI/100 g of carbohydrates (sugars and starches). A low-GL diet therefore can be achieved either by reducing the carbohydrate intake or by reducing the GI of the carbohydrates consumed.

Glycemic glucose equivalent

The glycemic glucose equivalent (GGE) is defined as "the weight of glucose equivalent in its effect to a given weight of food" and is calculated as

$$GGE = food\ wt\ (g) \times (\%\ available\ CHO) \times \text{GI for that food/GI for glucose}$$

where the percentage of available carbohydrates refers to the amount of available carbohydrates in 100 g of food. The GGE has been advocated as a more accurate predictor of glycemic response of a complex meal, but the validity of the GGE remains in question.

Overall, it has been suggested that the term "glycemic index" should be used when testing foods based on available carbohydrates, whereas the terms "glycemic load," "relative glycemic effect," or "glycemic glucose equivalent" should be used to classify the glycemic impact of foods based on the total carbohydrates or serving size.

Factors Influencing the Glycemic Index in Humans

The GI of a particular food can be affected by a number of factors, many of which are of relevance to the horse (see also[23,26,28]). Important factors include the following:

- The type of starch: for example, more amylopectin results in increased GI; more amylose results in reduced GI.
- The rate of digestion of carbohydrate within a particular feed: for example, extruding or puffing starch increases the glycemic response, whereas parboiling can reduce the GI. The degree of destructuring in the mouth and stomach influences how much of the starch granules remain embedded in the food matrix and therefore their accessibility to pancreatic amylases. Interactions between starch and proteins/lipids and fibers within the food influence also their accessibility to amylase. In white bread, for example, the gelatinized starch granules are embedded in a relatively thin protein network, and therefore the starch is readily accessible.
- The rate of gastric emptying, which in turn is influenced by the nature of the food: for example, high organic acids reduce gastric emptying.
- The nature of the monosaccharides absorbed: for example, in humans absorption of fructose and galactose is not associated with an increase in blood glucose concentrations.
- The insulin response elicited by the feed: for example, the proteins in milk and other dairy products elicit particularly high insulin responses.
- The effect of dietary fiber: inclusion of soluble viscous fiber (eg, guar or β-glucans) may increase the viscosity of the digestive medium, thereby limiting the diffusion and hence the absorption of glucose through epithelial cells, the result is a reduced GI.
- The presence of resistant starch: more resistant starch means a reduced GI.
- The presence of certain antinutritive factors, for example, those that inhibit amylase activity reduce GI.
- The nature of the previous meal: for example, a low-GI barley meal given as the evening meal significantly reduced the GI (as well as the insulin index) of white wheat flour given as the breakfast meal; the response to a morning glucose load was lower if a low-GI lentil dinner had been fed, rather than a high-GI meal (glucose), the night before.

- The time of day and the timing of any physical activity before the test.
- The method used for determination of AUC.

Relevance to the horse

The type and amount of starch- and sugar-containing feed that is ingested by the horse should, as in humans, influence the blood glucose and insulin responses in the horse. There are, perhaps, three major differences, however. First, there may be fermentation of available carbohydrate in the stomach of the horse. The extent of this fermentation depends on the individual's gastric flora, the nature of the feed, and the rate of gastric emptying. The end products of such fermentation are lactic acid and short-chain fatty acids rather than glucose, and the overall effect is to reduce the available carbohydrates reaching the small intestine. Second, in the horse the ingestion of meals containing large amounts of starch and sugar may increase the risk of digestive disturbance. Large starch meals may overwhelm small intestinal amylolytic capacity, with delivery of undigested material to the hindgut, rapid fermentation of the starch, and the potential for disturbance to the hindgut environment. Therefore, high-GL diets may cause short-term problems unrelated to any long-term metabolic influence of the feed GI. Additionally, a low glycemic response per se may not be the desired response if it means most of the starch has bypassed the small intestine (eg, as with high-amylose cereal grains such as corn).

In humans, fructose has a smaller influence on serum insulin concentrations than glucose and has no influence on plasma glucose concentrations. In the horse, however, there was no appreciable difference in the insulin or glucose concentrations when fructose, glucose, or a mixture was fed to resting animals, although there were some minor differences when these carbohydrates were fed between two exercise bouts.[29] Another study compared the effects of higher quantities of fructose and glucose, and it was suggested that in resting horses glucose does result in significantly higher glycemic and insulinemic responses than fructose. Fructose feeding during exercise resulted in lower but still marked glycemic responses, although there was no differential effect on the exercise-associated insulin response.[30]

Factors Influencing Glycemic Responses in Horses

The following list provides a nonexhaustive summary of studies that have examined factors affecting the glycemic responses to a feed in horses. It should be emphasized that there are a great deal of conflicting data in this area, in large part because of differences in trial design and methodology used for determination of GI or glycemic response.

Type of cereal grain

Sweet feed, oats, and corn produced higher glycemic responses than barley, flaked rice bran, loose beet pulp, loose soy hulls, and flaked wheat bran.[31]

The AUC for glucose in Thoroughbreds fed cracked corn, oat groats, and rolled barley providing approximately 2 g (starch and sugar) per kg body weight[32] were not significantly different, although barley was the lowest at 468 ± 42 mM/min compared with 519 ± 106 mM/min for the corn and 514 ± 43 mM/min for the oats. This apparent difference was decreased, however, when the glucose AUC was adjusted for actual hydrolyzable carbohydrate ingestion. Using glucose as the reference, the GI was 63% for corn and oat groats and 57% for barley. The authors noted that ingestion of corn resulted in the largest fluctuations in plasma glucose.

Sweet feeds and whole oats showed the greatest glycemic response, whereas alfalfa and sweet feed plus corn oil showed the lowest response in

Thoroughbred horses when the results of feeding 0.75 kg, 1.5 kg, and 2.5 kg of each feed per body weight were combined. No significant differences were found in the glucose AUC for whole oats and cracked corn.[33]

No differences were seen in the glycemic response in Standardbreds fed whole oats, barley, or corn at a moderate starch intake (between 1.2 to 1.5 g starch/kg body weight).[34,35]

Amount of feed

Increases in glycemic response were found when the feed intake was increased from 0.75 kg to 1.5 or 2.5 kg per meal for sweet feed, a high-fiber mix, or sweet feed plus oil. This pattern was not seen with whole oats (highest AUC at 1.5 kg intake), however. With cracked corn, similar results were observed for the medium and high intakes, and glycemic response was higher with both the medium and high intakes than with the low intake. For alfalfa, the medium intake resulted in a lower glycemic response than the low intake, which in turn was lower than with the high intake.[33]

There are conflicting data on the dose–response relationship when feeding oat starch. In one study, the GI was lower for 2.5 kg/body weight of whole oats than for 1.5 kg/body weight.[31] Conversely, another study observed an increase in glycemic response when the amount of oat starch was increased from 1.2 to 2 to 4 g starch/kg body weight.[34,35]

When the same amount and type of feed was given either in two (2.6 kg/meal), three (1.75 kg/meal), or four (1.3 kg/meal) meals per day, the larger concentrate meals fed twice a day resulted in modestly higher glycemic responses than the three or four daily meals. Although there were significant differences with respect to glucose AUC, it can be questioned whether these differences are clinically important (1253.7 mg/dL, 1168.7 mg/dL, and 1176 mg/dL for the two, three, and four meals/day schedules, respectively).[36]

Effect of feed processing

When the glycemic response of ground or steam-processed corn was compared with that of cracked corn, the highest GI (expressed relative to cracked corn) was for steam-flaked corn fed at 2 g/kg body weight/meal.[37]

No difference was found following mechanical or thermal processing of oats, barley, or corn with a moderate starch intake (between 1.2 and 1.5 g starch/kg body weight per meal), but a difference was found when the starch intake was increased to 2 g starch/kg body weight.[34,35]

In a study looking at the effects of different processing procedures for barley, the lowest degree of gelatinization was found in whole barley (14.9%), and the highest degree was in popped barley (95.6%). There was no difference in the glycemic response to whole barley and popped barley, however (levels of resistant starch were not determined).[38] Because the difference in the mean glucose AUC between the feeds was less than 5% of the highest AUC, however, effective ranking of the diets was not possible.

Different glycemic responses were found when the same quantity of starch was fed as a pellet or a sweet feed.[39]

No difference in postprandial glycemic response was found in weanling Standardbred horses fed the same ration either as alfalfa hay cubes and a grain mix (50:50) fed separately or the same mix ground and pelleted.[40]

Effect of adding fiber to the meal

No difference was observed in the postprandial AUC for glucose when 100% alfalfa, 100% corn, or a combined corn/alfalfa diet was fed to horses.[41]

Feeding long hay before or with a sweet feed resulted in a reduction of the glycemic response.[42]

Feeding up to 35% of short-chop lucerne (alfalfa) mixed with oats or sweet feed did not influence the glucose AUC.[43,44]

The addition of alfalfa chaff before, with, or after a meal of oats did not affect glycemic and insulin responses.[45]

The glycemic response within a particular forage type can vary considerably; in some legumes, such as alfalfa, starch content is highly variable (see[46]).

Effect of adding amylolytic enzymes

The addition of both α-amylase and amyloglucosidase to steam-rolled triticale significantly increased the peak plasma glucose responses when compared with glycemic responses elicited by the amyloglucosidase and control (triticale only) diets.[47] This study was not a crossover trial, however. The average plasma glucose concentration over the 5-hour sampling period also was significantly higher for horses fed the α-amylase and the α-amylase plus amyloglucosidase diets than for horses on the amyloglucosidase or control diets, but no differences among treatments were detected for peak or average plasma insulin concentrations. Interestingly, horses fed α-amylase had a significantly reduced average glucose response during the second sampling period (day 6 of feeding) compared with that observed during the first sampling period (day 3 of feeding). This difference was not seen with the α-amylase plus amyloglucosidase diet.[47]

Relationship between insulin and glucose responses

There are conflicting data on the relationship between glycemic and insulinemic response. Rankings for glycemic and insulinemic responses were similar when mature Quarter Horses were fed mixed diets of whole barley and oats; sugar beet pulp (soaked), grass meal, and soybean oil; rice bran and grass meal; or rice bran, grass meal, sugar beet meal, and soybean oil.[48] Other studies comparing responses to different types and amounts of starch have observed different rankings for glycemic and insulinemic indices.[34,35]

From the preceding discussion, it is readily apparent that many factors affect glycemic responses to meal ingestion in horses, and currently it is not possible to predict responses accurately based on knowledge of feed type and chemical composition. In a study[31] that examined the glycemic responses to 10 common equine feeds, it was noted that variation in the actual calories of each feed offered (4–6 Mcal of digestible energy), time to complete feed ingestion (15–300 minutes), feed refusal (14%, 31%, and 37% for soy hulls, rice bran, and beet pulp, respectively), feed processing, as well as the content and form of the starch and sugar probably contributed to the variation in the data. Additionally, if glucose is used as the reference material for determination of GI, it is important to note that many factors influence the response to an oral glucose load, including prior diet,[49] physiologic state (eg, reproductive status),[50–52] and clinical conditions such as obesity and insulin resistance.[53] Together, these findings suggest that many of the factors identified as influencing the GI in humans also are likely to affect responses in horses, including the type and amount of dietary carbohydrate fed and individual animal factors. A unique consideration in the horse is the impact of different feeds on the hindgut. Although a particular feed may elicit a low glycemic response, this characteristic does not rule out the possibility of adverse effects in the cecum and large colon; the feeding of meals rich in resistant starch (unprocessed corn or barley) is a prime example. Convenient and reliable methods for determining the impact of a feed on the hindgut microbial community are needed.

At present the validity and practical application of the GI concept in horses is uncertain, and more work is required.[54] Feed manufacturers should be strongly encouraged to test diets advocated to elicit a low GI or glycemic response to confirm this claim. Progress in this area also will require development of a standardized methodology for evaluating glycemic response in the horse.[54]

SUMMARY

There is mounting evidence that health benefits may be associated with the provision of low-GI foods to both humans and the horse. These health benefits have been linked to the slow rate of digestion and reduced postprandial insulin responses in low-GI foods, coupled with factors such as reduced fluctuations in blood glucose or differences in gut hormone responses. There are problems, however, in applying the low-GI concept to feed formulation and the development of dietary recommendations for horses, particularly in situations where there is no evidence in support of low-GI claims. Currently, the tools needed to predict glycemic response from feed formulation are not available; knowledge of chemical composition and data from actual feeding trials are needed to guide feeding recommendations. Currently, it is recommended that certain groups of horses (eg, growing horses, old horses, and those prone to laminitis and the equine rhabdomyolysis syndrome) be fed diets that have been shown to produce a low (or moderate) glycemic response, or at least diets that are likely to produce a high glycemic response, should be avoided.

REFERENCES

1. McIntosh B, Kronfeld D, Geor R, et al. Circadian and seasonal fluctuations of glucose and insulin concentrations in grazing horses. In: Proceedings of the 20th Equine Science Symposium. Maryland: Equine Science Society; 2007. p. 100–1.
2. Kronfeld DS, Harris PA. Equine grain-associated disorders. Compendium on Continuing Education for the Practicing Veterinarian 2003;25:974–82.
3. Kronfeld D, Treiber K, Hess T, et al. Insulin resistance in the horse: definition, detection and dietetics. J Anim Sci 2005;83:E22–33.
4. Trieber KH, Kronfeld DS, Geor RJ. Insulin resistance in equids—possible role in laminitis. J Nutr 2006;136:2094S–8S.
5. Harris PA. Energy requirements of the exercising horse. Annu Rev Nutr 1997;17: 185–210.
6. Cairns AJ, Pollock CJ. Fructan biosynthesis in excised leaves of *Lolium temulentum L.* Chromatographic characterisation of oligofructans and their labelling patterns following 14CO2 feeding. New Phytol 1998;109:399–405.
7. Pollock CJ, Cairns AJ. Fructan metabolism in grasses and cereals. Annu Rev Plant Physiol Plant Mol Biol 1991;42:77–101.
8. Longland A, et al. Starch, sugar and fructans: what are they and how important are they in diets for horses. In: Harris P, Hill SH, Elliott J, editors. Proceedings of the 1st WALTHAM – RVC laminitis conference. Newmarket (UK): Equine Veterinary Journal. p. 7–14.
9. Turner LJB, Humphreys MO, Cairns AJ, et al. Comparison of growth and carbohydrate accumulation in seedlings of two varieties of Lolium perenne. J Plant Physiol 2001;158:891–7.

10. Graham H. Digestibility of plant carbohydrates and associated components in pig diets. In: Plant carbohydrates and associated components: analytical methods and nutritional implications in monogastrics animals and man, NJF Seminar, Herning, Denmark; 1990. p. 502–5.
11. Available at: www.dairyone.com. Accessed February 2009.
12. de Fombelle A, Veiga L, Drogoul C, et al. Effect of diet composition and feeding pattern on the prececal digestibility of starches from diverse botanical origins measured with the mobile nylon bag technique. J Anim Sci 2004;82: 3625–34.
13. Cummings JH, Beatty ER, Kingman SM, et al. Digestion and physiological properties of resistant starch in the human large bowel. Br J Nutr 1996;75:733–47.
14. Tharanathan RN. Food derived carbohydrates—structural complexity and functional diversity. Crit Rev Biotechnol 2002;22(1):65–84.
15. Chatterton NJ, Harrison PA, Bennett JH, et al. Carbohydrate partitioning in 185 accessions of graminae grown under warm and cool temperatures. J Plant Physiol 1989;143:169–79.
16. Pollock CJ, Lloyd EJ. The effect of low temperature upon starch, sucrose and fructan synthesis in leaves. Ann Bot 1987;60:231–5.
17. Pollock CJ, Lloyd EJ, Stoddart JL, et al. Growth, photosynthesis, and assimilate partitioning in Lolium temulentum exposed to chilling temperatures. Physiol Plantarum 1983;59:257–62.
18. NRC (National Research Council). Nutrient requirements of horses. 6th revision. Washington, DC: National Academy Press; 2007.
19. Aston LM. Glycemic index and metabolic disease risk. Proc Nutr Soc 2006;65: 125–34.
20. Jenkins D, Wolever R, Taylor R, et al. Glycemic index of foods: a physiological basis for carbohydrate exchange. Am J Clin Nutr 1981;34:362–6.
21. Feskens EJM, Du H. Dietary glycemic index from an epidemiological point of view. Int J Obes 2006;30:S66–71.
22. Sahyoun NR, Anderson AL, Tylavsky FA, et al. Dietary glycemic index and glycemic load and the risk of type 2 diabetes in older adults. Am J Clin Nutr 2008;87: 126–31.
23. Foster-Powell K, Holt SH, BrandMiller JC. International table of glycemic index and glycemic load values. Am J Clin Nutr 2002;76:5–56.
24. Granfeldt Y, Wu X, Bjorck I. Determination of glycemic index some methodological aspects related to the analysis of carbohydrate load and characteristics of the previous evening meal. Eur J Clin Nutr 2006;60:104–12.
25. Wolever TMS. Physiological mechanisms and observed health impacts related to the glycemic index: some observations. Int J Obes 2006;30:S72–8.
26. Brouns F, Bjock I, Frayn KN, et al. Glycemic index methodology. Nutr Res Rev 2005;18:145–71.
27. Brand-Miller J, Thomas M, et al. Physiological validation of the concept of glycemic load in lean young adults. J Nutr 2003;133:2728–32.
28. Fardet A, Leenhardt F, Lioger D, et al. Parameters controlling the glycemic response to breads. Nutrition 2006;19:18–25.
29. Bullimore SR, Pagan JD, Harris PA, et al. Carbohydrate supplementation of horses during endurance exercise: comparison of fructose and glucose. J Nutr 2000;120:1760–5.
30. Vervuert I, Coenen M, Bichmann M. Comparision of the effects of fructose and glucose supplementation on metabolic responses in resting and exercising horses. J Vet Med A Physiol Pathol Clin Med 2004;51(4):171–7.

31. Rodiek AV, Stull CL. Glycemic index of ten common horse feeds. J Equine Vet Sci 2007;27(6):205–11.
32. Jose-Cunilleras E, Taylor LE, Hinchcliff KW. Glycemic index of cracked corn, oat groats and rolled barley in horses. J Anim Sci 2004;82:2623–9.
33. Pagan JD, Harris PA, Kennedy MAP, et al. Feed type and intake affects glycemic response in thoroughbred horses. Equine Nutrition and Physiology Symposium Proceedings 1999;16:149–50.
34. Vervuert I, Coenen M, Bothe C. Effects of oat processing on the glycemic and insulinaemic responses in horses. Journal of Animal Physiology and Animal Nutrition 2003;87:96–104.
35. Vervuert I, Coenen M, Bothe C. Effects of corn processing on the glycemic and insulinaemic responses in horses. Journal of Animal Physiology and Animal Nutrition 2004;88(9):348–55.
36. Steelman SM, Michael-Eller EM, Gibbs PG, et al. Meal size and feeding frequency influence serum leptin concentrations in yearling horses. J Anim Sci 2006;84:2391–8.
37. Hoekstra KE, Newman K, Kennedy MAP, et al. Effect of corn processing on glycemic responses in horses. Proc 16th Equine Nutr Phys Symp 1999:144–8.
38. Vervuert I, Coenen M, Bothe C. Effects of mechanical or thermal barley processing on glucose and insulin profiles in horses. Proceedings of the 9th ESVCN congress Grugliasco 2005;118.
39. Harbour LE, Lawrence LM, Hayes SH, et al. Concentrate composition, form and glycemic response in horses. Proc 18th Equine Nutr Phys Symp 2003:329.
40. Andrew JE, Kline KH, Smith JL. Effects of feed form on growth and blood glucose in weanling horses. J Equine Vet Sci 2006;26:349–55.
41. Stull CL, Rodiek AV. Responses of blood glucose, insulin and cortisol concentrations to common equine diets. J Nutr 1988;118(2):206–13.
42. Pagan JD, Harris PA. The effects of timing and amount of forage and grain on exercise response in Thoroughbred horses. Equine Vet J 1999;Suppl 30:451–8.
43. Harris PA, Sillence M, Inglis R, et al. Effect of short (< 2cm) lucerne chaff addition on the intake rate and glycemic response of a sweet feed. Pferdeheilkunde 2005; 21:88–9.
44. Harris PA, Sillence M, Inglis R, et al. Effect of short (<2cm) lucerne chaff addition on the intake rate and glycemic response to an oat meal. Proceedings of the 19th Equine Science Society Symposium 2005;151–2.
45. Vervuert I, Voigt K, Hollands T, et al. The effect of mixing and changing the order of feeding oats and chopped alfalfa to horses on: 1. Glycaemic and insulinaemic responses, and 2. Breath hydrogen and methane production. Proceedings of the 46th Congress of the British Equine Veterinary Association. Edinburgh, September 12–15, 2007.
46. Kronfeld D, Rodiek A, Stull C. Glycemic indices, glycemic loads and glycemic dietetics. J Equine Vet Sci 2004;24(9):399–404.
47. Richards N, Choct M, Hinch GN, et al. Examination of the use of exogenous a-amylase and amyloglucosidase to enhance starch digestion in the small intestine of the horse. Anim Feed Sci Technol 2004;114:295–305.
48. Zeyner A, Hoomeister C, Einspanier Gottschalk JA, et al. Glycemic and insulinaemic responses of quarter horses to concentrates high in fat and low in soluble carbohydrates. Equine Vet J 2006;Suppl 36:643–7.
49. Jacobs KA, Bolton JR. Effect of diet on the oral glucose tolerance test in the horse. J Am Vet Med Assoc 1982;180(8):884–6.

50. Williams CA, Kronfeld DS, Stanier WB, et al. Plasma glucose and insulin responses of Thoroughbred mares fed a meal high in starch and sugar or fat and fiber. J Anim Sci 2001;79:2196–201.
51. Hoffman RM, Kronfeld DS, Cooper WL, et al. Glucose clearance in grazing mares is affected by diet pregnancy and lactation. J Anim Sci 2003;81:1764–71.
52. Cubitt TA, George LA, Staniar WB, et al. Glucose and insulin dynamics during the estrous cycle of thoroughbred mares. Proceedings of the 20th Equine Science Symposium. Maryland, 2007.
53. Jeffcott LB, Field JR, McLean JG, et al. Glucose tolerance and insulin sensitivity in ponies and standardbred horses. Equine Vet J 1986;18:97–101.
54. Vervuert I, Coenen M. Glycemic index of feeds for horses. Pferdeheilkunde 2005; 21:79–82.

Pasture-Associated Laminitis

Raymond J. Geor, BVSc, MVSc, PhD

KEYWORDS

- Pasture • Laminitis • Nonstructural carbohydrates
- Fructans • Obesity • Insulin resistance
- Grazing management

Laminitis is a painful and debilitating condition of horses and ponies that has major economic and welfare implications.[1,2] In a US survey, apart from colic, laminitis was the most common reason for a horse or pony to be presented for veterinary treatment.[3] Furthermore, 13% of horse owners or operations reported problems with laminitis in their horses over the previous 12-month period, with approximately 5% of those horses affected by laminitis dying or being euthanized.[3] Several conditions have been associated with laminitis, notably gastrointestinal disease (eg, surgical colic, colitis), retained placenta or metritis, and severe infections (eg, pleuropneumonia). Nevertheless, there is general consensus among veterinarians and horsemen that dietary factors, particularly the ingestion of certain plant carbohydrates in pasture forage (but also in other equine feeds), play a major role in laminitis. Indeed, survey studies have indicated that most laminitis cases occur in horses and ponies kept at pasture (hence, the term *pasture-associated laminitis*). In one survey in the United Kingdom, 61% of laminitis cases occurred in animals kept at pasture,[4] whereas the results of the 1998 National Animal Health Monitoring System (NAHMS) laminitis study demonstrated that 46% of cases were associated with grazing on pasture.[3]

This article reviews current knowledge on the epidemiology and pathogenesis of pasture-associated laminitis, including the role of forage carbohydrates and metabolic predispositions. Countermeasures to decrease risk of laminitis in susceptible animals are also discussed, with emphasis on strategies to reduce the intake of carbohydrates involved in the triggering of the condition. Nutritional management of metabolic risk factors for laminitis (eg, obesity, insulin resistance [IR]) is discussed elsewhere in this issue (see the article by Geor and Harris elsewhere in this issue).

Department of Large Animal Clinical Sciences, D-202 Veterinary Medical Center, College of Veterinary Medicine, Michigan State University, East Lansing, MI 48824, USA
E-mail address: geor@cvm.msu.edu

Vet Clin Equine 25 (2009) 39–50
doi:10.1016/j.cveq.2009.01.004 vetequine.theclinics.com
0749-0739/09/$ – see front matter

EPIDEMIOLOGY AND RISK FACTORS

Anecdotal observations have indicated that pasture-induced laminitis occurs at times of rapid grass growth and the accumulation of certain carbohydrates (fructans, starches, and sugars) in pasture forage (during the spring and early summer and during the fall, particularly after rainfall). Surprisingly, few studies have examined the effect of time of year on the incidence of laminitis. Some reports[3–5] have indicated increased risk during spring and summer, whereas others have failed to demonstrate an association between season and the occurrence of acute laminitis.[6,7] The latter studies involved referral populations that may not have accurately reflected disease incidence in the general population, however. In the 1998 NAHMS survey study, laminitis accounted for approximately 20% of foot problems in the winter, whereas approximately 40% of these problems were attributed to laminitis in the spring and summer.[3] A 3-year retrospective study of pasture-kept horses and ponies in a specific region of the United Kingdom found that approximately 20% (291 of 1451) of the total population had at least one episode of laminitis.[5] This study also provided evidence to support the clinical observation that the disease tends to be recurrent in certain individuals. Specifically, 35% of the animals diagnosed with laminitis had repeated episodes over the total study period, with many animals diagnosed multiple times within the same year. The highest prevalence (2.39%) and incidence (16 cases per 1000 animals) occurred in May. There was a statistically significant positive association between hours of sunshine and incident laminitis, but laminitis prevalence and incidence were not associated with regional rainfall or ambient temperature. Presumably, this association between hours of sunshine and incident laminitis reflects altered nutritional intake (ie, increased consumption of forage carbohydrates during periods of bright sunshine that promote plant photosynthesis and carbohydrate accumulation) rather than the direct effect of exposure of horses to sunlight. The role of forage carbohydrates in the pathogenesis of pasture-induced laminitis is discussed elsewhere in this article in the section on pathogenesis of pasture laminitis.

Another important aspect of pasture laminitis is the clinical observation that certain horses or ponies tend to be affected more than others, with susceptible animals often prone to recurrent episodes. This raises the possibility that there are phenotypic or genetic factors that confer susceptibility or resistance to disease. The mechanisms underlying this predisposition are not fully understood, and this area is currently under investigation by several research groups. Nevertheless, there is gathering evidence implicating metabolic factors, particularly obesity, IR, and hyperinsulinemia, as major predisposing conditions for pasture laminitis.[8] Individual variation in tissue (eg, laminar epithelium, digital vasculature) response to trigger factors or in hindgut bacterial flora and their response to dietary substrates also may play a role, but there is minimal information in these areas. Differences in appetite and forage intake are other possible factors.

Clinical observations have long suggested that horses and ponies with a particular phenotype are predisposed to pasture-associated laminitis.[9] These animals fit the description of an "easy keeper," are often overweight or obese (or have regional adiposity, such as a cresty neck), and may be persistently hyperinsulinemic. The term *equine metabolic syndrome* (EMS) has been adopted to describe horses and ponies with evidence of generalized or regional adiposity, hyperinsulinemia, and subclinical (ie, hoof founder rings) or overt laminitis.[10–12] The link between IR and laminitis is supported by results of observational cohort studies in ponies. In an inbred herd of Welsh and Dartmoor ponies, the clustering of IR, hyperinsulinemia, obesity, and hypertriglyceridemia was associated with increased risk of pasture laminitis.[8] The term *prelaminitic metabolic syndrome* (PLMS) was used to describe the phenotype associated with laminitis risk. The PLMS criteria predicted 11 of 13 cases of clinical laminitis observed in May of the same year, with an odds ratio of 10.4 (ie, ponies with this insulin-resistant phenotype were at approximately 10 times higher risk for development of laminitis). A subsequent study of this population of ponies confirmed that the presence of obesity (generalized or regional, such as a cresty neck) or hyperinsulinemia (insulin >32 mU/L when sampled on winter pasture) was a useful predictor of laminitis episodes when ponies were exposed to spring pasture.[13]

Another study of outbred ponies in the United Kingdom confirmed the association between IR and pasture laminitis and provided evidence of hypertension in the high-risk ponies.[14] Interestingly, signs of this metabolic syndrome (ie, IR and hypertension) were evident in summer but not in winter, suggesting that consumption of summer pasture forage may induce abnormal metabolic responses leading to the expression of the prelaminitic phenotype.[14] It is worth mentioning that insulin sensitivity is markedly lower in ponies compared with horse breeds,[8,15] potentially explaining the apparent higher susceptibility of pony breeds to pasture laminitis reported in some epidemiologic studies.[4,5]

There are minimal published data on the possible association between IR and pasture-induced laminitis in horses. Nonetheless, the EMS phenotype has been described in several breeds, notably Morgans, Paso Finos, Arabians, and Norwegian Fjords,[10,11] and many of these horses are out on pasture when laminitis is first detected.[12] IR also may contribute to laminitis predisposition in pituitary pars intermedia dysfunction (PPID), also known as equine Cushing's disease. In clinical reports, chronic insidious-onset laminitis has been described in more than 50% of horses or ponies that have PPID.[16] Hyperglycemia, hyperinsulinemia, and glucose intolerance, findings consistent with IR, have been described in horses that have PPID.[17] Interestingly, in one report, hyperinsulinemia was associated with poor long-term survival in horses suspected of having PPID.[18]

There is evidence that obesity or regional adiposity predisposes horses and ponies to laminitis. In a prospective case-control study of 258 cases seen at six veterinary teaching hospitals, a cresty neck was found in significantly more cases than controls.[19] Ponies at higher risk for pasture laminitis had a higher body condition score (>7) compared with animals without a history of laminitis.[13] Regional adiposity, particularly a cresty neck, also was common in these animals. Mechanical trauma attributable to the increased load on the feet is one theory linking obesity with laminitis risk, but the increased risk for laminitis in obese equids is more likely related to other factors, such as IR and inflammation, which are consequences of obesity.[20–22] Several studies have demonstrated an association between adiposity and IR in horses.[11,13,22] It is important to recognize that not all obese horses are insulin resistant and, conversely, that IR can occur in nonobese animals. Therefore, clinical evaluation of adiposity alone is not sufficient for assessment of risk for pasture-associated laminitis.

Several researchers have proposed that one or more genetic polymorphisms underlie the metabolic syndrome that predisposes to pasture laminitis.[8,14] In the aforementioned study of Welsh and Dartmoor ponies, pedigree analysis suggested a dominant mode of inheritance for the PLMS phenotype, supporting the possibility of a genetic basis for the IR and laminitis predisposition in this population.[8] Further studies in more outbred populations are required to confirm these findings. It is possible that these susceptible ponies have a "thrifty genotype," however, in which the IR is, at least in part, an adaptive strategy for survival in nutritionally sparse environments. This strategy may go awry when these animals are exposed to high-calorie diets, however, with development of obesity, exacerbation of IR and hyperinsulinemia, and increased risk for laminitis. A similar scenario may contribute to the suggested increased susceptibility of easy-keeper horses (eg, Morgan, Arabian, Paso Fino, and Spanish mustang breeds) to EMS and pasture-associated laminitis.[10,12]

PATHOGENESIS OF PASTURE LAMINITIS

Pasture-associated laminitis clearly has a nutritional basis, but the exact mechanism(s) that links the consumption of pasture forage to development of laminar failure is not known. In broad terms, the ingestion of pasture forage may trigger laminitis by means of induction of digestive or metabolic disturbances. At certain times of the year, pasture forage is rich in nonstructural carbohydrates (NSCs), including simple sugars, starches, and fructans.[23] Rapid fermentation of these carbohydrates in the hindgut (cecum and colon) may cause intestinal disturbances, triggering a chain of events that culminates in laminitis.[1,23] Additionally, there is gathering evidence that intake of feeds rich in these carbohydrate fractions may exacerbate IR and hyperinsulinemia in predisposed animals, with a lowering of the threshold for laminitis.[8,12]

Much of our current knowledge of the pathogenesis of pasture-associated laminitis has been extrapolated from experimental models in which the disease is induced by the administration of large doses (~17 g/kg body weight [bwt]) of starch or oligofructose (7.5–12 g/kg bwt).[24,25] In both circumstances, it is thought that the delivery of a large proportion of undigested rapidly fermentable substrate (starch or fructan) to the hindgut initiates changes in the bacterial flora, with proliferation of gram-positive organisms, especially lactic acid-producing lactobacilli and streptococci, leading to a decrease in the intraluminal pH and an increase in intestinal permeability.[25–27] These alterations in the hindgut environment are thought to result in the production and absorption of various substances (eg, vasoactive amines, exotoxins, endotoxins) that initiate a systemic inflammatory response triggering development of laminitis.[1,26,28] The relevance of these experimental models to understanding pasture-associated laminitis has been questioned, partially because of their extreme nature (ie, extremely large dose of carbohydrates administered as a bolus). Nonetheless, it is possible that similar, albeit less severe, intestinal events are involved in the development of laminitis in horses and ponies consuming pasture forages rich in sugars, starches, or fructans (or overconsuming cereal grains and sweet feeds).

Nonstructural Carbohydrate Accumulation in Pasture Plants: Implications for Laminitis

At certain times of the year, the quantity of pasture NSCs ingested by grazing equids may approach or exceed the amount of starch or fructan known to induce laminitis when administered as a single dose.[23,29] Pasture plants contain varying levels of simple sugars, fructans, and starch. The vegetative tissues of temperate (cool season or C3) pasture grasses, such as perennial ryegrass or fescue, accumulate fructan as the primary storage carbohydrate, with most fructan stored in the stem until required by the plant as an energy source.[23,29] In contrast, starch is the storage carbohydrate of the seed of temperate grasses and the seed and vegetative tissues of legumes (eg, clover) and warm season (C4) grasses, such as Bermuda.[29] The type of fructan varies among grass species. The fructan in perennial ryegrass has a lower molecular weight (shorter chain length) when compared with that in timothy or orchard grass species. In vitro studies have shown more rapid fermentation of the lower molecular weight fructans in ryegrass, suggesting that this species may pose the highest risk for pasture-associated laminitis.[23]

A large number of environmental factors influence the accumulation of starches and fructans in pasture plants; these include the intensity and duration of sunlight, temperature (ambient and soil), soil fertility, water availability, and nitrogen status.[23,29] Studies in several northern European countries have shown fructan content of perennial ryegrass to vary between less than 100 g/kg dry matter (DM) and greater than 400 g/kg DM depending on the season and growing conditions.[29] In general, pasture NSCs are highest in spring, lowest in midsummer, and intermediate in the fall. For example, in pastures (tall fescue and Kentucky bluegrass mix) at Virginia Tech's Middleburg Agricultural Research and Extension Center, NSC content is highest in April and May (>15%–20% DM [ie, 150–200 g/kg]), intermediate in the fall, and lowest in midwinter and summer (<5%–7% DM).[30,31] There also can be marked daily fluctuations that coincide with patterns of energy storage (photosynthetic activity) and use, however. Thus, pasture NSCs tend to increase during the morning, reaching maximal values in the afternoon and then declining overnight. Therefore, horses grazing in the afternoon, when compared with nighttime or the morning, may ingest between two and four times as much NSCs. Stress conditions that restrict plant growth (and therefore energy demands) result in accumulation of NSCs. These stress conditions include low temperatures, killing frosts, applications of nonlethal herbicides, and low soil fertility.[23,29]

For horses with 24-hour access to pasture, daily forage intake likely ranges between 2% and 3% bwt (as DM), or 10 to 15 kg DM intake for a 500-kg horse.[23] Thus, NSC intake would range between 0.75 and 1.5 kg/d DM and between 2.25 and 4.5 kg/d DM for, respectively, pastures with an NSC content of 100 g/kg DM and those with an NSC content of 300 g/kg DM. The higher end of forage NSC intake approaches the amount of starch or fructan known to induce digestive disturbances and laminitis, albeit consumed over a 12- to 17-hour period rather than as a single bolus. Nevertheless, it is possible that the dosage of NSCs (eg, as fructan) required to trigger digestive and metabolic disturbances in susceptible animals (ie, a horse or pony with an insulin-resistant phenotype) is considerably lower than that needed to induce disease reliably in healthy experimental animals. Another possibility is that susceptible horses and ponies have differences in their gut flora compared with animals less prone to laminitis, with heightened hindgut fermentative responses to a given load of NSCs and increased production of laminitis trigger factors. The decrease in fecal pH associated with the feeding of the fructan inulin (3 g/kg bwt per day) did not differ between normal ponies and those predisposed to laminitis,[28] however.

Role of Insulin Resistance and Hyperinsulinemia

A second potential mechanism linking the consumption of pasture forage NSCs to laminitis is exacerbation of IR and hyperinsulinemia in predisposed animals.[8,12,32] Certainly, there is evidence that adaptation of weanling or mature horses to concentrates rich in starch and sugar results in a decrease in insulin sensitivity.[33] Preliminary studies of healthy grazing horses have shown a strong relation between pasture NSC content and circulating insulin concentrations,[31] with exacerbation of IR and hyperinsulinemia in laminitis-prone ponies when they are grazing spring pasture rich in NSCs.[8,32] In a single herd of Welsh and Dartmoor ponies kept at pasture, some of which were resistant to insulin and prone to recurrent pasture laminitis, serum insulin concentrations markedly increased during the months of April and May, and this occurrence coincided with an increase in pasture grass NSC content.[32] Furthermore, several ponies with the PLMS phenotype developed laminitis 7 to 10 days after exacerbation of hyperinsulinemia was detected. Similarly, feeding inulin (to simulate intake of fructan from spring grass) to ponies elicits an exaggerated insulin response in animals predisposed to laminitis.[34] It is possible that episodes of profound hyperinsulinemia induce laminitis in grazing horses or ponies, which is supported by results of a recent study in which acute laminitis was experimentally induced in healthy nonobese ponies by infusing exogenous insulin for up to 72 hours to achieve a serum insulin concentration of approximately 1000 mU/L.[35] It is also worth noting that endotoxemia secondary to disturbances in the hindgut microenvironment could exacerbate preexisting IR and hyperinsulinemia in association with increased NSC intake from pasture forage. In healthy horses, intravenous administration of lipopolysaccharide (20 ng/kg bwt) decreased insulin sensitivity and increased the pancreatic insulin response to a glucose load.[36]

IR also may lower the threshold for disease in the face of other conditions that trigger laminitis (eg, hindgut disturbances associated with rapid fermentation of starch or fructan ingested in pasture forage [or other feedstuffs rich in these carbohydrate fractions], which invoke a systemic inflammatory response or alter digital vascular hemodynamics). Insulin is a vasoregulatory hormone, invoking vasodilatation through pathways similar to those of insulin-mediated glucose metabolism.[37,38] In insulin-resistant states, insulin's ability to counteract endothelin-1–associated vasoconstriction may be compromised because of decreased nitric oxide synthesis, whereas compensatory hyperinsulinemia might stimulate increased endothelin-1 production.[37] Insulin also modulates inflammatory responses, and there is evidence from studies in human patients and experimental animals to suggest that the microvascular dysfunction (eg, platelet and leukocyte adhesion, leukocyte emigration) associated with sepsis or other inflammatory stimuli is exacerbated in insulin-resistant states.[39] Similarly, in horses and ponies with an insulin-resistant phenotype (ie, EMS), a proinflammatory state could amplify impairments to lamellar or digital vascular function associated with carbohydrate overload from pasture, thereby lowering the threshold for laminitis.

COUNTERMEASURES TO PASTURE LAMINITIS IN HIGH-RISK ANIMALS

From the preceding discussion, it is evident that countermeasures to pasture-associated laminitis must focus on two areas: (1) mitigation of metabolic predispositions (IR and obesity) in high-risk horses and ponies and (2) strategies for limiting intake of NSCs from pasture and other feedstuffs (ie, minimizing exposure to the dietary conditions known to trigger laminitis in these susceptible animals). Horses and ponies with a history of laminitis or physical characteristics suggestive of EMS or PPID should be carefully evaluated, including assessment of body condition and the presence of abnormal fat deposits in addition to screening tests for IR (eg, measurement of basal serum insulin concentration or assessment of glucose and insulin dynamics by the intravenous glucose tolerance test or the combined glucose-insulin test). Horses with IR or hyperinsulinemia require interventions to improve insulin sensitivity, including strategies for induction of weight loss (eg, restriction in dietary energy intake, increased physical activity) and possibly use of pharmacologic agents (eg, levothyroxine sodium, metformin) that increase insulin sensitivity or promote weight loss.[12,40–43] A more detailed discussion on these aspects is presented elsewhere in this issue (see the article by Geor and Harris elsewhere in this issue). The remainder of this section focuses on strategies for limiting intake of NSCs from pasture (and other feedstuffs) by equids at high risk for pasture laminitis.

Analysis of Forage and Feed Carbohydrates

Plants contain structural carbohydrates (cell wall constituents, including cellulose, hemicellulose, lingocellulose, and lignin) and NSCs. The NSC fraction includes simple sugars (monosaccharides and disaccharides), starches, oligosaccharides (including fructans), and soluble fibers (gums, mucilages, and pectins). Much of the discussion on forage carbohydrates and laminitis risk has focused on fructans, but other components of NSC, especially the simple sugars and starches, also may be important.[8,23,29] Therefore, an ideal forage analysis system would provide an accurate breakdown of all NSC components. Commercial forage testing laboratories use a number of different analytic techniques and terminologies to describe the different carbohydrate fractions, leading to some confusion in the equine community. For example, NSC has been defined in three ways:

1. NSC by difference, according to the following equation using values from proximate nutrient analysis:
   NSC = 100 – (crude protein % + nutrient detergent fiber % + moisture % + fat % + ash %)
   This NSC value represents sugars, starch, and fructans but also includes certain pectins, gums, and mucilages.
2. NSC by analysis, wherein NSC = water-soluble carbohydrates (WSCs) + starch (measured by enzymatic assay)
3. NSC by analysis, wherein NSC = ethanol-soluble carbohydrates (ESCs) + starch (enzymatic assay).

The WSC fraction includes simple sugars (eg, glucose, sucrose, fructose) and oligofructoses (ie, fructans), whereas the ESC fraction is an estimate of simple sugars only. Techniques are available for direct measurement of fructans in forage samples (eg, chromatography); however, to date, these methods have not been adopted by commercial laboratories. Fructans can be estimated by subtracting ESCs from WSCs, but it should be understood that this is only a rough estimate, because some fructans (especially the shorter chain oligofructoses) may be included in the ESC fraction.

Some owners and farm managers have used periodic assessments of pasture NSCs to determine the periods of highest risk when susceptible animals should have restricted or no access to pasture. It must be recognized that carbohydrate storage in pasture plants is a highly dynamic process,[23,29] however, and measurement of samples collected at a single time point may not reflect the range of values possible throughout the day. Conversely, measurement of the carbohydrate fractions in hay and other feedstuffs is recommended for selection of feeds suitable for laminitis-prone horses and ponies. This author prefers to measure WSCs, ESCs, and starch in forage and feed samples. These data provide information on the glycemic and insulinemic potential of the forage or feed (ie, ESCs, starches) in addition to the potential for the feed to be subject to rapid fermentation, all of which is relevant to the feeding management of insulin-resistant laminitis-prone horses and ponies.

Decisions on Pasture Turnout and Strategies to Limit Intake of Nonstructural Carbohydrates

Because pasture-associated laminitis occurs at pasture, the most obvious way to avoid the condition is to prevent access to pasture and to feed forage alternatives that are low in the carbohydrates known to be involved in triggering the disease. Complete elimination of pasture access is not always necessary, however, and many horses or ponies that have had one or more episodes of pasture laminitis can return to grazing activity provided that there has been successful implementation of countermeasures to obesity and IR. Decisions regarding whether and to what extent affected animals can be allowed access to pasture must be made on a case-by-case basis; however, in general:

- The horse or pony should be held off pasture until there has been complete resolution of the acute laminitis episode and, when indicated, diagnostic testing for IR and PPID. If there is no evidence of EMS or PPID, a gradual reintroduction to pasture may be considered. Start with 1 to 2 hours of grazing once or twice per day or with turnout for longer periods if the horse is fitted with a grazing muzzle. More caution may be required when pasture is green and growing rapidly (eg, in spring).
- Obese insulin-resistant horses should be held off pasture for a longer period (eg, 2–3 months), allowing time for implementation of management changes (ie, dietary restriction, increased physical activity) that result in improved insulin sensitivity. Even then, it is advisable to restrict severely or avoid any grazing during periods in which the pasture forage NSC content is likely to be high (eg, spring and early summer, after summer and fall rains that cause the grass to turn green, pastures that have been frosted or drought stressed [both can result in fructan accumulation]).[23,29]
- Some insulin-resistant horses and ponies with history of repeated episodes of laminitis require permanent housing in a dry lot because they seem to be susceptible to further episodes of laminitis in the face of even small variations in pasture availability and nutrient content.

Although restricting grazing to 1 to 2 hours at a time seems a reasonable strategy to limit NSC intake, in reality, there is minimal information on the quantity of pasture a horse or pony may be able to ingest during these short periods of grazing activity. One preliminary study (cited in Ref. [23]) indicated that ponies may ingest up to 40% of their typical daily DM intake as grass during 3 hours of turnout. Therefore, restricted grazing may not adequately limit daily intake of NSCs and rapidly fermentable carbohydrates, particularly at times of the year when pasture forage sugar or fructan content is high.

As mentioned, on sunny days, NSC content tends to increase during the morning, reaching maximal values in the afternoon and declining overnight. In one study of spring pasture in northern Virginia,[31] the nadir in forage NSC content occurred between 4:00 AM and 5:00 AM (~15% NSCs on DM basis), with the highest values between 4:00 PM and 5:00 PM (~22%–24% NSCs on DM basis). Furthermore, serum insulin concentrations in mares grazing on this pasture displayed a similar circadian pattern that was strongly related to the NSC content.[31] These observations support the common recommendation to turn susceptible animals out late at night or early in the morning with removal from pasture by midmorning. Again, this approach may not be foolproof in spring, because the NSC content of early-morning pasture, although lower when compared with the same pasture in the afternoon, may not be safe for susceptible animals.

The following points summarize current advice regarding strategies for avoiding high NSC intakes by horses and ponies at risk for pasture laminitis:

- Animals predisposed to laminitis should be denied access to grass pastures during the growing season.
- At other times of the year, limit the amount of turnout time each day (eg, 1–3 hours) and turn animals out late at night or early in the morning, removing

them from pasture by midmorning at the latest (because NSC levels are likely to be at their lowest late at night through early morning).

- Alternatively, limit the size of the available pasture by use of temporary fencing to create small paddocks or use a grazing muzzle.
- Avoid pastures that have not been properly managed by regular grazing or cutting, because mature stemmy grasses may contain more fructan (it is stored in the stem).
- Do not turn horses out onto pasture that has been exposed to low temperatures in conjunction with bright sunlight, such as occurs in the fall after a flush of growth or on bright cool winter days, because cold temperatures reduce grass growth, resulting in the accumulation of fructan.
- Do not allow animals to graze on recently cut stubble, because fructan is stored predominantly in the stem.

Alternative Feeds

Animals denied access to pasture for most or all of the day require provision of alternative feedstuffs. Horses at maintenance require approximately 2.0% of their bwt as forage or forage plus supplement to meet daily nutrient requirements. Grain and sweet feeds should not be fed, and the feeding of other "treats," such as carrots and apples, should be discouraged. Forage (as hay or hay substitute, such as chop, chaff, or haylage) should be the primary, if not sole, energy-providing component of the ration. Mature grass hay (ie, with visible seed heads and a high stem-to-leaf ratio) has higher fiber and lower NSCs when compared with immature hay and is suitable forage for the obese horse or pony. Alfalfa hay or other legumes, such as clover, are less preferred because, on average, these forages have higher energy and NSC content when compared with grass hay. An NSC content of less than 10% (as-fed basis) has been recommended.[12] Caution is required when feeding significant amounts of poorly digestible and highly silicated forages; anecdotally, this practice increases the risk for impaction colic in some animals. Ensiled forages generally have lower NSC content than hay made from the same crop. Despite the generally lower NSC content of haylage compared with hay, however, the high palatability of some haylages may result in higher total NSC intake. Ideally, the results of proximate nutrient analysis, including direct measurement of starch, WSCs, and ESCs, should be reviewed before selection of the hay.

Forage-only diets do not provide adequate protein, minerals, or vitamins. Therefore, this author recommends supplementing the forage diet with a low-calorie commercial ration balancer product that contains sources of high-quality protein and a mixture of vitamins and minerals to balance the low vitamin E, copper, zinc, selenium, and other minerals typically found in mature grass hays. These products are often designed to be fed in small quantities (eg, 0.5–1.0 kg/d); they can be mixed with chaff (hay chop) to increase the size of the meal and extend feeding time, which may alleviate boredom in animals provided a restricted diet. In some areas, forage-based low-calorie feeds complete with vitamins and minerals are available commercially; this type of feed offers convenience and may be used as a substitute for hay or fed as a component of the ration along with hay.

REFERENCES

1. Bailey SR, Marr CM, Elliott J. Current research and theories on the pathogenesis of acute laminitis in the horse. Vet J 2004;167:129–42.

2. Allen D. Overview of the pathogenesis of laminitis—models and theories. American Association of Equine Practitioners Equine Laminitis Research Meeting and Panel; 2004. Louisville (KY); 2004. p. 5–19.
3. USDA-NAHMS. Lameness and laminitis in US horses (monograph). In: United States Department of Agriculture National Animal Health Monitoring System. April 2000. #N318.0400.
4. Hinckley K, Henderson I. The epidemiology of equine laminitis in the UK. Warwick (UK): 35th Congress of the British Equine Veterinary Association; 1996. p. 62.
5. Katz L, DeBrauwere N, Elliott J, et al. The prevalence of laminitis in one region of the UK. 40th British Equine Veterinary Association Congress; 2001. p. 199.
6. Slater MR, Hood DM, Carter GK. Descriptive epidemiological study of equine laminitis. Equine Vet J 1995;27:364–7.
7. Polzer J, Slater MR. Age, breed, sex and seasonality as risk factors for equine laminitis. Prev Vet Med 1996;29:179–84.
8. Treiber KH, Kronfeld DS, Hess TM, et al. Evaluation of genetic and metabolic predispositions and nutritional risk factors for pasture-associated laminitis in ponies. J Am Vet Med Assoc 2006;228:1538–45.
9. Coffman JR, Colles CM. Insulin tolerance in laminitic ponies. Can J Comp Med 1983;47:347–51.
10. Johnson PJ. The equine metabolic syndrome: peripheral Cushing's syndrome. Vet Clin North Am Equine Pract 2002;18:271–93.
11. Frank N, Elliott SB, Brandt LE, et al. Physical characteristics, blood hormone concentrations, and plasma lipid concentrations in obese horses with insulin resistance. J Am Vet Med Assoc 2006;228:1383–90.
12. Frank N. Endocrinopathic laminitis, obesity-associated laminitis, and pasture-associated laminitis. San Diego (CA): Proceedings of the 54th American Association of Equine Practitioners meeting; 2008. p. 341–6.
13. Carter RA, Treiber KH, Geor RJ, et al. Prediction of incipient pasture-associated laminitis from hyperinsulinemia, hyperleptinemia and generalized and localized obesity in a cohort of ponies. Equine Vet J 2008;40. DOI:10.2746/042516408X342975.
14. Bailey SR, Habershon-Butcher JL, Ransom KJ, et al. Hypertension and insulin resistance in a mixed-breed population of ponies predisposed to laminitis. Am J Vet Res 2008;69:122–9.
15. Rijnen KE, van der Kolk JH. Determination of reference range values indicative of glucose metabolism and insulin resistance by use of glucose clamp techniques in horses and ponies. Am J Vet Res 2003;64:1260–4.
16. Donaldson MT, Jorgensen AJ, Beech J. Evaluation of suspected pituitary pars intermedia dysfunction in horses with laminitis. J Am Vet Med Assoc 2004;224:1123–7.
17. Garcia MC, Beech J. Equine intravenous glucose tolerance test: glucose and insulin responses of healthy horses fed grain or hay and of horses with pituitary adenoma. Am J Vet Res 1986;47:570–2.
18. McGowan CM, Frost R, Pfeiffer DU, et al. Serum insulin concentrations in horses with equine Cushing's syndrome: response to a cortisol inhibitor and prognostic value. Equine Vet J 2004;36:295–8.
19. Alford P, Geller S, Richardson B, et al. A multicenter, matched case-control study of risk factors for equine laminitis. Prev Vet Med 2001;49:209–22.
20. Hutley L, Prins JB. Fat as an endocrine organ: relationship to the metabolic syndrome. Am J Med Sci 2005;330:280–9.
21. Wild SH, Byrne CD. ABC of obesity: risk factors for diabetes and coronary heart disease. Br Med J 2006;333:1009–11.

22. Vick MM, Adams AA, Murphy BA, et al. Relationships among inflammatory cytokines, obesity and insulin sensitivity in the horse. J Anim Sci 2007;85: 1144–55.
23. Longland AC, Byrd BM. The importance of pasture nonstructural carbohydrates in equine laminitis. J Nutr 2006;136:2099S–102S.
24. Eades SC, Stokes AM, Johnson PJ, et al. Serial alterations in digital hemodynamics and endothelin-1 immunoreactivity, platelet-neutrophil aggregation, and concentrations of nitric oxide, insulin and glucose in blood obtained from horses following carbohydrate overload. Am J Vet Res 2007;68:87–94.
25. van Eps AW, Pollitt CC. Equine laminitis induced with oligofructose. Equine Vet J 2006;38:203–8.
26. Elliott J, Bailey SR. Gastrointestinal derived factors are potential triggers for the development of acute equine laminitis. J Nutr 2006;136:2103S–7S.
27. Milinovich GJ, Trott DJ, Burrell PC, et al. Changes in equine hindgut bacterial populations during oligofructose-induced laminitis. Environ Microbiol 2006;8: 885–98.
28. Crawford C, Sepulveda MF, Elliott J, et al. Dietary fructan carbohydrate increases amine production in the equine large intestine: implications for pasture-associated laminitis. J Anim Sci 2007;85:2949–58.
29. Longland AC. Starch, sugar and fructans: what are they and how important are they in diets for horses? In: Harris PA, Hill SJ, Elliott J, et al, editors. The latest findings in laminitis research. The First WALTHAM–Royal Veterinary College Laminitis Conference. Suffolk (UK): Equine Veterinary Journal Limited; 2007. p. 7–14.
30. Cubitt TA, Staniar WB, Kronfeld DS, et al. Environmental effects on nutritive value of equine pastures in Northern Virginia. Pferdeheilkunde 2007;23:151–4.
31. Byrd BM, Treiber KH, Staniar WB, et al. Circadian and seasonal variation on pasture NSC and circulating insulin concentrations in grazing horses. J Anim Sci 2006;84(Suppl 1):330–1 [abstract].
32. Treiber KH, Carter RA, Harris PA, et al. Seasonal changes in energy metabolism of ponies coincides with changes in pasture carbohydrates: implications for laminitis. J Vet Intern Med 2008;22:735–6 [abstract].
33. Kronfled DS, Treiber K, Hess T, et al. Insulin resistance in the horse: definition, detection and dietetics. J Anim Sci 2005;83:E22–31.
34. Bailey SR, Menzies-Gow NJ, Harris PA, et al. Effect of dietary fructan and dexamethasone on the insulin response of ponies predisposed to laminitis. J Am Vet Med Assoc 2007;231:1365–73.
35. Asplin KE, Sillence MN, Pollitt CC, et al. Induction of laminitis by prolonged hyperinsulinaemia in clinically normal ponies. Vet J 2007;174:530–5.
36. Toth F, Frank N, Elliott SB, et al. Effects of an intravenous endotoxin challenge on glucose and insulin dynamics in horses. Am J Vet Res 2008;69:82–8.
37. Kim JK, Montagnani M, Koh KK, et al. Reciprocal relationships between insulin resistance and endothelial dysfunction: molecular and pathophysiological mechanisms. Circulation 2006;113:1888–904.
38. Cosentino F, Luscher TF. Endothelial dysfunction in diabetes mellitus. J Cardiovasc Pharmacol 1998;S54–61.
39. Singer G, Granger DN. Inflammatory responses underlying the microvascular dysfunction associated with obesity and insulin resistance. Microcirculation 2007;14:375–87.
40. Geor RJ. Metabolic predispositions to laminitis in horses and ponies: obesity, insulin resistance and metabolic syndromes. J Equine Vet Sci 2008;28: 756–61.

41. Harris PA, Geor RJ. Nutritional countermeasures to laminitis. In: Harris PA, Hill SJ, Elliott J, et al, editors. The latest findings in laminitis research. The First WALTHAM–Royal Veterinary College Laminitis Conference. Suffolk (UK): Equine Veterinary Journal Limited; 2007. p. 29–37.
42. Harris PA, Bailey SR, Elliott J, et al. Countermeasures for pasture-associated laminitis. J Nutr 2006;136:2114S–21S.
43. Durham AE, Rendle DI, Newton JE. The effect of metformin on measurements of insulin sensitivity and beta cell response in horses and ponies with insulin resistance. Equine Vet J 2008;40:493–500.

Dietary Management of Obesity and Insulin Resistance: Countering Risk for Laminitis

Raymond J. Geor, BVSc, MVSc, PhD[a,*], Patricia Harris, MA, PhD, VetMB, MRCVS[b]

KEYWORDS

- Laminitis • Equine metabolic syndrome
- Insulin sensitivity • Nonstructural carbohydrates • Exercise

It has long been recognized that obesity and insulin resistance (IR) are associated with increased risk for laminitis in horses and ponies. Furthermore, in a recent informal survey of equine practitioners, these metabolic or endocrine abnormalities were listed as the most common predisposing factors for clinical cases of laminitis within their practices.[1] These anecdotal impressions are supported by the results of observational studies that demonstrate a link between an insulin-resistant phenotype and predisposition to laminitis, particularly the pasture-associated form of the disease.[2–7] The term *equine metabolic syndrome* (EMS) has been used to describe the clustering of obesity (generalized or regional), IR, and prior or current laminitis.[8,9] Diet seems to play an important role in the triggering of laminitis in horses or ponies with this phenotype, particularly the ingestion of pasture forage or other feeds (eg, cereal grains, sweet feeds) high in nonstructural carbohydrates (NSCs; simple sugars, starches, or fructans).[2,7,9]

Obesity seems to be a key risk factor, and most cases of obesity are associated with an imbalance between energy intake and expenditure. An individual's energy requirements obviously are affected by several external factors, such as environmental conditions and the level of exercise being undertaken (including activity during any turnout), in addition to internal factors, such as life stage and genetics. Many horses and ponies spend much of the day in confinement housing (stalls or small drylots), with occasional use in riding activities. In these circumstances, daily energy requirements are often no higher than maintenance levels; yet, many are fed much more

[a] Department of Large Animal Clinical Sciences, D-202 Veterinary Medical Center, College of Veterinary Medicine, Michigan State University, East Lansing, MI 48824, USA
[b] WALTHAM Centre for Pet Nutrition, Freeby Lane, Waltham-on-the-Wolds, Melton Mowbray, Leicestershire LE14 4RT, UK
* Corresponding author.
E-mail address: geor@cvm.msu.edu (R. J. Geor).

Vet Clin Equine 25 (2009) 51–65
doi:10.1016/j.cveq.2009.02.001 vetequine.theclinics.com

than this. Similarly, animals turned out to pasture at certain times of the year might consume several times their energy or calorie requirement.[10]

This article reviews the association between obesity, IR, and laminitis in horses and ponies and discusses dietary countermeasures for reduction in risk for laminitis in susceptible animals.

OBESITY, INSULIN RESISTANCE, AND METABOLIC SYNDROME

Obesity

There is no universally accepted definition of obesity in horses and ponies. According to the body condition scoring system developed by Henneke and colleagues,[11] horses with a body condition score (BCS) of 8 (fat) or 9 (extremely fat) are obese, whereas animals with a BCS of 7 are considered overweight. One limitation of BCS systems for assessment of obesity is the failure to detect differences in regional adiposity that may signify increased risk for disease. In human beings, visceral (abdominal) adiposity is more closely linked to risk for diabetes and cardiovascular disease than generalized obesity and measurement of waist circumference is a better indicator of abdominal fat accumulation than is body mass index.[12,13] In equids there may be a similar association between regional adiposity and disease risk. For example, neck crest adiposity is negatively associated with insulin sensitivity in horses and ponies.[4,7] It should also be noted that the Henneke BCS system, which was developed in quarter horses, may not be appropriate for ponies and other breeds that have a different pattern of fat distribution.

The 1998 National Animal Health Monitoring System (NAHMS) study estimated that 4.5% of the horse population in the United States was overweight or obese.[14] The accuracy of this estimate may be questioned, however, because it was based on owner reporting rather than the results of physical examination. In a recent prospective study of 300 randomly selected mature horses, 57 (19%) were classified as obese (BCS of 7.5–9.0) (C.D. Thatcher and colleagues, unpublished data, 2007), a prevalence far higher than the NAHMS study estimate. In a study of 319 pleasure riding horses in Scotland, 32% were obese (BCS of 6 on a six-point scale) and a further 35% were considered fat (BCS of 5).[15]

Insulin Resistance

The metabolic actions of insulin maintain whole-body glucose homeostasis and promote efficient glucose use. Insulin stimulates glucose uptake into skeletal muscle and adipocytes and glycogen synthesis in muscle and liver, with simultaneous inhibition of gluconeogenesis in liver to assist with regulation of glucose homeostasis.[16] With regard to insulin action on glucose metabolism, the maximal effect of insulin defines "insulin responsiveness," whereas the insulin concentration that elicits a half-maximal response defines "insulin sensitivity."[17] IR is usually defined as decreased sensitivity or responsiveness to insulin-mediated glucose disposal or inhibition of hepatic glucose production.[18] In human beings, IR plays a central role in the pathophysiology of type 2 diabetes mellitus and is highly associated with other important health problems, including obesity, hypertension, and a cluster of metabolic and cardiovascular abnormalities termed the *metabolic syndrome*.[19,20] In horses and ponies, as in human beings, obesity seems to be an important causative factor,[21] although it is important to recognize that not all obese horses are insulin resistant and that IR can occur in nonobese animals.[6,7,9] Studies in people and in animal models have demonstrated that obesity induces a chronic inflammatory state and that this inflammation plays an important role in the pathogenesis of IR.[20] Similarly, Vick and colleagues[22] reported associations between obesity and blood mRNA expression of tumor necrosis factor-α and interleukin-1β in horses, suggesting that systemic inflammation may play a role in the IR of obesity. Some equids with pituitary pars intermedia dysfunction (PPID) are insulin resistant, and this condition may predispose to laminitis, which is a common occurrence in PPID.[23,24] In one report, hyperinsulinemia was associated with poor long-term survival in horses suspected of having PPID.[25] Diet is another factor that modifies insulin sensitivity. Studies in healthy horses have shown that chronic adaptation to sweet feeds rich in NSCs (starch and sugars) results in decreased insulin sensitivity,[26] and the effect of dietary NSCs on insulin sensitivity may be magnified in equids with preexisting IR.

Metabolic Syndrome

In human medicine, metabolic syndrome is a set of diagnostic criteria identifying individuals at high risk for morbidity associated with IR, primarily type 2 diabetes and cardiovascular disease.[13,27] Although the criteria for diagnosis of metabolic syndrome vary, the core components are obesity (especially visceral), IR, dyslipidemia, and hypertension. Several mechanisms likely contribute to the association between the metabolic syndrome cluster and increased risk for cardiovascular disease, but a common view is that IR plays a central role in the development of pathologic manifestations.[19] In horses and ponies susceptible to recurrent laminitis, an insulin-resistant phenotype resembling the human metabolic syndrome has been described.[1–7] Descriptions of this laminitis-predisposed phenotype have varied but have included a clustering of obesity (generalized or regional), IR, hyperinsulinemia, hyperleptinemia, mild hypertriglyceridemia, and current or historical (eg, founder lines) evidence of laminitis.[1–9] Johnson[8] proposed use of the term *equine metabolic syndrome* to describe horses and ponies with this phenotype, whereas Treiber and colleagues[2] coined the term *prelaminitic metabolic syndrome* (PLMS) for identification of a set of risk factors in Welsh and Dartmoor ponies that predict increased risk for pasture-associated laminitis. The EMS phenotype has been described in several breeds but may be more common in ponies, Morgans, Paso Finos, Arabians, saddlebreds, and Norwegian Fjords.[8,9]

It has been proposed that horses and ponies with EMS or PLMS have a "thrifty genotype," in which, at least in part, the IR is an adaptive strategy for survival in nutritionally sparse environments. This strategy may fail when these animals are exposed to high-carbohydrate diets, however, with development of obesity, exacerbation of IR, and increased risk for laminitis.[2,3] Native UK pony breeds, for example, retain strong seasonality with respect to their appetite, and under "feral" conditions, they tend to gain weight during the summer months when food is abundant before losing it again during the winter. Such cyclic changes may not occur when food intake and quality are maintained during the winter, resulting in continued obesity or even progressive weight gain.[28]

INSULIN RESISTANCE, OBESITY, AND RISK FOR LAMINITIS

The idea that IR increases risk for laminitis is not new. More than 25 years ago, studies reported lower insulin sensitivity in ponies that experienced recurrent laminitis compared with healthy controls based on blood glucose responses during insulin[29] or glucose[30] tolerance tests. These observations have been supported by more recent studies that have sought to characterize the phenotype of ponies and horses apparently predisposed to recurrent laminitis.[1–7,31] In Welsh and Dartmoor ponies, an insulin-resistant phenotype was associated with a 10-fold higher risk for development of laminitis when grazing spring pasture when compared with non–insulin-resistant ponies.[2] In this population, generalized obesity, regional accumulation of neck crest adipose tissue ("cresty neck"), hyperinsulinemia, and hyperleptinemia were predictors of laminitis in ponies exposed to spring pasture.[7] Episodes of laminitis in these ponies are preceded by exacerbation of hyperinsulinemia, an interesting observation in light of the recent finding that prolonged periods (48–72 hours) of hyperinsulinemia result in laminitis in otherwise healthy ponies.[32]

Although obesity has been associated with laminitis in some studies, it has not been established whether this condition directly increases risk for laminitis or if the increased risk is attributable to other factors, such as IR and inflammation, that are consequences of obesity.[21,22] Indeed, researchers in the United Kingdom have identified nonobese ponies with an insulin-resistant phenotype that are prone to recurrent laminitis. Furthermore, seasonal and dietary factors affect the expression of the phenotype associated with laminitis risk.[5,6] In summer, but not in winter, laminitis-prone ponies had higher serum insulin concentrations when compared with age- and BCS-matched control ponies, suggesting that consumption of summer pasture (high in NSCs, including fructans) may induce expression of the metabolic syndrome phenotype that includes hyperinsulinemia.[6] Similarly, laminitis-prone ponies demonstrated exaggerated increases in serum insulin concentrations in response to the feeding of inulin, a type of fructan.[5] Thus, an increase in dietary NSCs induces expression of hyperinsulinemia (and possibly exacerbates IR) in laminitis-prone ponies. As mentioned, the feeding of high-starch diets to healthy horses results in decreased insulin sensitivity.[26] These observations underscore the need for control of NSC intake in insulin-resistant horses and ponies.

The mechanism that triggers episodes of laminitis in horses and ponies with an insulin-resistant phenotype has not been determined. The recent finding that laminitis can be induced in healthy ponies by maintaining supraphysiologic circulating insulin concentrations (serum insulin ~ 1000–1100 mU/mL) for 2 to 3 days suggests that hyperinsulinemia could play a direct role in the pathogenesis of laminitis.[32] Thus, it is reasonable to hypothesize that laminitis may be triggered in a chronically insulin-resistant horse or pony under conditions that exacerbate IR or hyperinsulinemia; such conditions would include grazing pasture with high NSC content (eg, during spring or when pastures are stressed by drought or frost),[2,7] consumption of other feeds rich in starch and sugars (eg, sweet feeds),[26] overfeeding that induces or worsens obesity,[21,22] the administration of corticosteroids,[33] or episodes of endotoxemia.[34] In support of this, Treiber and colleagues[35] have observed a marked increase in the serum insulin concentrations of laminitis-prone ponies during the transition from winter to spring in association with an increase in forage water-soluble carbohydrates (WSCs; which include simple sugars and fructans), with the most profound increases observed in ponies that subsequently developed laminitis. Similarly, Bailey and colleagues[5] reported exacerbation of hyperinsulinemia in laminitis-prone ponies, but not control ponies, in response to an increase in dietary fructan.

Disturbances to hindgut fermentation and bacterial flora, as occurs in the starch or fructan overload model of laminitis,[36–38] may be primary in the triggering of disease in animals with and without an insulin-resistant phenotype. The threshold for induction of laminitis may be lower in insulin-resistant horses and ponies when compared with animals with normal insulin sensitivity, however.[9] With carbohydrate overload, there are major alterations within the hindgut, including proliferation and lysis of streptococcal species, a decrease in pH, and an increase in intestinal permeability.[36,37] The latter promotes entry of endotoxins, other bacterial components, and vasoactive substances into circulation,[38] with initiation of a systemic and lamellar inflammatory response that triggers laminitis.[39] It is possible that these inflammatory responses are heightened in insulin-resistant animals with an existing proinflammatory state, or, viewed another way, the quantity of starch or fructan required to trigger lamellar inflammation that results in clinical laminitis may be lower in these susceptible animals.

IMPLICATIONS FOR LAMINITIS AVOIDANCE

From the preceding discussion, it is clear that IR, hyperinsulinemia, and obesity are associated with increased risk for development of laminitis. Recognition of these predisposing factors justifies (1) clinical evaluation of IR in horses or ponies with a history of recurrent laminitis or clinical signs suggestive of metabolic (eg, obesity, cresty neck) and endocrine (ie, PPID) abnormalities associated with heightened risk for laminitis and (2) instigation of countermeasures to IR and obesity such that the risk for future episodes of laminitis can be reduced.

Evaluation of Insulin Resistance

Insulin sensitivity or IR can be assessed by dynamic evaluation of glucose and insulin responses or by simple analysis of steady-state (ie, resting) blood glucose and insulin concentrations. There are advantages and disadvantages of both approaches. "Gold standard" dynamic tests, such as minimal model analysis of a frequently sampled intravenous glucose tolerance test (FSIGTT) and the euglycemic-hyperinsulinemic clamp (EHC), provide direct and specific measurement of insulin-mediated glucose disposal (mostly into the primary insulin-sensitive tissues, skeletal muscle, and adipose tissue).[18,40] These dynamic procedures are probably more sensitive for detection of IR when compared with static resting measurements. These tests are laborious and impractical in clinical settings, however. The simplest approach in clinical practice is to measure "resting" (basal) insulin and glucose concentrations for screening evaluation of IR. IR in horses and ponies is often characterized by hyperinsulinemia and normoglycemia indicative of compensated IR, wherein the glucose homeostasis is maintained by increased insulin secretion from the pancreas.[2,3,9] Although more work is needed to determine appropriate cutoffs, serum insulin concentrations of greater than 20 mU/L or greater than 30 mU/L (wherein 1 mU/L = 1 μU/mL) have been used to define hyperinsulinemia and to diagnose IR.[9] These somewhat arbitrary cutoff values were based on measurements using the radioimmunoassay manufactured by Diagnostic Products Corporation (Siemens Healthcare, Deerfield, Illinois). Different laboratories use different assay systems, however, and the agreement among these assays varies. It is therefore important to use a single laboratory for measurement of insulin concentrations, preferably one with appropriately developed equine reference ranges. It is also important to recognize that within an individual animal, there can be marked interday variation in serum insulin concentrations. Additionally, in the authors' experience, hyperinsulinemia (defined using the previously cited cutoffs) is not a universal finding in horses and ponies with IR and a history of laminitis, particularly when they are maintained on a low-NSC diet before sampling. In these cases, dynamic evaluation of glucose tolerance and insulin sensitivity often reveals the IR.

When measuring resting insulin and glucose concentrations, standardization of sampling and analytic procedures is critical for reliable interpretation of results, because a large number of animal and environmental factors can affect these measurements. Stress associated with a change in housing, feeding, or sampling procedures may affect results. Most importantly, diet composition, particularly the NSC (starch and sugars) content of feeds and forages, can have a marked impact on insulin concentration.[2,35] The authors have observed marked fluctuations in insulin concentrations (values increasing from 10–20 mU/L to >80–100 mU/L) in horses and ponies grazing pasture with high NSC content. Similarly, grain, concentrate, and even hay feeding is attended by variable hyperinsulinemia that may persist for several hours.

A suggested sampling protocol is as follows. All feed should be withheld for a minimum of 8 hours before sampling (from late evening), with blood drawn between 7:00 and 10:00 AM. For animals maintained at pasture, removal from pasture to a drylot or stall is recommended, especially during periods of active forage growth (eg, spring) when the high-sugar content of pasture forage can affect resting blood glucose and insulin concentrations. In laminitic animals, testing should be delayed until after resolution of the acute laminitic episode, because the associated pain and stress exacerbate hyperinsulinemia.

Repeat evaluation of resting insulin concentration or application of a dynamic test of glucose tolerance or insulin sensitivity is warranted for evaluation of IR in animals with borderline initial results (eg, resting insulin <20 mU/L) but other clinical or historical findings indicative of EMS or PPID. The combined glucose-insulin test developed by Eiler and colleagues[41] has been advocated for use in these circumstances. This test requires insertion of an intravenous catheter but is much less laborious when compared with the EHC or FSIGTT procedure. After collection of a baseline sample, glucose (50% dextrose solution, 150 mg/kg) and then insulin (regular insulin, 0.10 units; Humulin R; Eli Lilly, Indianapolis, Indiana) are injected by means of the catheter. Subsequent blood samples are collected at 1, 5, 15, 35, 45, 60, 75, 90, 105, 120, and 150 minutes after glucose and insulin infusion for measurement of glucose concentrations. Blood glucose concentrations can be measured with a handheld glucometer; alternatively, samples may be collected for subsequent laboratory analysis. With this test, a diagnosis of IR is rendered when plasma glucose does not return to baseline (preinfusion) values within 35 minutes.[41] Pretesting dietary management should be as described previously.

Dietary Management

IR and hyperinsulinemia have been strongly associated with risk for laminitis. Presumably then, improvement in insulin sensitivity and mitigation of hyperinsulinemia lessen risk for laminitis. In many cases, the IR is related to obesity and a reduction in adiposity is needed for improvement in insulin sensitivity. Particularly in the "easy keeper" breeds prone to obesity, the goal should be to achieve and maintain a moderate BCS (4–6 on the nine-point scale). Other aspects of management include avoidance of feedstuffs that may exacerbate IR and hyperinsulinemia (elimination of grain and sweet feeds from the diet plus restricted access to pasture when NSC content is likely to be high). Use of pharmacologic agents for medical therapy of IR (eg, levothyroxine, metformin) is indicated in refractory or severe cases. Use of supplements (eg, magnesium, chromium picolinate) touted to enhance weight loss or improve insulin sensitivity is a further consideration in overall dietary management.[42]

Induction of weight loss in obese animals

In horses and ponies, as in people, "eating less" and "exercising more" are key strategies for weight loss. Some general considerations include the following:

1. Owner or trainer recognition that the horse or pony is overweight or obese. As the old adage states, "Beauty is in the eye of the beholder," and different equestrian disciplines and breeds have adopted different accepted "norms" in body condition. Nonetheless, the effectiveness of any weight loss program critically depends on the willingness of the owner or caregiver to "buy into" the plan.

2. Evaluation of the current feeding program and housing. This includes a thorough evaluation of what feed is being provided (including supplementary feed, hay, pasture quality, and time allowed for grazing) and in what quantities.
3. Assessment of the weekly workload and soundness for exercise. How many hours per week is the horse or pony engaged in structured physical activity (eg, riding)? Many obese insulin-resistant equids receive little structured exercise. Information on current activity level and soundness for exercise forms the basis for development of recommendations for physical activity.
4. Set realistic goals for weight loss and regularly monitor progress. In the authors' experience, there is wide variation in the response of obese horses and ponies to weight loss treatment programs. In some, there is a substantial loss of body weight and adiposity after 2 to 3 months of diet restriction and increased physical activity. In others, progress can be frustratingly slow and further adjustments to diet and the level of physical activity may be needed for satisfactory improvement. As a guide, an effective weight loss regimen for a mature light-breed horse should result in the loss of approximately 25 to 30 kg over a 4- to 6-week period. This decrease in body weight may be accompanied by the loss of approximately 1 unit of BCS. Initial weight loss may occur by means of reduction in abdominal fat or the size of the gastrointestinal tract, however, and further weight loss may be required to achieve a noticeable decrease in BCS (A. Dugdale, personal communication, 2009). Body weight (measured directly or by use of a weight tape) and body condition (and perhaps mean neck circumference) should be assessed regularly (eg, every 2–4 weeks) during the weight reduction program so that progress can be monitored and the program amended as required.
5. Make all dietary changes gradually and avoid prolonged periods of feed withholding. Abrupt starvation in obese ponies, donkeys, and miniature horses (especially pregnant animals) carries the risk for hyperlipemia.
6. Develop an appropriate weight maintenance program once the target weight and body condition have been achieved. This includes monthly assessment of body weight and condition to ensure that the feeding program is appropriate to the current level of physical activity and other environmental influences on energy requirements (eg, ambient conditions).

In human beings, the combination of caloric restriction and regular physical activity can result in more substantial weight loss when compared with either strategy alone. Studies in people also have demonstrated that physical activity is beneficial even when weight loss does not occur, however, as evidenced by improvements in IR, blood lipid profile, and markers of inflammation, all of which are risk factors for cardiovascular disease. Similarly, a study in a small number of obese mares demonstrated improvements in insulin sensitivity without a change in body weight after 7 days of round-pen exercise (15–20 min/d).[43] Accordingly, a program of regular exercise is likely to be beneficial in the management of obese insulin-resistant (but sound) horses and ponies. In the authors' experience, weight reduction and subsequent control are improved when dietary restriction is combined with a program of riding or longeing. For example, start with two to three exercise sessions per week lasting 20 to 30 minutes per session and then build to four to five times per week with a gradual increase in the intensity and duration of exercise.

Caloric restriction is of paramount importance in the management of obese insulin-resistant equids. Several different dietary strategies can be applied depending on the present and desired body condition and other individual circumstances. A certain amount of trial and reassessment is invariably required to achieve the goal weight and condition in an individual animal. Key considerations are the quantity and composition of the ration. Removal from pasture (eg, to a large drylot) is necessary for adequate control of dietary intake. Some nutritionists and veterinarians have recommended restrictive grazing as a means to decrease caloric intake in overweight equids. A recent study in obese pony mares reported no change in body weight when ponies were provided access to pasture (during the day or at night) for 12 hours per day, however, likely because of increased forage consumption during the restricted grazing period.[44] In a separate study, it was estimated that ponies could consume 40% of their daily dry matter intake during 3 hours of pasture turnout.[45] Strategies that allow turnout while minimizing forage intake include application of grazing muzzles (attached to a breakaway halter), strip grazing behind other horses, mowing the pasture and removing clippings before providing access, putting a deep layer of wood chips over a small paddock, or using drylots or indoor schools. It is important to ensure that horses wearing grazing muzzles are able to consume adequate water. Some horses do not tolerate grazing muzzles, and they can alter herd dynamics.

In general, rations for obese insulin-resistant horses should be high in fiber and low in NSCs (see the section on feeding insulin-resistant horses). As a first step toward calorie restriction and weight loss, grain and other concentrated sources of calories (eg, commercial sweet feeds, feeds containing added fats) should be totally removed from the diet. Excessive feeding of other "treats," such as carrots and apples, also should be curtailed. Forage (as hay or hay substitute [eg, chop, chaff, haylage]) should be the primary, if not sole, energy-providing component of the ration. In some areas, forage-based low-calorie feeds complete with vitamins and minerals are available commercially; this type of feed offers convenience and may be used as a substitute to hay or fed as a component of the ration along with hay. In a recent study of obese ponies provided an ad libitum forage diet during summer and winter, voluntary intake (dry matter basis) was approximately 2% of body weight and BCS was virtually unchanged during the study period.[28] As a general guide, therefore, hay or hay substitute should initially be provided at no more than 1.5% of current body weight per day (ie, 17.5 lb [8 kg] for a 1200-lb [550-kg] horse), with subsequent further reductions in feed amount depending on the extent of weight loss. It is preferable not to decrease forage provision to less than 1.0% of target body weight; feeding smaller amounts of forage may increase risk for hindgut dysfunction, stereotypical behaviors (eg, wood chewing), ingestion of bedding, or coprophagy. The ration should be divided into three to four feedings per day. Strategies to prolong feed intake time should be considered, such as use of haynets with multiple small holes.

Feeding insulin-resistant horses

The primary goal in the feeding management of insulin-resistant horses and ponies (obese or nonobese) is avoidance of feeds rich in NSCs (starches, sugars, or fructans) that may increase risk for laminitis by exacerbation of IR and hyperinsulinemia or by disturbances to the hindgut microbial community that may trigger events leading to laminitis. This requires knowledge of the carbohydrate composition of feedstuffs for horses; the reader is referred to another article in this issue for a review of methods used for analysis and reporting of carbohydrate fractions in feeds (see the article by Harris and Geor elsewhere in this issue), but the general rules for feeding management of insulin-resistant horses include the following:

1. No grain or sweet feeds (ie, feedstuffs rich in starch or sugars). The starch content of oats, barley, and corn is, respectively, approximately 45% to 55%, 60% to 65%, and 65% to 75%. Sweet feeds contain grains plus molasses, and the NSC content

of some of these feeds can approach 30% to 40%. Provision of these feeds to insulin-resistant equids is likely to exacerbate IR or hyperinsulinemia.
2. Restricted or no access to pasture. At certain times of the year, pasture forage NSC content may approach 30% to 40% of dry matter. In susceptible animals, ingestion of this NSC-rich forage increases risk for development of laminitis.
3. A diet based on grass hay (or hay substitute) with low (<10%) NSC content.
4. Feeding for maintenance of body weight and BCS. Weight gain exacerbates IR, so it is important to avoid overfeeding. Regular evaluation of body weight or BCS is the best way to assess the adequacy of energy provision.

As discussed elsewhere in this issue (see the article by Geor), horses and ponies that have had recent episodes of laminitis and are insulin resistant should be denied access to pasture until there is improvement in insulin sensitivity. After improvement in insulin sensitivity, there can be a gradual reintroduction to pasture (eg, restricted grazing time [1–2 hours per day], strip grazing, turnout with a grazing muzzle). Even after improvement in insulin sensitivity, it is advisable to restrict or avoid any grazing during periods when pasture forage NSC content is likely to be high, such as during spring and early summer, after summer or fall rains that cause the grass to turn green, and when pastures have been subjected to drought or frost stress, all of which are conditions that favor fructan accumulation. Some equids remain persistently hyperinsulinemic despite weight loss and use of other dietary approaches to improve insulin sensitivity and seem to be intolerant of even small fluctuations in pasture or preserved forage nutrient composition. These animals may have to be permanently housed off pasture and fed preserved forage known to be low in NSCs.

The diet should be based on grass hay. Mature hay (ie, hay with visible seed heads and a high stem-to-leaf ratio) is preferred, especially in obese insulin-resistant horses, because of its lower digestible energy and NSC content when compared with less mature hay. Alfalfa hay or other legumes, such as clover, are less preferred, because, on average, these forages have higher energy and NSC content when compared with grass hay. Ensiled forages generally have lower NSC content than hay made from the same crop. Despite the generally lower NSC content of haylage compared with hay, however, the high palatability of some haylages may result in higher total NSC intake. Ideally, the results of proximate nutrient analysis, including direct measurement of starch and sugars (ie, NSC content), should be reviewed before selection of the hay. An NSC content of less than 10% is recommended. In the absence of data on hay NSC content, some nutritionists have recommended soaking hay in water for 30 to 60 minutes before feeding to leach WSCs (sugars and fructans). Recent work has suggested that under typical management conditions, this practice is unlikely to result in substantial change in the WSC content of most hay types, however.[46]

Forage-only diets do not provide adequate protein, minerals, or vitamins. Supplementing the forage diet with a low-calorie commercial ration balancer product that contains sources of high-quality protein and a mixture of vitamins and minerals to balance the low vitamin E, vitamin, copper, zinc, selenium, and other minerals typically found in mature grass hays is therefore recommended. These products can be fiber based or may be designed to be fed in small quantities (eg, 0.5–1.0 kg/d fed as is or mixed with hay chop [chaff]). Such fiber-based low-energy feeds can help to extend feeding time, and therefore help to alleviate boredom in animals provided a restricted diet.

Not all insulin-resistant horses and ponies are obese; in some of these animals, a ration of mostly hay may not meet energy requirements, particularly when some weight gain is desired or the animal is competing in athletic events. One approach is to add nonmolassed sugar beet pulp to the ration (eg, 0.5–1.5 lb/d). Beet pulp is rich in highly digestible fibers, provides more digestible energy when compared with most hay types, and does not elicit a marked glycemic or insulinemic response unless molasses is added at the time of processing. Beet pulp shreds should be soaked (in a volume of water three- to fourfold higher than that of the beet pulp) before feeding. The energy density of the ration also can be increased by feeding vegetable oil (eg, mixed with sugar beet pulp shreds or with hay cubes that have been softened in water). Corn and soy oils are commonly used in equine rations but need to be fresh and nonrancid and introduced gradually to the ration. One standard cup (~ 225 mL or 210 g) of vegetable oil provides 1.7 Mcal of digestible energy. Depending on energy requirements, ½ to 1 cup of oil can be fed once or twice daily (up to a maximum of ~ 100 mL per 100 kg of body weight). Smaller amounts (eg, ¼ cup once daily) should initially be fed, with a gradual increase over a 7- to 10-day period. Supplemental antioxidant (vitamin E, 100–200 IU, per 100 mL of added oil) should be provided. Stabilized rice bran (~ 20% fat) is another option for increasing the energy density of the diet, provided that the calcium/phosphorus ratio of the final ration is considered.

Another approach to dietary management of the lean or working insulin-resistant horse is provide a commercial feed along with hay. Most feed companies now offer products with lower starch and sugar content (<20%–25% NSCs) when compared with traditional sweet feeds (40%–50% NSCs) or cereal grains. Digestible fibers (sugar beet pulp or soy hulls) and vegetable oils are included in place of starch-rich ingredients, and energy density is similar or even higher when compared with sweet feeds. In theory, these lower NSC feeds result in lower postfeeding glycemic and insulinemic responses and carry lower risk for disturbances in hindgut function associated with the rapid fermentation of starch or sugars. Nevertheless, it is the authors' experience that the glycemic or insulinemic responses cannot reliably be predicted from the formulation (or assessment of NSC content) and that actual measurement of postfeeding glucose and insulin concentrations in horses is currently required to verify that the feed is "low-glycemic." These products are often marketed for use in horses and ponies at high risk for laminitis, including those that have IR or PPID. To the authors' knowledge, there have been no published controlled studies in target populations; therefore, data are not available to support or refute these medical claims. Nonetheless, these feeds are convenient for clients and the principle is sound; provided that these feeds do actually result in low postfeeding glucose and insulin responses, they are likely to be useful when fed according to manufacturers' recommendations.

Regular monitoring of serum insulin concentration, body weight, and BCS is recommended. Resting insulin concentration should be measured 7 to 10 days after the initiation of a new diet and at regular intervals thereafter. Similarly, it is advisable to evaluate insulin concentrations in horses or ponies that have been reintroduced to pasture. A substantial increase in serum insulin (>10–15 mU/L) may indicate exacerbation of IR, attributable to the feed directly or because of weight gain. In both circumstances, further changes in the composition or quantity of the ration may be needed.

Dietary supplements

Several supplements are marketed with claims for improved insulin sensitivity or reduced risk for laminitis, but evidence of efficacy is scant. Many products contain magnesium, chromium, or cinnamon. The streptogramin antibiotic "virginiamycin" has been successfully used to prevent pasture-induced laminitis, purportedly by preventing the overgrowth of gram-positive cecal bacteria.[38] This product has only limited availability (eg, not available in the United States, only available in Europe under special license), however, and, anecdotally, is not effective in all cases. The feeding of a protected hindgut buffer product (sodium bicarbonate) mitigated decreases in the fecal pH associated with pasture grazing,[47] but there are no data on efficacy for prevention of laminitis.

Chromium Chromium is thought to potentiate insulin action by means of activation of insulin receptor kinase or inhibition of insulin receptor tyrosine phosphatase.[48,49] Studies in people have shown that suboptimal intake of chromium (trivalent form) contributes to IR in type 2 diabetes and metabolic syndrome. Moreover, some but not all studies have shown improvement in glucose tolerance in insulin-resistant human patients provided a chromium supplement.[48] Accordingly, supplemental chromium (2.5–5.0 mg/d) has been fed to insulin-resistant horses and ponies. In a recent German study, overweight (BCS of 7.6 ± 0.8) hyperinsulinemic ponies were fed a yeast product with or without chromium together with hay for 4 weeks. An oral starch tolerance test (STT) was performed at the beginning and end of the supplementation period. Peak insulin responses during the STT were modestly lower in the supplemented versus nonsupplemented ponies[50]; however, the study design was not ideal, and further studies are needed to determine the effect of chromium supplementation on insulin sensitivity in horses or ponies with IR.

Magnesium Magnesium is an electrolyte (because it is a substance that exists as a positively charged particle in aqueous solution) and a mineral (because it forms part of the ash produced by combustion at high temperatures) that is required in several-gram quantities by horses each day.[51] It is absorbed mainly in the small intestine, and renal pathways are primarily responsible for its removal from the body, although small amounts are present in sweat. Some studies in human beings have demonstrated an association between magnesium status and IR in type 2 diabetes.[52,53] One hypothesis is that magnesium deficiency results in defective insulin receptor tyrosine kinase activity and exaggerated intracellular calcium concentration, both of which impair insulin action.[52] A review of randomized double-blind controlled trials that evaluated the effects of magnesium supplementation in patients who had type 2 diabetes concluded that supplementation may be effective in reducing fasting plasma concentrations and increasing high-density lipoprotein cholesterol but only in patients with actual magnesium deficiency, which was determined by measurement of intraerythrocytic concentrations.[53]

There are no data on the magnesium status of obese or insulin-resistant horses or ponies. Nonetheless, insulin-resistant animals are often fed a magnesium supplement (eg, magnesium oxide, 10–20 g, which provides magnesium, ~ 5–10 g). The magnesium requirement of a mature horse at maintenance is 7.5 g/d and is typically provided by the core diet.[49] Studies are required to determine whether higher level magnesium supplementation is beneficial for management of IR. In the meantime, it is advisable to ensure that rations for insulin-resistant equids at least meet minimum requirements (7.5 g/d).

MEDICAL THERAPY FOR INSULIN RESISTANCE

Levothyroxine sodium (Thyro L; Lloyd Inc., Shenandoah, Iowa) and metformin have been used as medical therapies for IR in horses and ponies.[9,54] Treatment with levothyroxine has been recommended for obese insulin-resistant horses or ponies in which more conservative approaches (ie, diet, exercise) have failed to effect adequate weight loss.[9] In healthy horses, a 6-month period of levothyroxine treatment resulted in weight loss and increased insulin sensitivity.[55] The recommended dosage for weight loss in mature horses is 48 mg/d (~ 4 teaspoons, administered in feed) for 3 to 6 months depending on clinical response. Treated animals should be gradually weaned from the drug when treatment goals have been attained; a recommended protocol involves decreasing the dosage from 48 mg/d to 24 mg/d for 2 weeks and then to 12 mg/d for a further 2 weeks.[9] Lower dose levothyroxine treatment (24 mg/d) has been recommended for management of persistently hyperinsulinemic but lean horses, but the effect of this treatment on insulin sensitivity has not been reported.

The biguanide metformin also has been used for therapy of IR in equids. In one report, treatment with metformin at 15 mg/kg administered per os twice daily (every 12 hours) resulted in a small decrease in the serum concentration of hyperinsulinemic horses and ponies.[54] In human beings, the primary action of metformin is to decrease hepatic gluconeogenesis, although it also may enhance tissue insulin sensitivity. Further studies are indicated to determine the pharmacokinetics, pharmacodynamics, and safety of metformin in horses.

SUMMARY

Alterations in diet and feeding management can be helpful in the management of obesity and IR. Caloric restriction, ideally combined with increased physical activity, to promote weight loss and improve insulin sensitivity is indicated for management of obese animals. In insulin-resistant animals with or without obesity, strict control of dietary NSC content (starches, sugars, and fructans), with elimination of grains and sweet feeds from the ration and restricted access to pastures that may be rich in NSC content, is currently recommended. Medical treatment with levothyroxine or metformin may be indicated in obese or insulin-resistant animals that do not respond to conservative dietary management.

REFERENCES

1. Geor R, Frank N. Metabolic syndrome—from human organ disease to laminar failure in equids. Vet Immunol Immunopathol 2008;doi:10.1016/j.vetimm.2008.11.012.
2. Treiber KH, Kronfeld DS, Hess TM, et al. Evaluation of genetic and metabolic predispositions and nutritional risk factors for pasture-associated laminitis in ponies. J Am Vet Med Assoc 2006;228:1538–45.
3. Treiber KH, Kronfeld DS, Geor RJ. Insulin resistance in equids—possible role in laminitis. J Nutr 2006;136:2094S–8S.
4. Frank N, Elliott SB, Brandt LE, et al. Physical characteristics, blood hormone concentrations, and plasma lipid concentrations in obese horses with insulin resistance. J Am Vet Med Assoc 2006;228:1383–90.
5. Bailey SR, Menzies-Gow NJ, Harris PA, et al. Effect of dietary fructans and dexamethasone administration on the insulin response of ponies predisposed to laminitis. J Am Vet Med Assoc 2007;231:1365–73.
6. Bailey SR, Habsershon-Butcher JL, Ransom KJ, et al. Hypertension and insulin resistance in a mixed-breed population of ponies predisposed to laminitis. Am J Vet Res 2008;69:122–9.
7. Carter RA, Treiber KH, Geor RJ, et al. Prediction of incipient pasture-associated laminitis from hyperinsulinemia, hyperleptinemia, and generalized and localized obesity in a cohort of ponies. Equine Vet J 2009;41:171–8.
8. Johnson PJ. The equine metabolic syndrome: peripheral Cushing's syndrome. Vet Clin North Am Equine Pract 2002;18:271–93.

9. Frank N. Endocrinopathic laminitis, obesity-associated laminitis, and pasture-associated laminitis. Proceedings of 54th Annual Convention of the American Association of Equine Practitioners. San Diego, CA, December 2008.
10. Harris PA, Stewart I. Weight control and management. Proceedings of the First British Equine Veterinary Association and WALTHAM Nutrition Symposia. Suffolk (UK): Equine Veterinary Journal Limited; 2005. p. 99–104.
11. Henneke DR, Potter GD, Kreider JL, et al. Relationship between condition score, physical measurements and body fat percentage in mares. Equine Vet J 1983;15: 371–2.
12. Lee S, Bacha F, Gungor N, et al. Waist circumference is an independent predictor of insulin resistance in black and white youths. J Pediatr 2006;148:188–94.
13. Alberti KG, Zimmet P, Shaw J. Metabolic syndrome—a new world-wide definition. A consensus statement from the International Diabetes Federation. Diabet Med 2006;23:469–80.
14. United States Department of Agriculture. NAHMS Equine '98. Part III. Management and health of horses. Available at: www.aphis.usda.gov/vs/ceah/cahm. Accessed August 5, 2008.
15. Wyse CA, McNie KA, Tannahil VJ, et al. Prevalence of obesity in riding horses in Scotland. Vet Rec 2008;162:590–1.
16. Saltiel AR, Kahn CR. Insulin signaling and the regulation of glucose and lipid metabolism. Nature 2001;414:799–806.
17. Kahn CR. Insulin resistance, insulin sensitivity, and insulin unresponsiveness: a necessary distinction. Metabolism 1978;27:1893–902.
18. Muniyappa R, Lee S, Chen H, et al. Current approaches for assessing insulin sensitivity and resistance in vivo: advantages, limitations and appropriate usage. Am J Physiol Endocrinol Metab 2008;294:E15–26.
19. Yudkin JS. Insulin resistance and the metabolic syndrome—or the pitfalls of epidemiology. Diabetologia 2007;50:1576–86.
20. Muoio DM, Newgard CB. Molecular and metabolic mechanisms of insulin resistance and β-cell failure in type 2 diabetes. Nat Rev Mol Cell Biol 2008;9: 193–205.
21. Carter RA, McCutcheon LJ, Burns TA, et al. Increased adiposity in horses is associated with decreased insulin sensitivity but unchanged inflammatory cytokine expression in subcutaneous adipose tissue. J Vet Intern Med 2008;22:735 [abstract].
22. Vick MM, Adams AA, Murphy BA, et al. Relationships among inflammatory cytokines, obesity, and insulin sensitivity in the horse. J Anim Sci 2007;85:1144–55.
23. Schott HC II. Pituitary pars intermedia dysfunction: challenges of diagnosis and treatment. Proc Am Assoc Equine Pract 2006;52:60–73.
24. Donaldson MT, Jorgensen AJ, Beech J. Evaluation of suspected pars pituitary intermedia dysfunction in horses with laminitis. J Am Vet Med Assoc 2004;224: 1123–7.
25. McGowan CM, Frost R, Pfeiffer DU. Serum insulin concentrations in horses with equine Cushing's syndrome: response to a cortisol inhibitor and prognostic value. Equine Vet J 2004;36:295–8.
26. Hoffman RM, Boston RC, Stefanovski D, et al. Obesity and diet affect glucose dynamics and insulin sensitivity in Thoroughbred geldings. J Anim Sci 2003;81: 2333–42.
27. Kahn R, Buse J, Ferrannini E, et al. for the American Diabetes Association and European Association for the Study of Diabetes. The metabolic syndrome: time for a critical appraisal: joint statement from the American Diabetes Association

and European Association for the Study of Diabetes. Diabetes Care 2005;28: 2289–304.
28. Dugdale AHA, Curtis GC, Knottenbelt DC, et al. Changes in body condition and fat deposition in ponies offered an ad libitum chaff-based diet. In: Proceedings of the 12th Congress of the European Society for Veterinary Clinical Nutrition; 2008. p. 39 [abstract].
29. Coffman JR, Colles CM. Insulin tolerance in laminitic ponies. Can J Comp Med 1983;47:347–51.
30. Field JR, Jeffcott LB. Equine laminitis—another hypothesis for pathogenesis. Med Hypotheses 1989;30:203–10.
31. Treiber KH, Hess TM, Kronfeld DS, et al. Insulin resistance and compensation in laminitis-predisposed ponies characterized by the minimal model. Pferdeheilkunde 2007;21:91–2.
32. Asplin KE, Sillence MN, Pollitt CC, et al. Induction of laminitis by prolonged hyperinsulinaemia in clinically normal ponies. Vet J 2007;174:530–5.
33. Tiley HA, Geor RJ, McCutcheon LJ. Effects of dexamethasone on glucose dynamics and insulin sensitivity in healthy horses. Am J Vet Res 2007;68:753–9.
34. Tóth F, Frank N, Elliott SB, et al. Effects of intravenous endotoxin on glucose and insulin dynamics in horses. Am J Vet Res 2008;69:82–8.
35. Treiber KH, Carter RA, Harris PA, et al. Seasonal changes in energy metabolism of ponies coincides with changes in pasture carbohydrates: implications for laminitis. J Vet Intern Med 2008;22:735–6 [abstract].
36. van Eps AW, Pollitt CC. Equine laminitis induced with oligofructose. Equine Vet J 2006;38:203–8.
37. Milinovich GJ, Trott DJ, Burrell PC, et al. Changes in equine hindgut bacterial populations during oligofructose-induced laminitis. Environ Microbiol 2006;8: 885–98.
38. Bailey SR, Marr CM, Elliott J. Current research and theories on the pathogenesis of acute laminitis in the horse. Vet J 2004;167:129–42.
39. Belknap JK, Giguere S, Pettigrew A, et al. Lamellar pro-inflammatory cytokine expression patterns in laminitis at the developmental stage and at the onset of lameness: innate vs. adaptive immune response. Equine Vet J 2007;39:42–7.
40. Firshman AM, Valberg SJ. Factors affecting clinical assessment of insulin sensitivity in horses. Equine Vet J 2007;39:567–75.
41. Eiler H, Frank N, Andrews FM, et al. Physiologic assessment of blood glucose homeostasis via combined glucose and insulin testing in horses. Am J Vet Res 2005;66:1598–604.
42. Harris PA, Bailey SR, Elliott J, et al. Countermeasures to pasture-associated laminitis in horses. J Nutr 2006;136:2114S–21S.
43. Powell DM, Reedy SE, Sessions DR, et al. Effect of short-term exercise training on insulin sensitivity in obese and lean mares. Equine Vet J 2002;(Suppl 34): 81–4.
44. Buff PR, Johnson PJ, Wiedmeyer CE, et al. Modulation of leptin, insulin and growth hormone in obese pony mares under chronic nutritional restriction and supplementation with ractopamine hydrochloride. Vet Ther 2007;7:64–72.
45. Ince JC, Longland AC, Moore-Colyer M, et al. A pilot study to estimate the intake of grass by ponies with restricted access to pasture. Proceedings of the British Society of Animal Science. York, England, April 2005.
46. Longland AC, Harker I, Harris PA. The loss of water-soluble carbohydrate and soluble protein from nine different hays submerged in water for up to 16 hours. In: Proceedings of the Equine Science Society, in press 2009.

47. Pagan JD, Lawrence TJ, Lawrence LA. Feeding protected sodium bicarbonate attenuates hindgut acidosis in horses fed a high-grain ration. Proceedings of 54th Annual Convention of the American Association of Equine Practitioners. Orlando, FL, December 2007.
48. Anderson RA. Chromium in the prevention and control of diabetes. Diabetes Metab (Paris) 2000;26:22–7.
49. Lau FC, Bagchi M, Sen CK, et al. Nutrigenomic basis of beneficial effects of chromium(III) on obesity and diabetes. Mol Cell Biochem 2008;317:1–10.
50. Verveurt I, Obwald B, Coenen M. Effects of chromium supplementation on metabolic profile in insulin resistant ponies. In: Proceedings of the 12th Congress of the European Society for Veterinary Clinical Nutrition; 2008. p. 40 [abstract].
51. Anon. National Research Council nutrient requirements of horses. 6th revised edition. Washington, DC: National Academies Press; 2007.
52. Barbagallo M, Dominguez A, Galioto A, et al. Role of magnesium in insulin action, diabetes and cardiovascular syndrome X. Mol Aspects Med 2003;24:39–52.
53. Song Y, He Y, Levitan EB, et al. Effects of oral magnesium supplementation on glycaemic control in Type 2 diabetes: a meta-analysis of randomized double blind controlled trials. Diabet Med 2006;23:1050–6.
54. Durham AE, Rendle DI, Newton JE. The effect of metformin on measurements of insulin sensitivity and beta cell response in 18 horses and ponies with insulin resistance. Equine Vet J 2008;40:493–500.
55. Frank N, Elliott SB, Boston RC. Effects of long-term oral administration of levothyroxine sodium on glucose dynamics in healthy adult horses. Am J Vet Res 2008;69:76–81.

The Role of Nutrition in Colic

Andy E. Durham, BSc, BVSc, CertEP, DEIM, MRCVS

KEYWORDS

• Equine • Epidemiology • Dietary starch • Digestion • Probiotics

Equine digestive anatomy and physiology evolved over more than 50 million years for an animal that had significant behavioral and dietary dissimilarities with the modern equid domesticated over the last few millennia.[1,2] The dietary demands of modern equine activities frequently require marked quantitative and qualitative dietary changes and feeding patterns compared with the evolutionary model. The contrast is marked when considering the feral equid continually browsing for fiber-rich, low-starch grasses, sedges, and shrubs that might slowly and gradually change in quality and quantity with the seasons versus the modern competition horse that may have two or three high-starch bolus feeds daily interspersed by limited forage and the possibility of abrupt and marked dietary changes provided by inexpert caregivers. The summary of ideal feeding practice, "to efficiently supply dietary ingredients in amounts that will meet the horse's nutrient needs, while still retaining the horse's normal feeding behavior,"[2] is almost inevitably compromised under most modern management systems that frequently exceed certain needs, fall short of others, and rarely closely mimic feeding patterns of horses predomestication. The imposition of modern diets and dietary management strategies for which the equine gastrointestinal tract is not evolutionarily adapted may well lead to intolerance manifesting as colic. Many diet-related variables have subsequently been recognized as risk factors for colic, such as cereal feeding, restricted grazing, and forage quality, although abrupt dietary changes have generally been found to outweigh the negative impact of specific qualitative dietary factors.[3]

Although significant regional and population differences may occur,[4,5] typically around 5 cases of colic are expected per 100 horses each year,[3,6] representing one of the most frequent and potentially serious conditions encountered in equine practice. The welfare implications of a common, painful, and sometimes fatal condition, and inconvenient interruption of training and competition schedules and financial losses estimated 10 years ago at more than $115 million per annum in the United States,[5,6] have inevitably led to considerable epidemiologic research and advice intended to moderate the incidence and severity of this familiar equine affliction.[3,7–10] In addition to regional and population differences in horses studied,

The Liphook Equine Hospital, Forest Mere, Liphook, Hampshire GU30 7JG, UK
E-mail address: andy@theleh.co.uk

Vet Clin Equine 25 (2009) 67–78
doi:10.1016/j.cveq.2008.11.003
vetequine.theclinics.com

interpretation of epidemiologic data may be further hindered by possibly differing or opposing effects of certain epidemiologic factors on specific disease subtypes associated with colic signs. Furthermore, association of certain covariables may potentially confound results and their interpretation. For example, a particular age group of a particular breed or type of horse may undergo a particular form of exertional activity while receiving a particular diet at a particular time of year associated with a particular style of management, any or all of which may have a causal (additive or opposing) relationship with diseases manifesting with abdominal pain.

CEREALS AND STARCHES

Carbohydrates invariably represent the major digestible energy source for horses across a wide range of diets[11] and have the best documented influence on colic risk in horses.[12] Various classification systems exist for partitioning dietary carbohydrates in equine diets but the system described by Hoffman and colleagues[13] is perhaps the most relevant when considering nutrition and colic. Three major fractions of carbohydrates were described comprising hydrolysable carbohydrates (CHO-H), which are readily digestible and absorbable in the equine small intestine subject to physiologic limitations (eg, monosaccharides, disaccharides, and some oligosaccharides and starches); rapidly fermented carbohydrates (CHO-F_R), which are readily and extensively fermented by microbial populations in the hindgut (eg, fructans, pectins, β-glucans, some oligosaccharides, and resistant starches); and slowly fermented carbohydrates (CHO-F_S), which are more gradually and incompletely fermented, usually by different microbial species (eg, hemicellulose, cellulose, lignins).[13] A large, diverse, and dominant population of fibrolytic bacteria (eg, *Clostridiaceae*, *Fibrobacter*, *Spirochaetaceae*) are normally found in the forage-fed equine hindgut that ferment CHO-F_S to short-chain fatty acids primarily comprising acetate, propionate, and butyrate.[14,15] A smaller population of saccharolytic species (eg, *Bacillus*, *Lactobacillus*, *Streptococcus*) also exists that hydrolyze CHO-F_R, along with any CHO-H that has escaped small intestinal digestion, primarily producing lactate and propionate.[12–14] The short-chain fatty acids absorbed from the large bowel contribute the major source of energy to forage-fed horses with acetate representing the largest individual substrate for oxidation.[11] Propionate is largely used for hepatic gluconeogenesis and butyrate may have a more local role in maintaining colonic enterocyte health.[11] Lactate is normally found at very low levels within colonic contents and, when present in larger concentrations, is associated with adverse effects on pH, microbial populations, and short-chain fatty acid absorption by the colon.[12]

Microbial population dynamics are markedly influenced by available dietary substrates and also pH changes consequent to their fermentation. Cecocolonic delivery of undigested CHO-H and CHO-F_R rapidly promotes bacterial multiplication and overgrowth of acidophilic *Streptococci* and *Lactobacilli*. Lactic acidosis decreases luminal pH from nearly neutral to as low as 6.0, markedly impairing survival of normal fibrolytic bacterial species and potentially leading to decreased CHO-F_S fermentation; decreased acetate production; impairment of mucosal barrier function; increased absorption of lipopolysaccharide, amines, and other noxious substances; dehydration of digesta; dysmotility; gaseous distention; colon displacement; and volvulus.[12,14,16–26] Interestingly, intraluminal colonic lactic acidosis, decreased fibrolytic bacteria, and increased acidophilic microbial species have been demonstrated not only in response to cereal feeding of horses, but have also been found within the large intestinal contents of horses with colic.[12]

Incomplete prececal digestion of starch is among the most important causal factors to consider in the association between diet and colic. Starches from different cereal sources have different proportions of straight-chain amylose and branched-chain amylopectin and differing relative digestibility. Oat and sorghum starch is more highly digestible than that in barley, wheat, or maize, although thermal processing techniques, such as micronization and popping, may also have a marked further beneficial influence.[27,28] Starch digestion occurs in two phases. First, α-amylase hydrolyzes amylose and amylopectin to disaccharides (maltose), trisaccharides (maltotriose), and larger oligosaccharides (α-dextrins), which are then further degraded by brush border enzymes.[29] Compared with other species the equine small intestine may be somewhat deficient in α-amylase, although it seems to possess good levels of disaccharidases.[30,31] The absorptive capacity of glucose by the equine small intestine improves following adaptation to high-starch feeds by up-regulation of the enterocyte glucose transporter protein sodium-glucose cotransporter isoform 1.[12] Because it is believed that sodium-glucose cotransporter isoform 1 up-regulation is dependent on exposure to monosaccharides rather than polysaccharides, this implies that starch digestion is indeed enhanced following dietary adaptation in horses as suggested by previous studies.[27] With relevance to colic in horses, however, there seems to be significant interindividual variation in α-amylase levels and it seems that adaptation is both limited and slow to develop.[12,32] Accordingly, incomplete prececal starch digestion is likely to occur in most horses fed to perform frequent and intense bouts of exercise. A study of racing Thoroughbreds in Australia reported a mean cereal intake of 7.3 kg/day (range, 3.8–13.2 kg/day),[33] which even when divided into several feeds is still expected to result in around half of the ingested starch arriving in the cecum.[34] Fecal pH was less than 6.2 in more than a quarter of horses in this study[33] consistent with a lack of adaptation to the diet and probable adverse cecocolonic health and function, as described previously.

The combination of relatively poor prececal starch digestibility and the dysfermentative effects of starches delivered to the large bowel suggest that equids are poorly suited to high-starch diets as frequently provided to competition horses.[12,34] Unsurprisingly, several studies have associated increased cereal feeding with colic risk. In one study comparing cereal-fed horses with grazing horses, those consuming only moderate quantities of concentrates (2.5–5 kg/day) were found to have an almost five times increased risk of colic (odds ratio [OR], 4.8; 95% confidence interval [CI], 1.4–16.6; P = .01) and the risk was increased further at higher levels of concentrate feeding (>5 kg/day: OR, 6.3; 95% CI, 1.8–22; P<.01).[35] Similarly, an approximately six times increased risk of colic was found in horses consuming more than 2.7 kg oats per day in another study (OR, 5.9; 95% CI, 1.6–22; P<.01).[36] A recent study of impaction colic in donkeys indicated that the risk of colic was more than doubled in those donkeys fed extra concentrate rations (OR, 2.2; 95% CI, 1.1–4.5; P = .03).[37] Pelleted feeds have been proposed to represent a particular colic risk in some studies,[7,35] although this has not been a consistent finding in all reports.[8,38]

Cereal feeding may have different effects on different causes of colic. One study found that concentrate intakes were significantly higher in horses diagnosed with duodenitis-proximal jejunitis than those with colic from other causes.[39] In contrast, enterolithiasis is one cause of colic that might actually benefit from modest colonic acidification because formation of enteroliths is suspected to be favored in an alkaline colonic environment enriched by protein-derived nitrogen and sulfur and also in minerals including calcium, magnesium, phosphorus, potassium, and sodium.[40–42]

Given the potential consequences of the limited capacity of the equine small intestine to hydrolyze starches, the practice of dividing cereal-based feeds into frequent, small meals is generally recommended as far as is reasonably practical.[43] Starch boluses fed at greater than 300 g/100 kg bodyweight have a marked effect on microbial populations with perhaps half of the ingested starch reaching the cecum,[23,28,34] and a guideline of no more than 200 g/100 kg bodyweight starch per meal (eg, approximately 2 kg of concentrate feed for a 500-kg horse) is frequently proposed.[24,28,44,45] In horses prone to colic, far lower starch boluses may be advisable because even when fed at 100 to 200 g/100 kg bodyweight per meal there is still frequently 40 g starch/100 kg bodyweight reaching the cecum.[28,34] The possible benefits of exogenous α-amylase added to high-starch equine diets is worthy of further investigation. In one study an increased glycemic response was seen in horses following incorporation of α-amylase (with or without further enzymes) to a high-starch diet suggesting increased prececal hydrolysis.[31] This effect was short-lived, however, and was not associated with significantly improved fecal pH or short-chain fatty acid concentrations as might have been expected.

When it is considered unlikely that a grass-forage diet modestly supplemented by cereal can provide enough energy for a working horse, then fiber-rich feeds, such as sugar beet pulp or alfalfa cubes, might be provided that contain similar digestible energy content to many cereal-based feeds but far less starch. Fat may then be supplemented to increase the energy density of the diet without the undesirable consequences of starch on the hindgut. Although vegetable oils have also been found to adversely affect cellulolysis in the equine hindgut, presumably as a consequence of bactericidal fatty acids,[46] this effect is far less disruptive than similar energy levels provided by starch-rich feeds and fat feeding has not yet been associated with colic in the horse.

GRAZING

Leguminous and subtropical grasses may store significant quantities of starch in their leaves in contrast to most temperate pasture grasses that store carbohydrate as fructans in the stems.[47] Although it is recognized that there is some prececal hydrolysis and fermentation of fructans,[11,47] this is quite limited compared with starches and fructans fit mainly into the CHO-F_R category.[13] Logical extrapolation of the dysfermentative effects of excess dietary starch might then lead to the assumption that grass might also contribute to colic risk in the horse, although additional important factors to consider are possibly differing rates of exposure of grass-fructan (or grass-starch) versus cereal-starch to the hindgut bacteria and also stable adaptation of fermentative bacterial populations to a particular continuous carbohydrate source. There is a marked contrast in probable bacterial population dynamics between trickle-feeding grass-fructans (or grass-starches) over perhaps 14 to 18 hours of grazing daily compared with bolus-feeding of concentrated cereal-starch in two meals perhaps lasting 10 minutes each during a 24-hour period. Nevertheless fructan can be consumed rapidly and in large quantities under certain climatic and management conditions leading to similar dysfermentative effects to undigested starch that reaches the cecum.[47]

Access to grazing has generally been regarded as offering some protection against colic, although this observation might be biased or confounded by associated factors, such as reduced observation of pastured horses, increased ambulatory activity, psychologic comfort, or climatic, seasonal, or other factors associated with a management decision to increase stabling. Nevertheless, a large study in Texas found that horses that were fully stabled or had recently reduced pasture access were at three times the risk of suffering colic (95% CI, 1.4–6.6; *P*<.01) after controlling for many other variables.[36] An even greater protective effect of grazing has also been proposed for specific colic subtypes, such as simple colon obstruction; epiploic foramen entrapment (EFE); and enterolithiasis cases, which are far more frequently reported in horses that spend little or no time at grass.[10,41,42,48,49] Although it might be argued that simple colon obstructions arise following stabling because of several other associated factors, such as the introduction of relatively dry forage rather than the withdrawal of grazing per se, multivariable analysis confirms the protective effect of access to pasture against enterolith formation and EFE even after controlling for alternative preserved forage intake.[42,49]

That is not to say, however, that grazing horses are at low risk of all types of colic. Fructan content of grasses and herbage can be markedly variable between different grasses, exacerbated by variable temperature and light exposure,[47,50] creating an increased likelihood of hindgut disturbance when grazing is changed or weather is changeable. Interestingly, equine grass sickness (EGS) and duodenitis-proximal jejunitis, two specific causes of colic that are unusual in being associated with increased grazing,[39,51,52] have both been etiologically linked with putatively altered enteric toxicoinfectious clostridial populations,[53,54] although the precise causal factors in these conditions remain uncertain. The further association between weather, season, and recent change of fields with risk of EGS also is consistent with a possible dietary influence on enteric bacterial populations.[51,52]

Grazing should generally be encouraged in preference to preserved forage for the benefit of gastrointestinal health but consideration should be given to introducing access to new grazing gradually and to allowing free access eventually to limit variable rates of consumption. Clearly, the balancing of other health and management issues is also a key to successful grazing policy and this has to be finally formulated on the basis of local conditions with respect to the quality and quantity of pasture and the characteristics of the individual horses concerned. Obese, laminitis-susceptible individuals or those considered to be at high risk of EGS, sand impactions, or duodenitis-proximal jejunitis may gain net health benefit from grazing restriction.

PRESERVED FORAGE

When grazing is restricted by availability or management requirements, then preserved forages should be regarded as the staple of equine diets. The quality within batches of preserved forage is likely to be less variable than grazing, although abrupt changes in forage type or even a change in batch of the same type of preserved forage still carries a significant risk of colic.[8,10,36] Particular types of forages have been found to be risk factors for particular types of colic. Poor quality hays that are especially high in less fermentable components of CHO-F_S increase the risk of ileal and colonic impactions,[36,38,55] whereas alfalfa hays higher in crude protein and minerals are associated with increased risk of enteroliths (alfalfa hay $\geq$50% of diet: OR, 4.7; 95% CI, 1.4–15.6; $P = .01$)[41,42] and fecoliths.[7] Colonic alkalinization resulting from alfalfa feeding has long been suspected to explain the significant association with enterolith formation exacerbated by the relatively high mineral content of alfalfa hay.[40] In contrast, oat and grass hays have been shown to reduce the risk of enterolith formation significantly over and above the associated benefit of decreased alfalfa feeding (oat hay $\geq$50% of diet: OR, 0.20; 95% CI, 0.07–0.62; $P<.01$; grass hay $\geq$50% of diet: OR, 0.22; 95% CI, 0.08–0.61; $P<.01$).[42] The buffering effect of the increased quantities of saliva consumed with prolonged mastication of preserved forage perhaps augmented by the greater buffering properties of alfalfa hays might also offer benefits to the health of the proximal gastrointestinal tract and may partly explain apparent protective effects against gastric ulceration and small intestinal strangulations.[7,56,57]

There is little evidence on which to base recommendations for fiber feeding in horses.[11] Where grazing is limited, a minimum of 1% to 1.5% bodyweight of preserved forage (as dry matter) is advisable.[2] Following gradual access to new forage supplies, free access should be considered in preference to intermittent provision of forage, and physical limitation of ingestion with narrow-weave haynets, double haynets, or "hay-bags" may be useful to simulate a natural trickle-feeding behavior.

Good dental care intuitively forms an integrated part of the dietary strategy offered to the horse with recurrent colic, although studies have not consistently found any beneficial effect of routine dental care on digestion, assimilation, or colic risk.[10,58–61] A recent study in donkeys with impaction colic, however, did identify dental disease as a very strong and highly significant risk factor for disease (OR, 29.7; 95% CI, 4–223.7; *P*<.01)[37] and dental examination and appropriate corrections seems to be advisable when presented with a case of impaction or recurrent colic.

DIETARY CHANGES

Whatever the exact dietary quality and quantity supplied to a horse, it seems that recent changes in diet represent an especially high risk for colic of various types,[8,10,35,36,49,51,55,58,62] an association that is most probably mediated by altered diet-adapted microbial populations. In an experimental study conducted in ponies, significant changes in hindgut bacterial flora and short-chain fatty acids concentrations promptly followed addition of 30% rolled barley to a hay-only diet.[18] Changes in diet have also been found to predispose to *Salmonella* shedding in hospitalized horses, further emphasizing a destabilizing effect on intestinal microflora.[63] In addition to the markedly increased risk of EGS in horses that have recently changed grazing, other studies have identified risk factors for general colic incidence including changing the batch or type of hay, changing the quantity or frequency of feeding, and erring from usual feeding times.[8,35,36] Although it is well accepted that abrupt dietary changes may lead to colic in horses, the common practice of feeding a few daily cereal-based meals interspersed by long periods of high-fiber forage intake (or no intake) of markedly differing nutritional quality represents marked intraday dietary change and probable significant diurnal variability in hindgut pH and bacterial populations and perhaps promotion of colic.[45]

The duration of the colic risk following dietary change varies between types of colic. In a study of horses with colic caused by simple colon obstruction and distention,[10] the risks of colic were greatest within a week of a change in forage (OR, 22; 95% CI, 2.8–170.4; *P*<.01) or concentrate (OR, 12; 95% CI, 2.7–54.4; *P*<.01), with the risks being reduced but still significant between 8 and 15 days of a dietary change (forage change OR, 4.9; 95% CI, 1.3–18.6; *P* = .02; concentrate change OR, 3; 95% CI, 1.0–8.9; *P*<.05). Diet changes more than 15 days previously were not significantly associated with colic risk.[10] A 2-week duration of colic risk following dietary change is also supported by several further studies of general colic incidence,[8,36,55,58] although other reports examining the temporal relationship between dietary change and risk of specific types of colic indicate that significantly increased risk of disease may exist for even longer after the change of diet. The risk of EFE was significantly increased for a period of 28 days following increased stabling (OR, 3.7; 95% CI, 1.4–9.7; *P*<.01).[49] Although the risk of EGS was found to be greatest within 2 weeks of a change of grazing (OR, 29.7; 95% CI, 66.7–130; *P*<.01), the increased risk of disease was still significant as long as 2 to 3 months following a field change (OR, 4.1; 95% CI,

1.0–16.6; $P<.05$).[51] Interestingly, several studies have found that a recent change in hay or forage is associated with higher risk of colic than a recent change in grain or concentrate.[8,10,36]

FURTHER FEED ADDITIVES

Many prebiotic and probiotic products are marketed for horses with gastrointestinal diseases and may have a reasonable evidence basis in some other species. The quality of commercially available probiotic products was scrutinized and questioned in one study that found that most products contained few, if any, viable or potentially beneficial organisms and sometimes potential pathogens were encountered.[64] In a further examination of a commercially available equine probiotic product claiming to contain lactobacilli, a pure growth of *Enterococcus gallinarum*, an occasional cause of antibiotic-resistant nosocomial infections in humans was obtained (A.E. Durham, unpublished data, 2008). An evidence-based approach to the design of appropriate equine bacterial probiotic products has thus far been unsuccessful.[65,66] In contrast, the investigation of yeast-containing probiotics including *Saccharomyces cerevisiae* and *Saccharomyces boulardii* has generally provided better quality supportive evidence in horses with gastrointestinal disease and they have been shown to protect against the adverse effects of starch overload[23,67] and also to reduce significantly the duration of diarrhea in clinical enterocolitis cases.[68]

In a recent study of risk factors for EFE it was found after multivariable analysis that access to a mineral-salt lick significantly reduced the risk of disease (OR, 0.3; 95% CI, 0.1–0.9; P = .03).[49] Given the triangular association between EFE, stereotypical behaviors, and gastrointestinal pH, the authors speculated that access to the salt lick stimulated increased salivation and the consequent gastrointestinal buffer perhaps offered some protection against EFE. Enterolithiasis, however, a condition that is unlikely to benefit from increased salivation (because colonic alkalinity seems to be a risk factor),[40] has also been found to be less likely in horses that are supplemented with minerals or vitamins (including mineral-salt licks or in-feed supplementation), although this finding did not reach statistical significance (enterolithiasis: OR, 0.5; 95% CI, 0.2–1.2; P = .11).[42] In the latter study, a further currently unexplained finding was that the only specific dietary variable other than alfalfa feeding that was associated with increased risk of enterolithiasis was the feeding of carrots (OR, 2.7; 95% CI, 1.0–7.6; P = .05).[42]

Psyllium is often fed to horses considered to be affected by or at risk from sand enteropathy.[69–71] One experimental study found that fecal output of sand that had been deposited surgically within the cecum of healthy ponies was not increased by 1 g/kg bodyweight psyllium when compared with an untreated control group.[72] Another study also failed to detect a beneficial effect of 0.5 g/kg bodyweight psyllium given daily when measuring fecal sand output following nasogastric dosing with sand.[73] In contrast, two more recent studies have provided support for the clinical use of psyllium in sand enteropathy cases. One study administered 1 kg of sand to healthy horses by nasogastric tube daily for 5 days and then administered either 1 g/kg psyllium combined with 2 L mineral oil, or 2 L mineral oil alone, from days 6 to 10. Fecal sand output was significantly greater in the group receiving the combined treatment from days 2 to 4 of administration.[74] A further study of a group of healthy horses with access to dry pasture or feedlot monitored fecal sand output for 7 days before and 35 days during administration of a psyllium-prebiotic-probiotic mixture containing approximately 0.5 g/kg bodyweight psyllium daily. Fecal sand output was significantly increased from 4 days after commencing treatment until the end of the study.[75]

SUMMARY

Equine gastrointestinal health seems best served by a slow and constant intake of a high-fiber, low-starch diet of even quality that maintains stability in fermentative fibrolytic bacterial species in the hindgut. Disruption and adverse dynamism of microbial populations may be especially promoted by dietary change when major feed ingredients are replaced or simply provided intermittently through the day. The demands of competition horses in particular often dictate that forage availability is restricted, energy-dense high-starch or high-fat boluses are ingested intermittently, and abnormally prolonged periods of total feed deprivation are common. The relative rarity of colic in domesticated horses (typically 95 in every 100 do not suffer colic during the course of a year) is a tribute to the adaptive capability of the equine gastrointestinal tract to the imposition of a diet that is frequently alien in respect of quality, quantity, and patterns of ingestion. Those individuals that do suffer from colic, however, especially if on a recurrent basis, should have their diet reviewed and adjusted toward that of their feral ancestors wherever and as far as possible.

REFERENCES

1. Houpt KA. Ingestive behaviour. Vet Clin North Am Equine Pract 1990;6:319–37.
2. National Research Council. Feeding behavior and general considerations for feeding management. In: Nutrient requirements of horses. 6th edition. Washington, DC: National Academies Press; 2007. p. 211–34.
3. Archer DC, Proudman CJ. Epidemiological clues to preventing colic. Vet J 2006; 172:29–39.
4. Uhlinger C. Investigations into the incidence of field colic. Equine Vet J Suppl 1992;13:16–8.
5. Tinker MK, White NA, Lessard P, et al. A prospective study of equine colic incidence and mortality. Equine Vet J 1997;29:448–53.
6. Traub-Dargatz JL, Kopral CA, Seitzinger AH, et al. Estimate of the national incidence of and operation-level risk factors for colic among horses in the United States, Spring 1998 to Spring 1999. J Am Vet Med Assoc 2001;219:67–71.
7. Morris DD, Moore JN, Ward S. Comparison of age, sex, breed, history and management in 229 horses with colic. Equine Vet J Suppl 1989;7:129–32.
8. Cohen ND, Gibbs PG, Woods AM. Dietary and other management factors associated with colic in horses. J Am Vet Med Assoc 1999;215:53–60.
9. Hillyer MH, Taylor FG, French NP. A cross-sectional study of colic in horses on thoroughbred training premises in the British Isles in 1997. Equine Vet J 2001; 33:380–5.
10. Hillyer MH, Taylor FG, Proudman CJ, et al. Case control study to identify risk factors for simple colonic obstruction and distension colic in horses. Equine Vet J 2002;34:455–63.
11. National Research Council. Carbohydrates. In: Nutrient requirements of horses. 6th edition. Washington, DC: National Academies Press; 2007. p. 34–43.
12. Shirazi-Beechey SP. Molecular insights into dietary induced colic. Equine Vet J 2008;40:414–21.
13. Hoffman RM, Wilson JA, Kronfeld DS, et al. Hydrolyzable carbohydrates in pasture, hay and horse feeds: direct assay and seasonal variation. J Anim Sci 2001;79:500–6.

14. Hintz HF, Argenzio RA, Schryver HF. Digestion coefficients, blood glucose levels and molar percentage of volatile acids in intestinal fluid of ponies fed varying forage-grain ratios. J Anim Sci 1971;33:992–5.
15. Daly K, Stewart C, Flint H, et al. Bacterial diversity within the equine large intestine as revealed by molecular analysis of cloned 16S rRNA genes. FEMS Microbiol Ecol 2001;38:141–51.
16. Goodson J, Tyznik WJ, Clin JH, et al. Effects of an abrupt diet change from hay to concentrate on microbial numbers and physical environment in the cecum of the pony. Appl Environ Microbiol 1988;54:1946–50.
17. Clarke LL, Roberts MC, Argenzio RA. Feeding and digestive problems in horses. Vet Clin North Am Equine Pract 1990;6:319–37.
18. de Fombelle A, Julliand V, Drogoul C, et al. Feeding and microbial disorders in horses: 1-effects of an abrupt incorporation of two levels of barley in a hay diet on microbial profile and activities. J Equine Vet Sci 2001;26:439–45.
19. Drogoul C, de Fombelle A, Julliand V. Feeding and microbial disorders in horses: 2: effect of three hay:grain ratios on digesta passage rate and digestibility in ponies. J Equine Vet Sci 2001;26:487–91.
20. Julliand V, de Fombelle A, Drogoul C, et al. Feeding and microbial disorders in horses: part 3—effects of three hay: grain ratios on microbial profile and activities. J Equine Vet Sci 2001;26:543–6.
21. Bailey SR, Rycroft A, Elliott J. Production of amines in equine cecal contents in an in vitro model of carbohydrate overload. J Anim Sci 2002;80:2656–62.
22. Bailey SR, Marr CM, Elliott J. Identification and quantification of amines in the equine caecum. Res Vet Sci 2003;74:113–8.
23. Medina B, Girard ID, Jacotot E, et al. Effect of a preparation of *Saccharomyces cerevisiae* on microbial profiles and fermentation patterns in the large intestine of horses fed a high fiber or a high starch diet. J Anim Sci 2002; 80:2600–9.
24. Hussein HS, Vogedes LA, Fernandez GC, et al. Effects of cereal grain supplementation on apparent digestibility of nutrients and concentrations of fermentation end-products in the feces and serum of horses consuming alfalfa cubes. J Anim Sci 2004;82:1986–96.
25. Lopes MA, White NA, Crisman MV, et al. Effects of feeding large amounts of grain on colonic contents and feces in horses. Am J Vet Res 2004;65:687–94.
26. Geor RJ, Harris PA. How to minimize gastrointestinal disease associated with carbohydrate nutrition in horses. In: Proceedings of the 52nd Annual Convention of the American Association of Equine Practitioners 2007. p. 178–85.
27. Kienzle E. Small intestinal digestion of starch in the horse. Rev Med Vet 1994;145: 199–204.
28. Julliand V, de Fombelle A, Varloud M. Starch digestion in horses: the impact of feed processing. Livest Sci 2006;100:44–52.
29. Gray GM. Starch digestion and absorption in nonruminants. J Nutr 1992;122: 172–7.
30. Dyer J, Fernandez-Castaño Merediz E, Salmon KS, et al. Molecular characterisation of carbohydrate digestion and absorption in equine small intestine. Equine Vet J 2002;34:349–58.
31. Richards N, Choct M, Hinch GN, et al. Examination of the use of exogenous a amylase and amyloglucoside to enhance starch digestion in the small intestine of the horse. Anim Feed Sci Technol 2004;114:295–305.
32. Buddington RK, Rashmir-Raven AM. Carbohydrate digestion by the horse: is it a limiting factor? Equine Vet J 2002;34:326–7.

33. Richards N, Hinch G, Rowe J. The effect of current grain feeding practices on hindgut starch fermentation and acidosis in the Australian racing Thoroughbred. Aust Vet J 2006;84:402–7.
34. Potter GD, Arnold FF, Householder DD, et al. Digestion of starch in the small or large intestine of the equine. Pferdeheilkunde 1992;1:107–11.
35. Tinker MK, White NA, Lessard P, et al. A prospective study of equine colic risk factors. Equine Vet J 1997;29:454–8.
36. Hudson JM, Cohen ND, Gibbs PG, et al. Feeding practices associated with colic in horses. J Am Vet Med Assoc 2001;219:1419–25.
37. Cox R, Proudman CJ, Trawford AF, et al. Epidemiology of impaction colic in donkeys in the UK. BMC Vet Res 2007;3:1–11. 10.1186/1746-6148-3-1.
38. Little D, Blikslager AT. Factors associated with development of ileal impaction in horses with surgical colic: 78 cases (1986–2000). Equine Vet J 2002;34: 464–8.
39. Cohen ND, Toby E, Roussel AJ, et al. Are feeding practices associated with duodenitis-proximal jejunitis? Equine Vet J 2006;38:526–31.
40. Hassel DM, Rakestraw PC, Gardner IA, et al. Dietary risk factors and colonic pH and mineral concentrations in horses with enterolithiasis. J Vet Intern Med 2004; 18:346–9.
41. Cohen ND, Vontur CA, Rakestraw PC. Risk factors for enterolithiasis among horses in Texas. J Am Vet Med Assoc 2000;216:1787–94.
42. Hassel DM, Aldridge BM, Drake CM, et al. Evaluation of dietary and management risk factors for enterolithiasis among horses in California. Res Vet Sci 2008;85: 476–80.
43. Harris PA. How should we feed horses - and how many times a day? Vet J 2007; 173:9–10.
44. Geor RJ. Diet, feeding and gastrointestinal health in horses. Proceedings of the 1st British Equine Veterinary Association and Waltham Nutrition Symposia 2005. p. 89–94.
45. Harris PA, Arkell K. How understanding the digestive process can help minimize digestive disturbances due to diet and feeding practices. Proceedings of the 1st British Equine Veterinary Association and Waltham Nutrition Symposia 2005. p. 9–14.
46. Jansen WL, Geleen SNJ, van der Kuilen J, et al. Dietary soyabean oil depresses the apparent digestibility of fibre in trotters when substituted for an iso-energetic amount of corn starch or glucose. Equine Vet J 2002;34:302–5.
47. Longland AC, Byrd BM. Pasture nonstructural carbohydrates and equine laminitis. J Nutr 2006;136:2099S–102S.
48. Dabareiner RM, White NA. Large colon impaction in horses: 147 cases (1985–1991). J Am Vet Med Assoc 1995;206:679–85.
49. Archer DC, Pinchbeck GL, French NP, et al. Risk factors for epiploic foramen entrapment colic in a UK horse population: a prospective case-control study. Equine Vet J 2008;40:405–10.
50. Longland AC, Cairns AJ. Fructans and their implications in the aetiology of laminitis. Proceedings of the 3rd Dodson and Horrell International Conference on Feeding horses 2000. p. 52–5.
51. Wood JLN, Milne EM, Doxey DL. A case-control study of grass sickness (equine dysautonomia) in the United Kingdom. Vet J 1998;156:7–14.
52. McCarthy HE, Proudman CJ, French NP. Epidemiology of equine grass sickness: a literature review (1909–1999). Vet Rec 2001;149:293–300.

53. Griffiths NJ, Walton JR, Edwards GB. An investigation of the prevalence of the toxigenic types of *Clostridium perfringens* in horses with anterior enteritis: preliminary results. Anaerobe 1997;3:121–5.
54. Hunter LC, Miller JK, Poxton IR. The association of *Clostridium botulinum* type C with equine grass sickness: a toxicoinfection? Equine Vet J 1999; 31:492–9.
55. Cohen ND, Peloso JG. Risk factors for history of previous colic and for chronic, intermittent colic in a population of horses. J Am Vet Med Assoc 1996;208: 697–703.
56. Nadeau JA, Andrews FM, Mathew AG, et al. Evaluation of diet as a cause of gastric ulcers in horses. Am J Vet Res 2000;61:784–90.
57. Lybbert T, Gibbs P, Cohen N, et al. Feeding alfalfa hay to exercising horses reduces the severity of gastric squamous mucosal ulceration. Proceedings of the 53rd Annual Convention of the American Association of Equine Practitioners 2007. p. 525–6.
58. Cohen ND, Matejka PL, Honnas CM, et al. Case-control study of the association between various management factors and development of colic in horses. Texas Equine Colic Study Group. J Am Vet Med Assoc 1995;206:667–73.
59. Reeves MJ, Salman MD, Smith G. Risk factors for equine acute abdominal disease (colic): results from a multi-center case-control study. Prev Vet Med 1996;26:285–301.
60. Ralston SL, Foster DL, Divers T, et al. Effect of dental correction on feed digestibility in horses. Equine Vet J 2001;33:390–3.
61. Carmalt JL, Townsend HGG, Janzen ED, et al. Effect of dental floating on weight gain, body condition score, feed digestibility, and fecal particle size in pregnant mares. J Am Vet Med Assoc 2004;225:1889–93.
62. Mehdi S, Mohammed V. A farm-based prospective study of equine colic incidence and associated risk factors. J Equine Vet Sci 2006;26:171–4.
63. Traub-Dargatz JL, Salman MD, Jones RL. Epidemiologic study of salmonellae shedding in the feces of horses and potential risk factors for development of the infection in hospitalized horses. J Am Vet Med Assoc 1990;196:1617–22.
64. Weese JS. Microbiologic evaluation of commercial probiotics. J Am Vet Med Assoc 2002;220:794–7.
65. Weese JS, Anderson ME, Lowe A, et al. Screening of the equine intestinal microflora for potential probiotic organisms. Equine Vet J 2004;36:351–5.
66. Weese JS, Rousseau J. Evaluation of *Lactobacillus pentosus* WE7 for prevention of diarrhea in neonatal foals. J Am Vet Med Assoc 2005;226:2031–4.
67. Jouany JP, Gobert J, Medina B, et al. Effect of live yeast culture supplementation on apparent digestibility and rate of passage in horses fed a high-fiber or high-starch diet. J Anim Sci 2008;86:339–47.
68. Desrochers AM, Dolente BA, Roy MF, et al. Efficacy of *Saccharomyces boulardii* for treatment of horses with acute enterocolitis. J Am Vet Med Assoc 2005;227: 954–9.
69. Bertone JJ, Traub-Dargatz JL, Wrigley RW, et al. Diarrhea associated with sand in the gastrointestinal tract of horses. J Am Vet Med Assoc 1988;193:1409–12.
70. Ragle CA, Meagher DM, Lacroix CA, et al. Surgical treatment of sand colic: results in 40 horses. Vet Surg 1989;18:48–51.
71. Ruohoniemi M, Kaikkonen R, Raekallio M, et al. Abdominal radiography in monitoring the resolution of sand accumulations from the large colon of horses treated medically. Equine Vet J 2001;33:59–64.

72. Hammock PD, Freeman DE, Baker GJ. Failure of psyllium mucilloid to hasten evaluation of sand from the equine large intestine. Vet Surg 1998;27:547–54.
73. Lieb S, Weise J. A group of experiments on the management of sand intake and removal in the equine. Proceedings of the 16th Equine Nutrition and Physiology Symposium 1999. p. 257.
74. Hotwagner K, Iben C. Evacuation of sand from the equine intestine with mineral oil, with and without psyllium. J Anim Physiol Anim Nutr (Berl) 2008;92:86–91.
75. Landes AD, Hassel DM, Funk JD, et al. Fecal sand clearance is enhanced with a product combining probiotics, prebiotics, and psyllium in clinically normal horses. J Equine Vet Sci 2008;28:79–84.

Nutrition and Dietary Management of Equine Gastric Ulcer Syndrome

Rilla E. Reese, BS[a], Frank M. Andrews, DVM, MS[b,*]

KEYWORDS

• Equine • Gastric ulcers • Equine gastric ulcer syndrome
• Nutrition • Diet • Dietary management

Equine gastric ulcer syndrome (EGUS) is a condition in horses characterized by ulcers in the terminal esophagus; proximal (squamous) stomach; distal (glandular) stomach; and proximal duodenum.[1] Diagnosis of EGUS is based on history, clinical signs, endoscopic examination, and response to treatment. All ages and breeds of horses are susceptible to EGUS, and current pharmacologic strategies focus on blocking gastric acid secretion and increasing stomach pH, which creates a permissive environment for ulcer healing. Long-term treatment with pharmacologic agents is expensive, however, and requires frequent daily handling of the horse. Recently, nutritional and dietary management factors have been identified to play an important role in gastric ulcers in horses. Diet and nutritional management can be used as an adjunct and follow-up to pharmacologic therapy to decrease ulcer severity and recurrence. This article focuses on nutritional and dietary factors that have been implicated to cause EGUS and how the horse diet can be managed to lessen ulcer severity and prevent recurrence of EGUS. Highlighted in this article are the basic anatomy and physiology of the equine stomach, current feed management practices that put the horse at risk for EGUS, and dietary strategies that can decrease ulcer severity and prevent recurrence once ulcers are successfully treated. Much is still unknown about the cause of EGUS, however, and contradicting studies are common, indicating that continued research is needed to clarify the cause and role of nutritional and dietary factors.

ANATOMY AND GASTRIC ACID SECRETION

Horses are predisposed to gastric ulcers because of their compound stomach. Most ulcers (80%) occur in the proximal-third of the stomach, which is lined by nonglandular

[a] Department of Animal Sciences and Large Animal Clinical Sciences, The University of Tennessee College of Veterinary Medicine, Knoxville, TN, USA
[b] Equine Health Studies Program, Department of Veterinary Clinical Sciences, School of Veterinary Medicine, Louisiana State University, Skip Bertman Drive, Baton Rouge, LA 70803, USA
* Corresponding author.
E-mail address: fandrews@vetmed.lsu.edu (F.M. Andrews).

Vet Clin Equine 25 (2009) 79–92
doi:10.1016/j.cveq.2008.11.004 vetequine.theclinics.com
0749-0739/08/$ – see front matter

stratified squamous epithelia. The distal two thirds of the stomach is lined by glandular mucosa that secrete protective mucus and bicarbonate, and hydrochloric acid (HCl), and pepsinogen for digestion.[2] This glandular region also has an extensive capillary network and undergoes rapid restitution of epithelium when injured. Approximately 20% of ulcers occur in this region, and many heal rapidly without therapeutic intervention. The nonglandular squamous mucosa is predisposed to acid injury because it lacks this substantial protective mucus and bicarbonate layer.[3]

Horses are continuous gastric HCl secretors, and acid exposure is thought to be the primary cause of EGUS.[4] Gastric acid secretion is stimulated by gastrin, histamine, and acetylcholine from the vagus nerve. Other acids (volatile fatty acids [VFA], bile acids, and lactic acid) and enzymes (pepsin) found in the stomach also contribute, however, to an acidic environment and low stomach pH. A recent study found that horses have a lower pH in the proximal stomach during early morning (1:00–9:00 AM), which suggests a circadian pattern for gastric acid secretion.[5] Prolonged exposure of the proximal stomach to a low pH environment is the likely cause of EGUS and is similar to gastroesophageal reflux disease in humans.

Synergistic action between VFA, lactic acid, bile acids, and HCl may cause acid damage to the nonglandular mucosa of the stomach, leading to EGUS.[6–8] Both HCl alone and in combination with VFA (pH $\leq$ 4) by-products of grain fermentation by resident stomach bacteria have been shown to inhibit nonglandular stomach mucosal cell sodium transport, resulting in cell swelling and eventual ulceration. The ulcerogenic effects of VFAs were dose-dependent, and the severity of the damage was related to VFA carbon chain length.[7–9] A recent study showed that D- and L-lactic acids, also by-products of bacterial fermentation of grain, when exposed to the nonglandular stomach mucosa in vitro in an acid environment, did not significantly alter barrier function or sodium transport through the tissues, when compared with VFA with similar PK_a.[10] The role of lactic acid in the cause of EGUS needs further investigation.

Bile acids, however, were shown to increase nonglandular mucosal cell permeability to hydrogen ions, which eventually leads to ulceration.[6] The effects of bile acids in EGUS are questionable, however, because they usually come from less acidic duodenal reflux and are nonulcerogenic at a pH greater than 4.[11] Also, the proteolytic enzyme pepsinogen, which is cleaved to pepsin at a pH less than 4, may act synergistically with HCl to result in acid damage. Although HCl and stomach pH have been incriminated as the main causes of EGUS, it is likely that a combination of HCl, organic acids, and pepsin act to cause injury to the gastric mucosa, causing EGUS.

RISK FACTORS FOR EQUINE GASTRIC ULCER SYNDROME

Although acid injury has been implicated in the cause of EGUS, several risk factors for its development have also been identified (**Table 1**).[12,13]

Exercise Intensity

Horses involved in training and racing are at high risk to develop EGUS.[14] Current prevalence figures show that 60% to 90% of performance horses have EGUS. A recent study showed that horses running on a high-speed treadmill have increased abdominal pressure and decreased stomach volume.[15] The authors' speculated that this activity allowed contraction of the stomach, resulting in reflux of the acid from the glandular mucosa into the nonglandular mucosa, leading to injury. Daily exercise may increase the exposure of the nonglandular mucosa to acid, explaining the increased prevalence of gastric ulcers in horses in training. Furthermore, an increase in serum gastrin concentration has been shown to occur in exercising horses.[16] This

Table 1
Physiologic factors affecting ulcer development

Aggressive Factors	Protective Factors: Nonglandular Mucosa	Protective Factors: Glandular Mucosa
Hydrochloric acid secretion	Epithelial restitution	Bicarbonate-mucus layer secretion
Organic acid production	Mucosal blood flow	Epithelial restitution
Pepsin conversion from pepsinogen	—	Mucosal blood flow
Duodenal reflux of bile acids	—	Prostaglandin E production

increase in serum gastrin may increase glandular HCl secretion, which in turn may lead to acid damage.

A recent study showed that sodium transport in the nonglandular mucosa was down-regulated in horses less than or equal to 5 years of age (the age of most racehorses) compared with horses greater than or equal to 12 years of age.[17] The inability of the nonglandular mucosal cells to up-regulate sodium transport may predispose them to cell swelling and eventual ulceration, which may be why young horses are more susceptible to EGUS.

Intermittent Versus Continuous Feeding

Horses grazing at pasture have a decreased prevalence of EGUS. During grazing, there is a continuous flow of saliva and ingesta that buffer stomach acid; stomach pH is greater than or equal to 4 for a large portion of the day. When feed is withheld from horses before racing or as with stabled horses, however, gastric pH drops rapidly, and the nonglandular mucosa is exposed to an acid environment. In contrast, a recent study showed that pastured pregnant and nonpregnant mares had a high prevalence of gastric ulcers.[18] The high prevalence of gastric ulcers in these pastured mares may be because horses consume less forage during evening hours than during daytime hours, which may result in less saliva production and a low pH environment in the proximal stomach. A recent study by Husted and colleagues[5] showed that proximal stomach pH was lower in the early morning hours (1:00–9:00 AM) regardless of housing (paddock or stable). This may be why both pastured and stabled horses are susceptible to EGUS, albeit by varying degrees. Still, intermittent feeding has been shown to cause and increase the severity of nonglandular ulcers in horses, and this concept has been used as a model consistently to produce EGUS in research settings.[19–21]

Stall Confinement

Alongside feeding practices, stall confinement has been implicated as a risk factor for EGUS. A recent study, however, showed that neither proximal nor ventral stomach pH changed significantly in horses housed in stalls alone, housed in stalls with a companion, or housed in a grass paddock.[6] Here again, pH in the proximal stomach was lower during the early morning hours regardless of housing, and feed intake was lowest during these hours. Other factors in stabled horses may increase their risk of developing EGUS. For example, stabled horses are bolus fed (two large meals daily). These meals are traditionally high in grains and consumed rapidly, which leads to a decrease in saliva production and less buffering of stomach contents. Also, high-grain diets may be fermented by resident stomach bacteria to VFA, which in an acid environment may lead to ulceration.[7–9,22]

High-Concentrate Diets

Size and composition of the grain meal is thought to have a profound effect on risk for developing EGUS. Serum gastrin concentrations are highest in horses fed a high-grain diet. These diets are high in digestible carbohydrates, which are fermented by resident bacteria, resulting in the production of VFA. In the presence of low stomach pH (≤ 4), VFA cause acid damage to the nonglandular squamous mucosa.[7–9,22] In a recent study, however, horses fed alfalfa hay and a pelleted concentrate diet had lower gastric ulcer scores than horses fed Coastal Bermuda hay.[23] Furthermore, a previous study showed that horses fed alfalfa hay and grain had a higher stomach pH and lower ulcer scores when compared with horses fed Brome grass hay without grain.[22] In this study, the authors speculated that calcium and protein, both high in the alfalfa hay–grain diet, buffered stomach contents, resulting in a protective effect on the nonglandular mucosa. Alfalfa hay when fed with or without concentrates may have a protective and antiulcer effect in horses.

Clinical Signs of Equine Gastric Ulcer Syndrome

Clinical signs associated with EGUS are numerous but often vague. Ulcers are more commonly diagnosed in horses showing overt clinical signs (**Table 2**).[1,24,25] In Thoroughbred horses in race training, gastric ulcers are associated with poor performance, poor hair coat, picky eating, and colic. Gastric ulcers were identified in 88% to 92% of horses with a client complaint of conditions associated with ulcers or horses showing subtle signs of poor health, compared with 37% to 52% identification in horses not showing symptoms. In addition to an increased prevalence of ulcer diagnosis in clinically affected horses, the severity of ulceration may be correlated with the severity of the symptoms.

DIAGNOSIS

Diagnosis of EGUS requires a thorough history, physical examination, and a minimum database. Identifying risk factors and clinical signs are helpful in making a diagnosis; however, gastroscopy is the only definitive diagnosis for gastric ulcers currently available. Standing gastroscopy procedures have been described in detail elsewhere in the literature and require at least a 2-m endoscope to visualize the nonglandular mucosa and margo plicatus and a 2.5- to 3-m endoscope to visualize the pylorus and proximal duodenum in most adult horses.[26,27] Use of a gastric ulcer scoring system allows clinicians to compare gastroscopic findings, monitor healing of ulcers, and evaluate efficacy of treatment.[1,28]

Currently, there are no hematologic or biochemical markers to diagnose EGUS. A recent report, however, showed that horses with gastric ulcers had lower red blood cell counts and hemoglobin concentrations than horses that did not have gastric

Table 2
Clinical signs and risk factors of adult horses developing equine gastric ulcer syndrome

Clinical Signs	Risk Factors
Acute colic	Stress
Recurring colic	Transportation
Excessive recumbency	High-grain diet
Poor body condition	Stall confinement
Partial anorexia	Intermittent feeding

ulcers.[29] Some horses with EGUS may be slightly anemic or hypoproteinemic, but in the authors' experience, red blood cell and hemoglobin concentrations are rarely outside of normal reference ranges.

Another presumptive diagnostic technique is the sucrose absorption test.[30] Urine sucrose concentrations were significantly higher for horses with gastric ulcer scores greater than 1. Using the sucrose permeability test, a urine sucrose concentration cutoff value of 0.7 mg/mL or higher revealed an apparent sensitivity of 83% and specificity of 90% for detecting ulcers in horses. This test may provide a noninvasive test to detect and monitor gastric ulcers. It requires sophisticated equipment, high-performance liquid chromatography, however, which may not be readily available to clinical practitioners.

In a recent study, a fecal occult blood test was found to be helpful in diagnosis of EGUS.[31] The positive predictive value of the fecal occult blood test in horses with EGUS was 90%; however, the negative predictive value was only 17%, suggesting that horses with a positive fecal occult blood test are likely to have a gastric ulcer, whereas a horse with a negative test is also likely to have a gastric ulcer. To improve the negative predictive value of the fecal occult blood test, investigators developed another test (SUCCEED Equine Fecal Blood Test) that uses specific equine monoclonal antibodies to both albumin and hemoglobin in an easy-to-use kit. A recent report showed a greatly improved predictive value of the negative test (72%), but the predictive value of a positive test was slightly lower (77%).[32,33] This new test may be helpful in diagnosing EGUS in horses, but should be used as part of a complete work-up. A false-positive fecal occult blood test may also result if a recent rectal examination has been performed or if the horse has a protein-losing enteropathy.

Unfortunately, laboratory techniques provide only presumptive diagnostic evidence of EGUS; if gastroscopy is not available and ulcers are strongly suspected, it may be worthwhile to start empiric treatment and observe for resolution of clinical signs. If the horse does not respond to treatment, referral to a facility with a gastroscope is indicated.

MANAGEMENT OF EQUINE GASTRIC ULCER SYNDROME

Pain relief, healing, and prevention of secondary complications are the primary goals of antiulcer therapy and management recommendations. The mainstay of pharmacologic treatment of EGUS is to increase stomach pH and suppress HCl acid secretion. Because of the high recurrence rate, effective acid control should be followed by nutritional and dietary management strategies to prevent ulcer recurrence.

Pharmacologic Therapy

Once EGUS is diagnosed, therapy should be initiated to achieve these goals. Some EGUS lesions heal spontaneously, but most require pharmacologic therapy to heal, especially while horses remain in athletic training.[1,34,35] The most accepted strategy to treat EGUS is acid-suppressive therapy. Currently, omeprazole (GastroGard, Merial Limited, Decatur, Georgia), a proton-pump inhibitor, is the only Food and Drug Administration–approved product for treatment and prevention of recurrence of EGUS. Other pharmacologic therapies have been used to treat EGUS with mixed success, however, and their suggested doses are listed in **Table 3**.

Duration of Pharmacologic Treatment

It is difficult to predict how long a nonglandular or glandular gastric ulcer takes to heal, but the recommended treatment time for most antiulcer medications is 28 days.

Table 3
Drug therapy for treatment of equine gastric ulcer syndrome

Drug	Dosage	Route of Administration	Dosing Interval
Omeprazole	0.5–1 mg/kg	Intravenously	Q 24 h
Omeprazole (GastroGard)	4 mg/kg (treatment) 1 mg/kg (prevention)	Orally	Q 24 h
Ranitidine	1.5 mg/kg	Intravenously	Q 6 h
Ranitidine	6.6 mg/kg	Orally	Q 8 h
Famotidine	0.3 mg/kg	Intravenously	Q 12 h
Famotidine	2.8 mg/kg	Orally	Q 12 h
Misoprostol	5 µg/kg	Orally	Q 8 h
Sucralfate	20–40 mg/kg	Orally	Q 8 h
AlOH/MgOH antacids	30 g AlOH/15 g MgOH	Orally	Q 2 h

Management changes in addition to pharmacologic therapy, however, may speed the healing of ulcers. For example, after a feed deprivation model of ulcer induction, ulcers were healed or nearly healed in horses after 9 days of pasture turnout,[20] whereas Thoroughbred horses treated with omeprazole while still in training took longer to heal: 57%, 67%, and 77% healing after 14, 21, and 28 days of treatment, respectively.[35] Horses with spontaneous occurring ulcers in a field trial treated with omeprazole showed 86% healing after 28 days of treatment.[36,37] The authors recommend endoscopic examination after 14 days of omeprazole therapy to determine if the ulcers are healed. If the gastric ulcers are healed, the dose can be reduced (1 mg/kg, orally, every 24 hours) to prevent recurrence of ulcers while the horse remains in race training.[38] If the ulcers are still present, the full 28-day course of omeprazole should be followed and the horse further evaluated after that time. When endoscopy is not available, horses should be treated for at least 28 days. It should be noted that clinical signs might resolve before complete healing has taken place. Signs of poor appetite, colic, or diarrhea usually resolve within a few days after initiating treatment, and the horse is expected to make improvements in body condition and attitude within 2 to 3 weeks.[39] Histamine type 2 antagonist therapy should be continued for at least 28 days, but healing may take longer than 40 days and may not be as effective as treatment with omeprazole paste.[40]

In general, it may take longer to treat large ulcers, more severe ulcers, and ulcers in the nonglandular mucosa.[41] In cases where clinical signs have resolved and the risk factors for ulcer development are low, spontaneous healing of ulcers may occur without further treatment. Spontaneous healing does not usually occur in horses that continue intensive training, however, and ulcers may reoccur in those successfully treated if therapy is discontinued.[35,38] If clinical signs attributed to EGUS have not resolved after 48 hours of treatment, the diagnosis or therapy should be reconsidered.

Environmental, Nutritional, and Dietary Management of Equine Gastric Ulcer Syndrome

Pharmacologic therapy may be necessary to heal both glandular and nonglandular gastric ulcers in horses, but once pharmacologic therapy is discontinued, the ulcer likely quickly returns if management changes are not instituted. Environmental, nutritional, and dietary management can be initiated during therapy to help facilitate ulcer healing and ultimately prevent ulcer recurrence. Intense or long-duration exercise, stall confinement, and diet are risk factors for EGUS. Managing these risk factors can decrease severity and prevent ulcer recurrence.

Modification of Exercise Intensity and Duration

In horses, intense exercise, racing, and race training has been shown to contribute to worsening of nonglandular gastric ulcers compared with horses kept at pasture or not in training. Also, endurance exercise has been shown to play a role in the cause of EGUS in horses. In one study, 67% of horses competing in 50- and 80-mile endurance rides had gastric ulcers.[42] In addition, repeated oral administration of hypertonic replacement electrolyte solutions to these horses was shown to increase the number and severity of gastric ulcers.[43] These oral hypertonic electrolyte replacement products should be used with caution in exercising horses and should be administered after exercise with a small grain or hay meal. Furthermore, training and exercise intensity should be reduced, when possible, until ulcers have healed.

Pasture Turnout

One study found that even giving a horse in a stall ad lib grass hay did not improve ulcers, whereas horses maintained on pasture rarely had gastric ulcers.[44,45] Pasture turnout is the best dietary method of controlling gastric ulcers. The diet fed to stalled horses can be modified, however, to decrease the risk of ulcers. Current dietary recommendations include providing continuous feeding of alfalfa hay or alfalfa hay mixed with good quality grass. Sweet feed should be kept to a minimum, and grains like barley or oats can be substituted to decrease its fermentation to VFAs.

Eliminate Bolus Feeding and Increase Forage and Fiber

Another effective method to decrease EGUS is to feed a high-forage diet continuously. Stabled horses are frequently fed two large meals daily, which results in lower saliva production and increases the rate and extent of intragastric fermentation and the gastric emptying rate. Diet composition, meal size, and feeding frequency have been identified to contribute to the cause of gastric ulcers in horses. In humans, ingestion of a high-protein meal is a stimulus for the release of gastrin and subsequent release of gastric acid.[44] In the horse, one study showed that the ingestion of a grain meal resulted in a higher gastrin stimulus than grass hay.[45] Horses fed hay versus withholding feed had similar acid output, but higher gastric pH. It was theorized that the salivary bicarbonate and the buffering effect of the hay were responsible for the higher pH.

The composition and frequency of feeding forage is important in preventing EGUS. In addition to providing constant access to feed to buffer gastric acidity, modifying the diet may help prevent ulcers. Although the gastric juice VFA concentrations were higher in horses fed an alfalfa-grain diet, they had higher gastric juice pH and lower ulcer scores than the same horses fed Brome grass hay.[22] In that study, no gastric hormones were measured, and it was hypothesized that the calcium in the alfalfa hay could have a direct effect on gastric secretions or that the protein was acting as a buffer for the pH. In a rat model, a diet of 2% calcium inhibited basal gastric secretion but not secretions in response to histamine stimulation.[46] Providing constant access to alfalfa hay likely helps to raise gastric pH.[22,23]

Horses fed straw as the only forage available were 4.4 times more likely to have a gastric ulcer severity score greater than or equal to 2 (0–5 scale) compared with hay feeding.[47] Also, horses fed straw were 5.7 times more likely to have a gastric ulcer severity score of greater than or equal to 2, compared with haylage feeding. Also, horses fed greater than 2 g/kg body weight (BW) of starch per day were likely to have a twofold increase in gastric ulcer severity score of greater than or equal to 2, compared with feeding haylage. Although the absolute fiber and grain requirements have not been determined for horses, current recommended levels of long-stem, high-quality forage are at 1 to 1.5 kg/100 kg of BW and 0.5 kg/100-kg BW concentrates.[9,48] Straw should not be fed as a sole source of forage.

Decrease Size and Increase Frequency of Concentrate Feeding

Serum gastrin concentrations are high in horses fed high-concentrate diets.[45] Gastrin is the only hormone known to stimulate secretion of hydrochloric acid, and rations that contain more readily available nutrients, such as pellets and sweet feed, produce a significant increase in postprandial gastrin concentrations. In particular, grain feeding was shown to delay gastrin secretion, which corresponded to an increase in gastric acid secretion after the stomach had emptied the grain contents.[49] In an empty stomach acid is more likely to be exposed to nonglandular mucosa and cause injury, similar to gastroesophageal reflux disease in people.

Also, high-concentrate diets are high in hydrolysable (water soluble) carbohydrates. Hydrolysable carbohydrates are readily fermented by resident stomach bacteria, resulting in the production of VFAs, which in the presence of a low stomach pH ($\leq$4) cause damage to the nonglandular squamous mucosa.[7–9,22]

The size of the grain meal may also affect the extent of intragastric fermentation, thereby affecting VFA production.[50] Métayer and colleagues[50] compared the gastric emptying rates in horses fed small (300 g/100 BW) versus large (700 g/100 BW) high-starch concentrate meals. Although the calculated rate of gastric emptying (grams per minute) was higher with the large meal, gastric emptying in terms of percent of the original meal was much slower. When horses are fed large, starch-rich meals, intragastric fermentation and VFA fermentation may be favored because of the large amount of fermentable carbohydrates and the longer retention time within the stomach. In the same study, when comparing the high- and low-starch meals, gastric emptying was significantly faster for horses consuming a meal lower in starch than one high in starch. Larger meal size and higher starch content were associated with gastric emptying in terms of percent of total original meal. A recent study showed that when grain was fed at 0.5 kg/100 kg BW, VFA concentrations were below threshold values for causing damage to nonglandular mucosa.[9] Grain or concentrates should not be fed in excess of 0.5 kg/100 kg BW every 6 hours.[22]

Antibiotics Versus Probiotics

Helicobacter pylori and other *Helicobacter* species have not been shown to cause EGUS, although *Helicobacter* DNA has been isolated from the glandular and nonglandular stomach mucosa in horses.[51,52] Instead, other resident, acid-tolerant bacteria (*Escherichia coli*, *Lactobacillus*, and *Streptococcus)* are suspected to cause EGUS, and a large population of these bacteria was isolated from the gastric contents of horses fed various diets in one study.[53] In rats, which have a compound stomach similar to horses, bacteria (*E coli*) rapidly colonized acetic acid-induced stomach ulcers and impaired ulcer healing.[54] In this study, oral antibiotic treatment with streptomycin or penicillin suppressed bacterial colonization of the ulcer and markedly accelerated ulcer healing compared with placebo-treated controls. Also, oral administration of lactulose resulted in increased *Lactobacillus* growth and colonization of the ulcer bed, which may facilitate ulcer healing. In a recent study in horses with spontaneously occurring gastric ulcers, an antibiotic (trimethoprim sulphadimidine) or a probiotic preparation containing *Lactobacillus agilis*, *L salivarius*, *L equi*, *Streptococcus equinus*, and *S bovis* administered orally decreased ulcer number and severity compared with untreated controls.[55] These data suggest that resident stomach bacteria are important in maintenance and progression of nonglandular gastric ulcers in horses. Treatment with antibiotic or probiotic preparations may facilitate ulcer healing after 2 weeks of treatment, but a full effect did not occur until after 4 weeks of treatment. Antibiotic treatment may be indicated in horses with chronic nonresponsive gastric ulcers, but more importantly, probiotic preparations containing *Lactobacillus* and *Streptococcus* may be helpful in prevention of gastric ulcers or may be used as an adjunct to pharmacologic treatment.

Dietary Supplements

A plethora of dietary supplements on the market for horses boast efficacy in treatment and prevention of gastric ulcers. Many of these products have not been tested in the horse, and to date, very little scientific evidence exists on their efficacy. Discussed next are several supplements that have some scientific testing or have ingredients that have been shown to be helpful in ulcer treatment and prevention.

Seabuckthorn Berry Extract

There is an increasing interest in the use of herbs and berries that may have therapeutic application in humans and animals. Berries and pulp from the seabuckthorn plant (*Hippophae rhamnoides*) are high in vitamins, trace minerals, amino acids, antioxidants, and other bioactive substances and have been used successfully to treat mucosal injury, including decubital ulcers, burns, and stomach and duodenal ulcers in humans.[56,57] In addition, seabuckthorn berries have been shown successfully to treat and prevent acetic acid-induced gastric ulcers in rats.[58] A recent study was completed to evaluate the efficacy of seabuckthorn berry pulp and extract (90 mL, fed twice daily; SeaBuck Complete, Seabuck, LLC, Midvale, Utah) on the treatment and prevention of gastric ulcers in horses.[59] This preparation of seabuckthorn berries did not significantly decrease nonglandular gastric ulcer scores in eight treated horses, compared with the untreated controls; however, this preparation prevented an increase in gastric ulcer scores following an alternating feed deprivation, ulcer induction model, compared with untreated control horses, which had a significant increase in gastric ulcer scores. Also, gastric ulcer scores in seven of the eight seabuckthorn-treated horses either stayed the same or decreased compared with just two of the eight untreated controls. Although this preparation of seabuckthorn berry did not heal ulcers in these horses, it may prevent nonglandular ulcers from getting worse during times of stress or feed deprivation.

Calcium Carbonate Supplements

Many supplements on the market contain calcium carbonate, a primary component of human antacid preparations (Tums, Rolaids). These products contain varying concentrations of calcium carbonate and various other herbs and coating agents. The author (FMA) performed a small study with an antacid preparation containing calcium carbonate (Neigh-Lox, Kentucky Performance Products, Versailles, Kentucky) to determine efficacy in treatment and prevention of gastric ulcers in horses (unpublished data, 2001). In that study, four healthy horses were fed hay and a small amount of grain top-dressed with 124.5 g of this calcium carbonate supplement twice daily for 3 weeks. Gastric juice pH increased to greater than or equal to 4 for 2 hours after feeding this supplement, when compared with control not supplemented. Also, in an in vitro study using Ussing chambers, this supplement, when added to VFA-damaged stomach tissue, resulted in recovery of sodium transport through nonglandular tissue. These data suggest that calcium carbonate preparations may have some efficacy in maintaining mucosal integrity, but because of the short duration effect on gastric juice pH, more frequent feedings may be necessary to prevent EGUS.

Oils (Corn Oil, Rice Bran Oil)

Dietary fats delay gastric emptying time in humans and other species.[60] In contrast to most species, gastric emptying rates are slower in horses fed a high-carbohydrate diet, compared with horses fed a high-fat diet, although these rates were not statistically significant.[61] Gastric relaxation was significantly greater in horses fed the high-carbohydrate diet, however, compared with horses fed the high-fat diet. Supplementation of dietary fat may not have a profound effect on gastric emptying in horses.

In another study,[62] ponies fitted with gastric canulas fed dietary corn oil (45 mL, orally, once daily) by dose syringe had a significantly lower gastric acid output and increased prostaglandin concentration in gastric juice. The authors' concluded that corn oil supplementation could be an economical approach to the therapeutic and prophylactic management of glandular ulcers in horses, especially those associated with the use of nonsteroidal anti-inflammatory drugs.

In contrast to the previous study, results from an evaluation of the antiulcerogenic properties of corn oil, refined rice bran oil, and crude rice bran oil (240 mL, once daily, mixed in grain) showed no statistical differences in nonglandular ulcer scores between the treatment groups.[63] Glandular ulcers were rare, however, in these horses. In this model, dietary oils did not prevent nonglandular gastric ulcers in these horses, suggesting that dietary oils may not be useful in treatment or prevention of nonglandular ulcers, but may be helpful in treatment or prevention of glandular ulcers.

Concentrated Electrolyte Pastes or Solutions

Repeated oral administration of hypertonic replacement electrolyte solutions, commonly given to endurance horses, has been shown to increase the number and severity of gastric ulcers.[43] These products should be used with caution in horses and may be best given after exercise with feed to minimize their effects on the gastric mucosa.

SUMMARY

EGUS is common in horses, and stomach acids and environmental, nutritional, and dietary factors are likely important causative factors. On initial diagnosis of EGUS, treatment should be started with effective pharmacologic agents. Prevention of ulcer recurrence depends primarily on environmental, nutritional, and dietary management. When possible, the following summary of important nutritional and dietary recommendations should be followed to lessen severity and prevent EGUS:

1. Keep the horse eating by providing a minimum of 1 to 1.5 kg/100 kg BW of long-stem, high-quality forage free-choice throughout the day and night.
2. Feed alfalfa hay or a mixture of alfalfa hay to help buffer stomach acid.
3. Feed grain and concentrates sparingly. Give no more than 0.5 kg/100 kg BW of grain or grain mixes (eg, sweet feed), and do not feed grain meals less than 6 hours apart.
4. Try corn oil or other dietary supplements, but feed hypertonic electrolyte pastes or supplements after exercise with a grain meal.
5. Consider therapeutic or preventative doses of effective pharmacologic agents (GastroGard or Ranitidine) in horses that are performing high-intensity exercise, traveling, or in a high-stress situation.

ACKNOWLEDGMENTS

The authors thank Ms. Misty Bailey for editing this manuscript.

REFERENCES

1. Anon. Recommendations for the diagnosis and treatment of equine gastric ulcer syndrome (EGUS). Equine Vet Educ 1999;1(2):122–34.
2. Murray MJ. Aetiopathogenesis and treatment of peptic ulcer in the horse: a comparative review. Equine Vet J Suppl 1992;13:63–74.
3. Ross IN, Bahari HMM, Turneberg LA. The pH gradient across mucus adherent to rat fundic mucosa in vivo and the effect of potential damaging agents. Gastroenterology 1981;81:713–8.
4. Cambell-Thompson ML, Merritt AM. Basal and pentagastrin-stimulated gastric secretion in young horses. Am J Phys 1990;259:R1259–66.
5. Husted L, Sanchez LC, Olsen SN, et al. Effect of paddock vs. stall housing on 24 hour gastric pH with the proximal and ventral equine stomach. Equine Vet J 2008; 40:337–41.
6. Berschneider HM, Blikslager AT, Roberts MC. Role of duodenal reflux in non-glandular gastric ulcer disease of the mature horse. Equine Vet J Suppl 1999;29:24–9.
7. Nadeau JA, Andrews FM, Patton CS, et al. Effects of hydrochloric, acetic, butyric and propionic acids on pathogenesis of ulcers in the non-glandular portion of the stomach of horses. Am J Vet Res 2003;64(4):404–12.
8. Nadeau JA, Andrews FM, Patton SC, et al. Effects of hydrochloric, valeric and other volatile fatty acids on pathogenesis of ulcers in the non-glandular portion of the stomach of horses. Am J Vet Res 2003;64:413–7.
9. Andrews FM, Buchanan BR, Smith SH, et al. In vitro effects of hydrochloric acid and various concentrations of acetic, propionic, butyric, or valeric acids on bioelectric properties of equine gastric squamous mucosa. Am J Vet Res 2006; 67(11):1873–82.
10. Andrews FM, Buchanan BR, Elliott SB, et al. In vitro effects of hydrochloric acid and lactic acid on bioelectric properties of equine gastric squamous mucosa. Equine Vet J 2008;40:301–5.
11. Argenzio RA. Comparative pathophysiology of non-glandular ulcer disease: a review of experimental studies. Equine Vet J Suppl 1999;29:19–23.
12. Murray MJ, Schusser GF, Pipers FS, et al. Factors associated with gastric lesions in Thoroughbred racehorses. Equine Vet J 1996;28(5):368–74.
13. Rabuffo TS, Orsini JA, Sullivan E, et al. Association between age or sex and prevalence of gastric ulceration in Standard bred racehorses in training. Am J Vet Med 2002;221(8):1156–9.
14. Vatistas NJ, Sifferman RL, Holste J, et al. Induction and maintenance of gastric ulceration in horses in simulated race training. Equine Vet J Suppl 1999;29:40–4.
15. Lorenzo-Figueras M, Merritt AM. Effects of exercise on gastric volume and pH in the proximal portion of the stomach of horses. Am J Vet Res 2002;63(11):1481–7.
16. Furr M, Taylor L, Kronfeld D. The effects of exercise training on serum gastrin responses in the horse. Cornell Vet 1994;84:41–5.
17. Abbott LL, Peretich AL, Dhar MS, et al. Role of sodium-potassium ATPase and sodium-hydrogen exchanger mRNAs in equine gastric ulcer syndrome. Proceedings of the 9th International Colic Research Symposium. Liverpool, England; 2008. p. 29–30.

18. Le Jeune SS, Neito JE, Dechant JE, et al. Prevalence of gastric ulcers in Thoroughbred broodmares in pasture. Proceedings of the 52nd Annual American Association of Equine Practitioners Meeting. San Antonio, December 2–6, 2006.
19. Murray MJ, Schusser GF. Measurement of 24-h gastric pH using an indwelling pH electrode in horses unfed, fed, and treated with ranitidine. Equine Vet J 1993;25: 417–21.
20. Murray MJ. Equine model of inducing ulceration in alimentary squamous epithelial mucosa. Dig Dis Sci 1994;12:2530–5.
21. Feige K, Furst A, Eser MW [Effects of housing, feeding, and use on equine health with emphasis on respiratory and gastrointestinal disease]. Schweiz Arch Tierheilkd 2002;144(7):348–55 [in German].
22. Nadeau JA, Andrews FM, Mathew AG, et al. Evaluation of diet as a cause of gastric ulcers in horses. Am J Vet Res 2000;61(7):784–90.
23. Lybbert T, Gibbs P, Cohen N, et al. Feeding alfalfa hay to exercising horses reduces the severity of gastric squamous mucosal ulceration. Proceedings of the 54th Annual Meeting of the American Association of Equine Practitioners meeting. Orlando, Florida, December 1–5, 2007.
24. Murray MJ, Grodinsky C, Anderson CW, et al. Gastric ulcers in horses: a comparison of endoscopic findings in horses with and without clinical signs. Equine Vet J Suppl 1989;7:68–72.
25. Vastista NJ, Snyder JR, Carlson G, et al. Epidemiological study of gastric ulceration in the Thoroughbred race horse: 202 Horses 1992–1993. Proceedings of the American Association of Equine Practitioners meeting, December 4–7, 1994.
26. Murray MJ, Nout YS, Ward DL. Endoscopic findings of the gastric antrum and pylorus in horses: 162 cases (1996–2000). J Vet Intern Med 2001;15:401–6.
27. Andrews FM, Reinemeyer CR, McCracken MD, et al. Comparison of endoscopic, necropsy and histology scoring of equine gastric ulcers. Equine Vet J 2002;34(5): 475–8.
28. MacAllister CG, Andrews FM, Deegan E, et al. A scoring system for equine gastric ulcers. Equine Vet J 1997;29:430–3.
29. McClure SR, Glickman LT, Glickman NW. Prevalence of gastric ulcers in show horses. Am J Vet Med 1999;215(8):1130–3.
30. O'Connor MS, Steiner JM, Roussel AJ, et al. Evaluation of sucrose concentration for detection of gastric ulcers in horses. Am J Vet Res 2004;65(1):31–9.
31. Pellegrini FL. Results of a large scale necroscopic study of equine colonic ulcers. J Equine Vet Sci 2005;25:113–7.
32. Carter S, Pellegrini FA. The use of novel antibody tools to detect the presence of blood in equine feces. Company Bulletin Freedom Health LLC 2006;1:1–3.
33. Pellegrini FL, Carter SD. An equine necroscopic study to determine the sensitivity and specificity of a dual antibody test. Company Bulletin Freedom Health LLC 2007;2:1–2.
34. Murray MJ, Haven ML, Eichorn ES, et al. The effects of omeprazole or vehicle on healing of gastric ulcers in thoroughbred Race horses. J Vet Intern Med 1995;9: A161.
35. Andrews FM, Sifferman RL, Bernard W, et al. Efficacy of omeprazole paste in the treatment and prevention of gastric ulcers in horses. Equine Vet J Suppl 1999;29: 81–6.
36. MacAllister CG, Sangiah S. Effect of ranitidine on healing of experimentally induced gastric ulcer in ponies. Am J Vet Res 1993;54(7):1103–7.

37. MacAllister CG, Sifferman RL, McClure SR, et al. Effects of omeprazole paste on healing of spontaneous gastric ulcers in horses and foals: a field trial. Equine Vet J Suppl 1999;29:77–80.
38. McClure SR, White GW, Sifferman RL, et al. Efficacy of omeprazole paste for prevention of recurrence of gastric ulcers in horses in race training. Am J Vet Med Assoc 2005;226(10):1681–4.
39. Murray MJ. Diagnosing and treating gastric ulcers in foals and horses. Vet Med 1991;8:820–7.
40. Lester GD, Smith RL, Robertson ID. Effects of treatment with omeprazole or ranitidine on gastric squamous ulceration in racing Thoroughbreds. Am J Vet Med Assoc 2005;227:1636–9.
41. MacAllister CG. Medical therapy for equine gastric ulcers. Vet Med 1995;11: 1070–6.
42. Nieto JE, Synder JR, Beldomenico P, et al. Prevalence of gastric ulcers in endurance horses: a preliminary report. Vet J 2004;167:33–7.
43. Holbrook TC, Simmons RD, Payton ME, et al. Effect of repeated oral administration of hypertonic electrolyte solution on equine gastric mucosa. Equine Vet J 2005;37:501–4.
44. Merki HS, Wilder-Smith CH, Walt RP, et al. The cephalic and gastric phases of gastric secretion during H2-antagonist treatment. Gastroenterology 1991;101: 599–606.
45. Smyth GB, Young DW, Hammon LS. Effects of diet and feeding on past-prandial serum gastrin and insulin concentrations in adult horses. Equine Vet J Suppl 1988;7:56–9.
46. Fisher H, Kaufman RH, Hsu HC, et al. Inhibition of gastric acid secretion in the rat by high calcium. Nutr Res 1990;10:1441–53.
47. Luthersson N, Hou Nielsen K, Harris P, et al. Risk factors associated with equine gastric ulceration syndrome in 201 horses in Denmark. Proceedings of the 9th International Equine Colic Research Symposium. Liverpool, England, June 15–18, 2008.
48. Geor RJ, Harris PA. How to minimize gastrointestinal disease associated with carbohydrate nutrition in horses. Proceedings of the American Association of Equine Practitioners meeting. Orlando, Florida, Decmber 1–5, 2007.
49. Sandin A, Girma K, Sjöholm B, et al. Effects of differently composed feeds and physical stress on plasma gastrin concentration in horses. Acta Vet Scand 1998;39:265–72.
50. Métayer N, Lhôte M, Bahr A, et al. Meal size and starch content affect gastric emptying in horses. Equine Vet J 2004;36:436–40.
51. Scott DR, Marcus EA, Shirazi-Beechey SSP. Evidence of Helicobacter infection in the horse. Proceedings of the American Society of Microbiologists. June 20–24, 2001.
52. Contreras M, Morales A, García-Amado MA, et al. Detection of *Helicobacter*-like DNA in the gastric mucosa of Thoroughbred horses. Lett Appl Microbiol 2007;45: 553–7.
53. Al Jassim RAM, Scott PT, Trebbin AL, et al. The genetic diversity of lactic acid producing bacteria in the equine gastrointestinal tract. FEMS Microbiol Lett 2006;248:75–81.
54. Elliott SN, Buret A, McKnight W, et al. Bacteria rapid colonize and modulate healing of gastric ulcer in rats. Am J Phys-GI 1998;275:425–32.

55. Al Jassim RAM, McGowan T, Andrews FM, et al. Role of bacteria and lactic acid in the pathogenesis of gastric ulceration. In: Rural industries research and development corporation final report. Brisbane, Queensland, Australia; 2008, p. 1–26.
56. Geetha S, Ram MS, Singh V, et al. Anti-oxidant and immunomodulatory properties of seabuckthorn (Hippophae rhamnoides) an in vitro study. J Ethnopharmacol 2002;79:373–8.
57. Beveridge T, Li TSC, Oomah BD, et al. Seabuckthorn products: manufacturing and composition. J Agric Food Chem 1999;47:3480–8.
58. Xing J, Yang B, Dong Y, et al. Effects of sea buckthorn (Hippophaë rhamnoides L.) seed and pulp oils on experimental models of gastric ulcer in rats. Fitoterapia 2002; 73:644–50.
59. Reese RE, Andrews FM, Elliott SB, et al. The effect of seabuckthorn berry extract (Seabuck Complete) on prevention and treatment of gastric ulcers in horses. Proceedings of the 9th International Equine Colic Research Symposium. Liverpool, England, June 15–18, 2008.
60. Sidery MB, Macdonald IA, Blackshaw PE. Superior mesenteric artery blood flow and gastric emptying in humans and the differential effects of high fat and high carbohydrate meals. Gut 1994;35:186–90.
61. Lorenzo-Figueras M, Preston T, Ott EA, et al. Meal-induce gastric relaxation and emptying in horses after ingestion of high-fat versus high-carbohydrate diets. Am J Vet Res 2005;66:897–906.
62. Cargile JL, Burrow JA, Kim I, et al. Effect of dietary corn oil supplementation on equine gastric fluid acid, sodium, and prostaglandin E_2 content before and during pentagastrin infusion. J Vet Intern Med 2004;18:545–9.
63. Frank N, Andrews FM, Elliott SB, et al. Effects of dietary oils on the development of gastric ulcers in mares. Am J Vet Res 2005;66:2006–11.

Nutrition of Critically Ill Horses

Elizabeth A. Carr, DVM, PhD*, Susan J. Holcombe, VMD, MS, PhD

KEYWORDS

- Equine • Nutrition • Enteral • Parenteral
- Critical illness

Horses evolved as grazing herbivorous animals, meeting energy and nutritional needs with forages, salts, and water. In most cases, feeding horses based on teleologic principles is best, unless the horse is unwilling or unable to eat. There are little data on feeding critically ill or hospitalized horses and its association or effect on morbidity and mortality or length of hospital stay. In humans, malnutrition in sick (but not critically ill) patients is associated with prolonged hospitalization and increased infection.[1,2] Despite the lack of unequivocal benefit on mortality, nutritional support in people is the standard of care and is becoming so in horses. Horses, like other animals, can be fed orally and, when that is not possible, intravenously or parenterally. Enteral feeding is less expensive, more physiologic, improves immunity (especially of the gut), and is somewhat easier and safer. However, in human medicine several meta-analyses have suggested that there may be little beneficial effect on outcome of enteral nutrition over parenteral nutrition despite higher complications rates with parenteral nutrition, and some have suggested that the nutrition supplied is more important than the route.[3–5] Nevertheless, current guidelines strongly recommend early use of enteral nutrition with parenteral nutrition reserved for human patients when sufficient nutrients cannot be supplied enterally.[5–7] Although data on horse nutrition is currently lacking, early enteral nutrition with parenteral supplementation when warranted is becoming the standard of practice.

Feed can be withheld from healthy, nonstressed horses for 2 to 3 days, but not from horses that are obese, sick, injured, cachectic, or from pony or miniature breeds. Nutritional support should be considered in patients with potentially increased metabolic rate, such as young growing animals, individuals presenting with a prior history of malnutrition or hypophagia, patients with underlying metabolic abnormalities that could worsen with food deprivation, and individuals with an illness such as severe trauma or sepsis that results in an increased energy demand. Underweight horses require nutritional support earlier. Obese or over-conditioned individuals, particularly pony breeds, miniature horses, donkeys, and lactating mares are at risk for developing

Department of Large Animal Clinical Sciences, College of Veterinary Medicine, Michigan State University, East Lansing, MI 48824, USA
* Corresponding author.
E-mail address: carreliz@cvm.msu.edu (E.A. Carr).

Vet Clin Equine 25 (2009) 93–108
doi:10.1016/j.cveq.2008.12.002
vetequine.theclinics.com
0749-0739/08/$ – see front matter

hyperlipemia and should receive nutritional support if their serum triglycerides are above normal values or to prevent hypertriglyceridemia from developing. Older horses, or individuals diagnosed with Equine Cushing's syndrome and the more recently described Peripheral Cushing's Syndrome, are insulin resistant and at greater risk for developing hyperlipemia, and fatty infiltration of the liver.

Two excellent reviews on feeding management of sick horses have been published in prior issues of the Veterinary Clinics of North America,[8,9] and the authors refer readers to these articles for more information on this topic.

SIMPLE STARVATION: PURE PROTEIN CALORIE MALNUTRITION

The average, healthy adult horse can tolerate food deprivation, referred to as a pure protein or calorie malnutrition or simple starvation, for 24 to 72 hours with little systemic effects. The assumption is that (as in humans) periods of starvation in normal, healthy horses are accompanied by neuroendocrine changes within the body that lower the metabolic rate, resulting in a decrease in nutrient needs that facilitates survival. A decline in blood glucose concentration occurs with food deprivation. Insulin activity decreases, and glucagon activity increases. Catecholamines and hormones associated with stress are down-regulated, which lower the metabolic rate. During brief periods of inappetence, hepatic glycogenolysis and gluconeogenesis maintain fairly normal blood glucose concentration. Glycogen stores are depleted quickly, and fatty acids become the primary energy source. Glucose-dependent tissues, such as the brain and erythrocytes, cannot use fatty acids initially, so hepatic gluconeogenesis using amino acids as substrates continues. Glycerol produced from lipid degradation, lactate from the Krebs cycle, and amino acids provided from muscle tissue breakdown continue to be used for gluconeogenesis to provide energy. Lipid mobilization is triggered by alterations in insulin/glucagon levels and the activity of hormone sensitive lipase. With time, the horse's body adapts to using ketone bodies derived from fatty acid metabolism for energy. The protein required for cardiac and respiratory function and enzyme activity is conserved. Resting energy expenditure is decreased because of a decreased metabolic rate produced by increases in circulating levels of growth hormone, glucagon, leptin, and cortisol, and a decrease in insulin and thyroid hormones. These hormone fluxes are an afferent stimulus for the hypothalamic response to starvation resulting in an increased drive to eat and a decrease in energy expenditure. Metabolism slows in an effort to conserve body fuels and the body survives primarily on fat stores—sparing lean tissue until such a time as refeeding occurs.

The effects of food deprivation on stressed catabolic animals are considerably different from those observed in healthy animals. Their resting metabolic rate is increased instead of decreased, and protein conservation does not occur because protein becomes the principal fuel source (catabolism). Hypermetabolism and catabolism are approximately proportional to the severity of disease and lead to accelerated wasting.[10–12] Some of the neuroendocrine changes that occur in these hypercatabolic patients include increased sympathetic nervous system stimulation and increased production of catecholamines leading to increased metabolic rate. This metabolic state is also the result of a complex interaction of inflammatory cytokines (interleukin [IL]-1, IL-2, IL-6; tumor necrosis factor α [TNF-α]; and γ-interferon) released at the site of injury, inflammation, or disease. Infusion of cytokines including IL-6 and TNF-α result in stimulation of corticotrophin, cortisol, epinephrine, growth hormone, and glucagon resulting in an increase in the resting metabolic rate and lipolysis.[13,14] TNF-α activation of nuclear factor kappa-beta (NFK-β) results in direct and indirect stimulation of proteolytic pathways.[15] The direct effect is related to the activation of the ubiquitin proteaseom pathway, whereas the indirect effects involve stimulation of the hypothalamo-pituitary-adrenal axis, with a concurrent increase in glucocorticoid secretion.[16] The released amino acids are used by the liver to produce acute phase proteins and gluconeogenesis.[16,17] Glucagon, glucocorticoids, epinephrine, and growth hormone are increased causing relative insulin resistance, dysregulation of glycemia, increased protein catabolism and nitrogen loss, and, ultimately, more rapid development of malnutrition.[18] A marked reduction in total body protein synthesis occurs because amino acids are used for energy. These horses have increased metabolic demands, are in a catabolic state, preferentially use protein for fuel, develop insulin resistance and glucose intolerance, become weak, and have poor wound healing and incompetent immune function.[19,20] Nitrogen loss during this catabolic response can be as high as 20 to 30 g/d—versus 4 to 5 g/d in a human experiencing simple starvation. A healthy human allowed access to water can survive approximately 3 months with food deprivation or pure protein calorie malnutrition. In contrast, the same individual with a critical illness would survive approximately 1 month, those with preexisting malnutrition less than two weeks. Clearly, nutritional support is warranted.

ENTERAL NUTRITION

While nutritional supplementation will reverse the catabolic processes occurring during simple starvation it will not completely reverse those occurring during metabolic stress because while tissue injury persists catabolic processes are maintained. In the critically ill patient, protein catabolism continues despite protein supplementation in the diet. However, nutritional supplementation will have benefits in minimizing the severity of protein loss; providing both essential and conditionally essential amino acids, vitamins, and minerals; and in decreasing morbidity associated with illness.

The phrase "if the gut works, use it" results from numerous animal and human studies that show enteral nutrition is superior to parenteral nutrition in supporting organ function, improving organ blood flow, patient weight gain, and immune function—principally because of its effect on the gastrointestinal mucosa. Enteral nutrition is a trophic stimulus for the gastrointestinal tract directly through the presence of nutrients and indirectly through stimulation of trophic hormones such as enteroglucagon. Early enteral nutrition is the initiation of enteral feeding within 48 hours after hospital admission. In a large clinical study of surgical and trauma patients early enteral nutrition significantly decreased morbidity and length of stay when compared with delayed enteral nutrition and parenteral nutrition.[21]

One of the important features of the gastrointestinal tract is the role of the intestinal epithelium as a barrier to invasion by pathogenic microorganisms. The barrier function of the bowel mucosa is maintained by the intake and processing of bulk nutrients along the digestive tract. Depletion of nutrients in the bowel lumen is accompanied by degenerative changes in the bowel mucosa, such as shortening of the microvilli and generalized disruption of the microvillus architecture.[22,23] Translocation of bacteria across the gastrointestinal mucosa has been documented during periods of bowel rest in intensive care patients and this has been attributed to mucosal disruption from lack of luminal nutrients.[24] Enteral nutrition, but not parenteral, has a protective effect against bacterial translocation across the intestinal wall and may help to prevent subsequent sepsis by maintaining the functional integrity of the bowel mucosa. Therefore, even if the gastrointestinal tract cannot be used to meet complete needs, small amounts of enteral feeding may be useful with partial parenteral supplementation.

Enteral nutrition can vary from normal feedstuffs, slurry diets composed primarily of normal feedstuffs and liquid diets containing component requirements (**Tables 1–4**). In horses with a decreased appetite the choices are limited to those diets that can be administered through a nasogastric tube. Slurries composed of complete pelleted diets offer the advantage that they are inexpensive and well-balanced for the maintenance requirements of an adult horse. They also contain fiber, which is beneficial to gastrointestinal activity, colonic blood flow, enzymatic activity, and colonic mucosal cell growth and absorption.[25] The major disadvantage of pelleted complete feeds is the difficulty of administration through a nasogastric tube. One kilogram of pelleted complete feed soaked in 6 L of water can be administered through a large bore nasogastric tube using a marine-supply bilge pump. If a bilge pump is not available, pulverizing the pellets before adding water may improve gravity flow. The horse should be checked for gastric reflux before feeding, and the slurry should be administered slowly with attention paid to the horse's attitude and reaction. Because the stomach volume of an adult (450 kg) horse is approximately 9 to 12 L, each feeding should not exceed 6 to 8 L. Placement of an indwelling esophagostomy feeding tube is a good option if prolonged feeding is expected in horses with dysphagia, oral or head and neck trauma, or prolonged anorexia with a functional gastrointestinal system. Cervical esophagostomy can be performed in the standing, sedated horse; has few potential complications; and permits prolonged extraoral feeding.[26]

The horse is restrained in a stanchion and sedated. A nasogastric tube is placed through the nose into the distal esophagus, if possible, to aid in identifying the esophagus. The hair on the mid cervical region (at the level of the fifth cervical vertebra) is clipped and prepared aseptically. Local anesthetic is injected for a length of 10 cm just ventral to the jugular vein. A 7 to 8 cm linear incision is made just ventral to the jugular vein. The sternocephalicus and brachiocephalicus muscles are separated and the deep fascia is incised. The esophagus will be palpable with the nasogastric tube in place. The carotid sheath is dorsal to the esophagus. Careful blunt dissection aids in separating the carotid sheath from the esophagus and allows the esophagus to be elevated toward the incision. A 1.5 to 2 cm linear incision parallel to the long axis of the esophagus is made to facilitate insertion of the feeding tube. The tube should be advanced into the stomach. A purse-string suture can be placed around the esophageal mucosa incorporating the nasogastric tube and the tube should be secured to the skin. Keep the end of the tube capped with a 10 to 12 mL syringe between feedings or administration of fluids. When esophagostomy feeding is no longer necessary, the tube can be pulled and the site will heal by second intention.

An alternative when prolonged enteral nutrition is required is a smaller bore, softer (polyurethane) tube. This is recommended for long term intubation though the smaller

Table 1
Nutritional content of selected complete feeds

	Equine Senior	Strategy	Purina Horse Chow
Crude protein	14%	14%	10%
Fat	4%	6%	2%
Fiber	16%	8%	30%
Kcal/kg feed	2695	3300	—

Table 2
Nutritional content of selected liquid diets

	Vital HN	Osmolite	Critical Care Meals/Packet
Kcal/L	1000	1008	1066
Protein	41.7 g/dL	40 g/dL	12%
Fat	10.8 g/dL	34 g/dL	1%
Carbohydrate	185 g/L	135.6 g/L	73%

diameter tube precludes the use of slurry diets. Human and equine liquid formulations are available and have been used as enteral nutrition support in horses.[27–30] Alternatively, diets prepared using specific components have been described.[31] Corn oil may be added to the diet to increase the caloric content. The use of human products in the full-size horse can be very expensive and have been associated with diarrhea. Liquid diets can be administered by way of continuous flow or bolus meal dosing, which recruits the gastro-colic reflex.

When instituting enteral feeding especially in a patient with prolonged anorexia it is recommended to start gradually—the goal is to achieve maintenance requirements over a period of days. There is no exact formula for achieving maintenance requirements as many factors (underlying illness, breed, duration of anorexia) will affect the individual's ability to tolerate larger volume enteral feeding. Rapid changes in intake, particularly with component feeding or high fat diets may be associated with colic or diarrhea.

HOW MUCH TO FEED?

Energy requirements should be calculated according to the size, age, condition, and metabolic stress of the horse. The daily energy expenditure is expressed as the basal energy expenditure, which is the heat production of basal metabolism in the resting and fasted state. Maintenance requirements for healthy adult horses are estimated to be 33 to 40kcal/kg/24h or about 18,000 kcal/d. This level of nutrition has been shown to maintain body weight in healthy, adult horses standing in stalls. There are no good estimates of increased requirements in horses following surgery, trauma, hemorrhage, or burns—even in human medicine this data is quite

Table 3
Composition of and feeding schedule for Naylor diet

Constituents	Day 1	Day 2	Day 3	Day 4	Day 5	Day 6	Day 7
Electrolyte mixture	230	230	230	230	230	230	230
Water (L)	21	21	21	21	21	21	21
Dextrose (g)	300	400	500	600	800	800	900
Dehydrated cottage cheese (g)	300	450	600	750	900	900	900
Dehydrated alfalfa meal (g)	2000	2000	2000	2000	2000	2000	2000
Energy (non-protein calories), kcal	7400	8400	9400	10400	11800	11800	12200

Data from Naylor JM, Freeman DE, Kronfeld DS, et al. Alimentation of hypophagic horses. Comp Cont Educ Vet 1992;6:S93,1984.

Table 4
Suggested formulas for equine parenteral nutrition

mL	0–8 h	8–16h	16–24+h	0–8 h	8–16+h
Dextrose 50%	1000	1000	1000	1000	1000
Lipid 20%	500	500	500	250	500
Amino acid 10%	1000	1000	1000	1000	1000
Isotonic fluids	4000	4000	4000	1500	1500
Multivitamin conc.	5	5	5	5	5
Total volume	6500	6500	6500	3750	4000
Rate (ml/hr)	500	750	1000	3–5 mL/kg/h	3–5 mL/kg/h
Bags/d	2	3	4	1	2
Kcal/bag	3000	3000	3000	2200	3000
Kcal/d	6000	9000	12,000	2200	3000

Adult: maintenance = 35–40 kcal/kg/d. 450 kg horse: 15,750–18,000 kcal/d. Foal: maintenance = 120–150 kcal/kg/d. 50 kg foal: 6000–7500 kcal/d.

variable. Overfeeding is fraught with complications. Therefore, attempting to meet basal energy needs in the critically ill horse is a useful goal. In humans, observational studies examining the association between amount of caloric intake and clinical outcomes suggest that providing between 25% to 66% of calculated energy requirements is optimal.[32] These observations are supported by animal studies showing restrictive energy intake is associated with decreased inflammatory cytokines, improved metabolic profiles, and better survival compared with increased amounts of calories.[33] Horse studies are lacking; therefore, the following recommendations are made.

The total energy of a feedstuff is divided into the digestible energy (DE) and the nondigestible energy. DEis further divided into metabolic energy (used to provide energy) and that which is lost, nonmetabolizable, such as gases produced and urea excreted in the urine. By convention, energy requirements are calculated in terms of digestible energy. The amount of DE needed to meet maintenance energy requirements (DE_m) of the mature, normally active, nonworking horse can be estimated using the following formulas:

$$\text{Horses} \leq 600\text{kg} : DE_m(\text{Mcal/day}) = 1.4 + (BW \times 0.03)$$

$$\text{Horses} \geq 600\ \text{kg} : DE_m(\text{Mcal/day}) = 1.82 + (BW \times 0.0383) - [0.000015 \times BW]$$

BW = body weight in kilograms

The resting energy requirement (DE_r) defines the amount of energy required for maintenance (neither weight gain nor loss) of the completely inactive animal and is determined using a metabolism stall in a thermoneutral environment. This is approximately 70% of maintenance energy and can be calculated using the formula: DE_r (Mcal/d) = (BW × 0.021) + 0.975. Clearly, DE^M of a horse can be affected by several factors including the age, size, and physical condition of the horse; the amount and type of activity; and environmental factors. Even when all these factors are controlled, individual variation occurs.

Energy requirements in the pregnant mare do not significantly increase until late gestation and are estimated to be 1.1, 1.13, and 1.2 times DE_m in the last 3 months of gestation. During lactation, energy demands peak over the first 3 months then decline toward weaning and can be calculated using the following formulas:

First 3 months of lactation

$$300\text{-}900\text{kg mares}: DE(Mcal/day) = DE_m + (0.03 \times BW \times 0.792)$$

$$200\text{-}299\text{kg mares}: DE(Mcal/day) = DE_m + (0.04 \times BW \times 0.92)$$

After 3 months of lactation:

$$DE(Mcal/kg) = DE_m + (0.02 \times BW \times 0.792) \text{for } 300\text{-}900 \text{ kg mares and,}$$

$$DE(Mcal/day) = DE_m + (0.03 \times BW \times 0.792) \text{for } 200\text{-}299 \text{ kg mares}$$

The energy and protein requirement for the critically ill horse is not known and likely varies depending on disease state, environment, and fitness level of the individual. However, it is likely to be close to the DE_r or DE_m. In humans, multipliers have been used to estimate the energy requirements in certain conditions including severe sepsis, trauma, or burn injuries. However, the increased metabolic demand of illness or surgical trauma and recovery is likely to be balanced by the inactivity of the patient during hospitalization. Consequently, these multipliers may overestimate the caloric requirement of certain illnesses. Exceptions include individuals with extreme trauma, burns, or severe sepsis; surgical conditions that require intestinal resection; and patients with large areas of devitalized tissue (clostridial myonecrosis patients undergoing multiple fasciotomies). When estimating the energy requirements of the majority of horses, DE_r are an acceptable target.

PROTEIN REQUIREMENT

In addition to energy requirements, it is important to ensure adequate protein intake to minimize protein catabolism. Maintenance requirements for crude protein in the adult horse can be estimated using the formula: crude protein grams = 40 × DE_m (Mcal/d). For example, a 500 kg horse with a DE_m of 16.5 Mcal/d would require 660 g of protein per day. Alternatively, protein requirements can be estimated to provide 0.5 g–1.5 g protein/kg horse/d (or 250–750 g/d) for the 500 kg horse. It is recommended to use the higher end of this estimate when calculating protein needs in a sick patient.

ASSESSMENT OF NUTRITIONAL SUPPORT

Body weight should be measured daily, if possible, to determine if nutritional support is adequate to maintain body weight. The most accurate method is to use a walk-on floor scale. A weight tape is a useful alternative when a scale is not available. Weight tapes are used to measure the girth just behind the elbow; the circumference correlates with pounds or kilograms. However, body weight in critically ill horses can fluctuate with changes in water balance. Diet and hydration status can alter body weight by as much as 5% to10%. For example, a 500 kg horse presented with colic may be 7% dehydrated at admission. At the time of exploratory celiotomy, the large colon may be emptied to facilitate correction of a surgical lesion. Rehydration of the above animal would result in a weight increase of 35 kg. The large colon and cecum can hold between 75 and 90 L of ingesta; removal of a portion of this content could result in a weight loss of 50 kg or more. Consequently, weight changes need to be considered in light of hydration status, feed intake and other procedures that may have occurred.

PARENTERAL NUTRITION

The most common indication for parenteral nutrition in horses is feed intolerance because the gastrointestinal tract function is impaired. In human patients and animal studies, parenteral nutrition has been found to improve wound healing, minimize muscle protein loss, decrease the weight loss usually seen in catabolic patients, and bolster immune function in patients that cannot tolerate oral nutrition. Disadvantages include the negative effects of withholding enteral nutrition on the gastrointestinal tract with resultant decrease in gut mass and structural protein, decreased motility and digestive function, and loss of mucosal integrity. Hyperosmolar parenteral nutrition solutions increase the risk of thrombophlebitis, particularly when using a peripheral vein; and the risk of catheter-related sepsis increases when using parenteral nutrition. Metabolic complications associated with parenteral nutrition include azotemia, hyperglycemia, hypercapnia, and hyperlipemia. All of these can be avoided with careful monitoring of serum values and recognition of underlying disease processes that may make the animal intolerant of certain components of parenteral solutions. In addition, the use of destabilized lipid emulsions has been associated with adverse consequences (see lipid section). Components used in formulating parenteral nutrition include protein in the form of amino acids, carbohydrates in the form of dextrose, and lipids in the form of long chain fatty acids; plus electrolytes, minerals, trace elements, and vitamins. Carbohydrates and lipids are used to meet the horse's energy needs, prevent breakdown of autologous protein for energy, and allow the administered protein to be used for wound healing and immune functions. Lipids and dextrose provide nonprotein calories—with lipids and dextrose providing 30% and 60% of the nonprotein calories, respectively—depending on patient tolerance and the type of metabolic disease. The amino acid solution is used to meet protein requirements.

Lipids

Lipid is the most calorically dense nutrient, providing 9 kcal/g of lipid. Lipids also provide essential fatty acids. Commercial lipid emulsions contain long-chain triglycerides that are derived from either soybean or safflower oil. Glycerol, a carbohydrate energy source, is added to make these emulsions isotonic; and a phospholipid is added to help stabilize the emulsion. Lipids are isosmotic, so the addition of lipids to the amino acids and dextrose solution will decrease its overall tonicity and, therefore, decrease the risk of thrombophlebitis. The metabolic clearance of lipids involves the hydrolysis of triglycerides by lipoprotein lipase. This enzyme is present in capillary endothelial cells. Endotoxemia and gram-negative infections cause a decrease in lipoprotein lipase levels; and bacterial endotoxin may induce macrophages and other white blood cells to release mediators that suppress the activity of lipoprotein lipase. Clinically, this is seen as intolerance to lipids, and persistent lipemia and hypertriglyceridemia. The stability of the lipid emulsion can be affected by pH, addition of other solutions, sunlight, and storage time. As the emulsion destabilizes, lipid droplets coalesce and polyunsaturated fatty acids are oxidized. Larger lipid droplets cannot be cleared by endothelial cell metabolism and are taken up by phagocytes. In addition, the production of these progressively larger lipid droplets can result in lipid embolization of smaller vessels. It is important to understand the factors that affect the stability of lipid emulsions and avoid using products that are old, or have evidence of destabilization.

Amino Acids

Normal, healthy adult horses require 0.7 to 1.5 g/kg/d of protein. This is likely increased in the critically ill patient. Supplementation of the branched-chain amino acids (valine, leucine, and isoleucine) decreases trauma and sepsis-induced muscle catabolism and improves nitrogen retention. Arginine is essential for wound healing, immune competence, and promoting a positive nitrogen balance; though it may be detrimental in critical illness, especially with ongoing inflammatory response, by increasing nitric oxide formation. This is still controversial and there is no equine data to support either supposition.[34] Clinically, deficits in glutamine in critically ill human patients correlate with mortality, making supplementation an obvious goal.[35] Data concerning critically ill horses is lacking, though plasma glutamine levels fell significantly following viral challenge in a group of horses.[36] Glutamine has tissue protective properties, anti-inflammatory and proimmunologic actions, provides metabolic support, and functions as an antioxidant-inducible nitric oxide synthase attenuator.[35] In a rat cecal ligation model, glutamine administration 1 hour after the onset of sepsis prevented development of acute respiratory distress and improved mortality in treated rats compared with placebo controls.[37] In human patients undergoing major abdominal surgery glutamine administration led to improved gastrointestinal permeability based on lactose–mannitol ratios.[38] In horses glutamine was shown to facilitate mucosal restitution following oxidant injury; though it seems that the jejunum uses glutamine more avidly than the colon in normal horses.[39,40] During catabolism, large amounts of amino acids are released from muscle. Glutamine is used as a fuel source by enterocytes, leukocytes, and macrophages; and for renal acid-base homeostasis.[35] Glutamine is also a cell-signaling molecule during illness and injury; regulates gene expression related to metabolism, signal transduction, cell defense and repair; and activates intracellular signaling pathways.[41] Glutamine preserves tissue metabolic function in the face of sepsis, shock, and ischemia–reperfusion injury; and attenuates the insulin resistance and subsequent hyperglycemia observed in these patients. It would seem appropriate to supplement critically ill horses with glutamine, though information regarding the amount, route, timing, and patient selection is still lacking.

Vitamin Requirements

Vitamins are divided into fat-soluble and water-soluble and are organic compounds important in many enzymatic functions and metabolic pathways. Fat-soluble vitamins include A, K, D and E. Water-soluble vitamins include B and C. The microbial population in the horse's large colon and cecum synthesizes Vitamin K and all the B vitamins with the exception of niacin. The horse produces Vitamins D, C, and niacin; whereas the precursors to vitamin A, beta carotene, and vitamin E must be ingested. The need for supplemental vitamin and mineral support will depend on the type and duration of supplementation. Fat-soluble vitamins are stored in body tissues and generally do not require supplementation for short periods of anorexia. Complete pelleted diets have vitamins and minerals added to meet the Nutritional Research Council requirements. When feeding a component diet or parenteral diet, vitamin and mineral supplementation is necessary. Antioxidant therapy is especially important in septic or endotoxemic patients. Selenium has been shown to be a potent antioxidant. Others include zinc, vitamin C, E, and beta carotene. Selenium down-regulates NFkB and limits the production of inflammatory cytokines.[42] Owing to reported anaphylactic or allergic reactions with intravenous administration, these vitamins should be given orally. Some of the intravenous multivitamin preparations can be added to parenteral nutrition. These products contain the fat-soluble vitamins A, D, and E that are solubilized in an aqueous medium, permitting intravenous administration. No adverse reactions have been reported following administration of these products. Vitamin C can be administered orally as 10 to 20 g of ascorbic acid once daily per 450-kg horse. Vitamin E can be supplemented orally at 500 units once daily per 450-kg horse. The B-complex vitamins include thiamin, folic acid, panthothenic acid, and niacin. Thiamin (vitamin B1) is a component of thiamin pyrophosphate, an essential cofactor in carbohydrate metabolism. Vitamin B complex can be added to the parenteral nutrition solution at 20 to 30 mL per 450-kg horse per day. Alternatively, water-soluble vitamins can be added to a separate bag of intravenous crystalloids to decrease the risk of contamination of the parenteral solution. Because water-soluble vitamins are light-sensitive, these fluids should be protected from light.

Resting energy requirements should be used when calculating parenteral nutrition volumes for adult animals. However, protein requirements should be determined using maintenance requirements or estimated using the formula: 0.5 g–1.5 g protein/kg BW/d. The higher end of this formula is recommended in sick, compromised patients. The ratio of nonprotein calories/nitrogen should be at least 100:1 in the final solution. Lipids should provide approximately 30% to 40% of the nonprotein calories whenever possible. The addition of lipids to parenteral nutrition is beneficial in patients with persistent hyperglycemia or hypercapnia, reducing the dependency on glucose as the principal energy source. The amount of fat used will depend on the amount of carbohydrate provided; with fat storage occurring in the presence of excess carbohydrate calories.

PREPARING THE PARENTERAL NUTRITION SOLUTION

Parenteral nutrition is usually administered to horses for short periods of time (3–10 days) as partial parenteral nutrition. Total nutritional requirements are generally not met. Lipids provide 9 kcal/g, protein 4 kcal/g, and dextrose 3.4 kcal/g. The initial goal is to provide approximately 30% to 40% of the calories with lipids and 60% to 70% with dextrose. If prolonged parenteral nutrition is required, lipid supplementation may be increased to as much as 60% of the total nonprotein calorie requirements. A 500 mL bottle of 20% lipid emulsion[a] contains 0.2 g/ml lipid × 9 kcal/g × 500 mL = 900 kcal. A 500 mL bottle of 50% dextrose[a] contains 0.5 g/mL of dextrose × 3.4 kcal/g × 500 mL = 850 kcal. One liter of 10% amino acid solution[a] contains 0.1 g/mL of amino acids × 4 kcal/g × 1000 mL = 400 kcal. Solutions composed of 5–8 g/kg/d of dextrose, 2 g/kg/d of amino acids, and 1 g/kg/d of lipid are well tolerated by horses. Five to 10 mL of a multivitamin solution can be added.[b]

ADMINISTERING PARENTERAL NUTRITION SOLUTIONS

Previously, it has been suggested that this high osmolality formulation should be given only into a central vein because of the risk of thrombophlebitis. Reports of successful administration by way of peripheral vessels are now common; and administration in horses by way of the jugular vein has been performed with few complications. To minimize the risk of thrombophlebitis, use nonthrombogenic catheters such as polyurethane catheters; and keep the catheter dedicated to the parenteral nutrition (ie, do not administer medications and fluids through the same port). If parenteral nutrition is to be administered following surgery, a second catheter can be placed in the opposite jugular vein or a double lumen catheter can be placed. Seven French, 20-cm, polyurethane, antimicrobial, double-lumen catheters are available

---

[a] Dextrose 50%, 500 ml, LiposynII 20%, 500 ml, Aminosyn 10%, 2000 ml (Abbott Laboratories, North Chicago, Illinois).

[b] Multivitamin concentrate, product # 4205 (American Pharmaceutical Partners, Inc., Los Angeles, California).

from several sources.[c,d] The parenteral nutrition can be administered through the 18-g portal while fluids and medications are administered through the 14-g portal. The parenteral nutrition should not be disconnected. If the horse is walked several times daily or removed from the stall for any reason, it is best to take the bag of parenteral nutrition with the horse. This decreases the risk of contamination and sepsis at the catheter site as well avoiding potential hypoglycemia due to sudden discontinuation of a glucose infusion. The fluid lines used for the parenteral nutrition should be changed every 24 hours.

Parenteral nutrition should be administered using an infusion pump. Postoperative abdominal surgery patients and horses with endotoxemia may have increased cortisol, adrenaline, and glucagon levels, resulting in glucose intolerance and hyperglycemia. Therefore, begin administering 25% to 30% of the calculated nutritional requirements per hour; and every 6 to 8 hours increase the administration rate by 25%, up to 75% to 100% of the horse's basal metabolic requirement. Monitor urine and blood glucose every 4 to 6 hours, and serum triglycerides and blood urea nitrogen (BUN) daily. If the renal threshold of glucose (200–220 mg/dL with normal renal function) is exceeded, glucosuria and osmotic diuresis ensues. The rate of infusion should then be decreased to a tolerated level or an insulin infusion started to maintain euglycemia. Previously, tight glucose control was recommended because maintaining glucose between 80 and 110 mg/dL in surgical ICU patients was associated with improved outcome.[43] The waters were muddied a bit by a study that showed only improved outcome in medical ICU patients that stayed in the ICU 3 or more days.[44] Other studies showed increased incidence of hypoglycemia in the tight glucose control groups, which was associated with increased mortality.[5] Current recommendations include avoidance of hyper- and hypoglycemia with tight glucose control.[5] Clearance of lipids can be impaired with gram-negative sepsis and endotoxemia. Monitoring serum triglycerides is important to prevent hyperlipemia, especially in miniature horses and ponies. Alternatively, one can monitor the appearance of the plasma for evidence of lipemia. However, significant hypertriglyceridemia can develop before visual detection of lipemic plasma—making this test relatively insensitive. In high-risk cases (miniature horses, ponies, and donkeys; or individuals with elevated serum triglycerides) it may be safest to avoid lipid administration and use a parenteral solution containing only carbohydrate and protein. Protein administration should be monitored by periodic determination of BUN; which will decrease if inadequate protein is provided, or may increase if excessive protein is provided. Also, decreased total protein (< 4.0 g/dL) or decreased albumen (<3.0 g/dL) may indicate inadequate protein intake. Electrolytes should be monitored at least once daily and the horse should be weighed, if possible, each day.

Once the horse tolerates enteral feeding, decrease the rate of parenteral nutrition administration slowly, by half every 6 to 8 hours, to avoid hypoglycemia due to elevated insulin levels in horses receiving parenteral nutrition.

HYPERLIPEMIA

Hyperlipemia occurs most commonly in predisposed breeds (ponies, miniature horses, and donkeys). Anorexia and illness result in increased fat mobilization (lipolysis) that exceeds the liver's capacity to clear triglycerides in the plasma. High levels of circulating triglycerides, packaged as very-low-density lipoproteins (VLDLs), are

[c] Double-lumen, 7 French catheter, #A1620 (MILA International, 7604 Dixie Hwy, Florence, Kentucky).
[d] Double-lumen, 7 French catheter, #AK-17702 (Arrow International, Inc., Reading, Pennsylvania).

taken up by tissues and organs resulting in organ dysfunction, and worsening clinical parameters. Hyperlipemia without grossly lipemic blood (severe hypertriglyceridemia) has also been recognized in horses associated with clinical illness or mandatory fasting; however, the severity and response to treatment in this group of individuals appears to be more favorable.

Control and resolution of hyperlipemia requires treatment of the underlying disease process, supportive care to correct metabolic derangements, and nutritional supplementation to attempt to reverse the negative energy balance and halt lipid mobilization. Most individuals with hyperlipemia are completely anorexic. However, if the gastrointestinal tract is functional, enteral supplementation can be very effective in controlling and resolving hyperlipemia. The advantages of enteral feeding include the benefit of maintaining intestinal integrity, motility, and function; and financial costs (compared with parenteral feeding). There are several complete pelleted diets available commercially that can be easily used to provide balanced nutrition. In addition, various other types of diets have been recommended—including liquid diets and component feeding.[27–30] Liquid or component feeds can be fed continuously through a small bore nasogastric tube; whereas pelleted diets require passage of a large bore tube and meal feeding. In full-size ponies and horses it is relatively simple to pass the larger tube and gavage feed multiple meals a day. The tube can be removed between feedings allowing the animal access to additional feed and water. It is recommended to begin gavage feeding with small meals and gradually increase to full feed over a period of 24 to 48 hours.

Parenteral nutrition (PN) has been successfully used to treat hyperlipemia in predisposed breeds and severe hypertriglyceridemia in others. Given the excess circulating VLDLs, partial PN excluding lipid, is generally recommended. In a recent report, a combination of 50% dextrose and 15% amino acids solution (1:1) was used to provide approximately 61% of daily energy requirement and 82% of daily protein requirement in the treatment of five ponies and one donkey with hyperlipemia.[45] Infusion of this solution was associated with hyperglycemia that was not easily controlled with insulin therapy. All patients had a prompt decrease in serum triglycerides following PN infusion.

In another retrospective report evaluating severe hypertriglyceridemia (defined as hyperlipemia without evidence of lipemic serum) in horses, successful resolution of hypertriglyceridemia was achieved with IV dextrose support alone.[46] In the authors' opinions, this has not been the case with hyperlipemia in predisposed breeds. In these cases it is recommended to provide PN that contains both protein and dextrose at levels as close to resting energy requirements as possible.

Survival in predisposed breeds with hyperlipemia has been shown to correlate with severity of hyperlipemia, making it difficult to determine the true benefit of enteral versus parenteral nutritional support.[47] In the authors' experience, we have had more rapid resolution of hyperlipemia using enteral nutrition compared with parenteral nutrition. However, regardless of the route, it is clear that early nutritional support is critical in the successful treatment of this syndrome.

NUTRITIONAL SUPPORT IN LIVER FAILURE

The liver is the largest organ in the body and has many functions including clearance of drugs and toxins, catabolism, conjugation and excretion of various substances, storage of vitamins and minerals, metabolism of carbohydrates and fats, and synthesis of proteins. In humans, chronic liver disease is commonly associated with malnutrition and cachexia. Likely causes of malnutrition and cachexia include decreased dietary intake and malabsorption due to functional changes in the intestine.

Other causes are alterations in bile acid secretion, decreased protein synthesis, and hypermetabolism of critical illness resulting in poor use of proteins, glycogen, and fat. Although horse data is lacking, these factors likely play a role in the metabolic changes seen in horses with acute and chronic liver disease. Therefore, early nutritional support formulated for the horse with liver dysfunction is likely to be beneficial in maintaining body mass and tissue protein.

It has been suggested that the major goals of nutritional support of the horse with liver dysfunction should be to (1) meet energy requirements, (2) meet them without exceeding dietary protein needs, (3) feed a diet that contains a high ratio of branched chain amino acids (BCAA) to aromatic amino acids, (4) feed low-fat and low-salt diets, and (5) feed high-starch diets.[12] A decrease in appetite is typical of horses with liver disease and likely the result of the underlying disease process, inflammatory cytokines, and changes in intestinal motility and absorption; also complicating disorders such as gastric ulcer disease. It is unclear if the human patient with chronic liver disease is truly experiencing a hypermetabolic state of critical illness as human studies show variable results. However, whether because of a hypermetabolic state or simply the result of liver dysfunction, human patients with chronic cirrhosis have increased energy expenditures, insulin resistance, and increased mobilization of lipids for fuel. In contrast, the patients with acute, fulminant hepatitis or liver failure are likely experiencing a hypermetabolic state of critical illness and will likely have even more severe protein breakdown and energy wasting. Again, despite the lack of data in the horse, it is likely that the horse with liver dysfunction will have an increased energy demand, insulin resistance, excessive lipid oxidation, and excessive protein catabolism.

The use of neomycin (to decrease ammonia producing bacteria) may blunt intestinal villi, worsening the malabsorption. Malabsorption of fat and fat-soluble vitamins can occur with severe cholestatic disorders. Deficiencies in water-soluble vitamins (vitamin B complex and vitamin C) are common in humans with cirrhosis; and supplementation may be beneficial. Supplementation of both vitamin E and selenium is recommended as deficiencies have been reported to increase the severity of toxic injury from copper and iron. Also, supplementation has been shown to improve liver antioxidant levels in response to oxidative stress.[48] Zinc deficiency is thought to play a role in hepatic encephalopathy in humans and supplementation has been reported to improve glucose use in humans with cirrhosis.

Ideally horses with liver dysfunction should be fed grass hay or grazed on late summer or fall pastures to avoid high-protein diets (legume hay or pasture and early spring grasses). Frequent small meals may help limit excessive hyperammonemia and prevent signs of hepatic encephalopathy. Feedstuffs high in BCAA and relatively low in protein content include corn, sorghum, beet pulp, and molasses. Parenteral amino acid preparations high in BCAA are available if parenteral nutrition is deemed necessary. Avoidance of supplements containing iron or copper is recommended as these can affect liver function.

Unfortunately, one of the limitations of feeding an appropriate diet is palatability and appetite as many horses with liver dysfunction have a poor appetite and are consequently more picky about what they will ingest. In this situation, maintaining adequate protein and calorie intake should be the primary goal and it may become necessary to feed less desirable feedstuffs. As clinical signs and severity of disease improve, a change toward a diet tailored to meet the above requirements can be implemented. In human patients with chronic liver disease, oral nutritional supplementation in the face of a reasonable appetite resulted in reduced hospitalization for infections and a trend toward improved survival.[49] Consequently, it may be beneficial to supplement horses orally even in the face of an apparently adequate appetite.

REFERENCES

1. Robinson G, Goldstein M, Levine GM, et al. Impact of nutritional status on DRG length of stay. JPEN J Parenter Enteral Nutr 1987;11:49–51.
2. Shukla VK, Roy SK, Kumar J, et al. Correlation of immune and nutritional status with wound complications in patients undergoing abdominal surgery. Am Surg 1985;51:442–5.
3. Simpson F, Doig GS. Parenteral vs. enteral nutrition in the critically ill patient: a meta-analysis of trials using the intention to treat principle. Intensive Care Med 2005;31:12–23.
4. Peter JV, Moran JL, Phillips-Hughes J, et al. A meta-analysis of treatment outcomes of early enteral versus early parenteral nutrition in hospitalized patients. Crit Care Med 2005;33:213–20.
5. Vincent JL. Metabolic support in sepsis and multiple organ failure: more questions than answers. Crit Care Med 2007;35(9):S436–40.
6. Heyland DK, Dhaliwal R, Drovers JW, et al. Canadian clinical practice guidelines for nutrition support in mechanically ventilated critically ill adult patients. JPEN J Parenter Enteral Nutr 2003;27:355–73.
7. Kreymann KG, Berger MM, Deutz NE, et al. ESPEN guidelines on enteral nutrition: intensive care. Clin Nutr 2006;25:210–23.
8. Magdesian GK. Nutrition for critical gastrointestinal illness: feeding horses with diarrhea or colic. Vet Clin North Am Equine Pract 2003;19(3):617–44.
9. Dunkel BM, Wilkins PA. Nutrition and the critically ill horse. Vet Clin North Am Equine Pract 2004;20(1):107–26.
10. Michie HR. Metabolism of sepsis and multiple organ failure. World J Surg 1996; 20:460–4.
11. Campbell IRT. Limitations of nutrient intake: the effects of stressors. Trauma, sepsis and multiple organ failure. Eur J Clin Nutr 1999;53:S143–7.
12. Lewis LD. Feeding and care of horses with health problems. In: Lewis LD, editor. Equine clinical nutrition feeding and care 2nd edition. Williams & Wilkins; Baltimore (MD): 1995. p. 289–99.
13. Stouthard JML, Romijn JA, Van der Poll T, et al. Endocrine and metabolic effects of interleukin-6 in humans. Am J Phys 1995;268:E813–9.
14. Van der Poll T, Romijn JA, Endert E, et al. Tumor necrosis factor mimics the metabolic response to acute infection in healthy humans. Am J Phys 1991;261: E457–65.
15. Bessey PQ, Watters JM, Aoki TT, et al. Combined hormonal infusion simulates the metabolic response to injury. Ann Surg 1984;200:264–81.
16. Hasselgren PO, Fischer JE. Counter-regulatory hormones and mechanisms in amino acid metabolism with special reference to the catabolic response in skeletal muscle. Curr Opin Clin Nutr Metab Care 1999;2:9–14.
17. Leverve X. Inter-organ substrate exchanges in the critically ill. Curr Opin Clin Nutr Metab Care 2001;4:137–42.
18. Gelfand RA, Mathews DE, Bier D, et al. Role of counter regulatory hormones in the catabolic response to stress. J Clin Invest 1984;74:2238–48.
19. Romijn JA. Substrate metabolism in the metabolic response to injury. Proc Nutr Soc 2000;59:447–9.

20. Langhans W. Peripheral mechanisms involved with catabolism. Curr Opin Clin Nutr Metab Care 2002;5:419–26.
21. Schroeder D, Gillanders L, Mahr K, et al. Effects of immediate postoperative enteral nutrition on body composition, muscle function and wound healing. JPEN J Parenter Enteral Nutr 1991;15:376–83.
22. Saito H, Trocki O, Alexander JW, et al. The effect of route of nutrient administration on the nutritional state, catabolic hormone secretion, and gut mucosal integrity after burn injury. JPEN J Parenter Enteral Nutr 1987;11:1–7.
23. Rokyta R, Matejovic M, Krouzecky A, et al. Enteral nutrition and hepatosplanchnic region in critically ill patients—friends or foes? Physiol Res 2003;52:31–7.
24. Hernandez G, Velasco N, Wainstein C, et al. Gut mucosal atrophy after a short enteral fasting period in critically ill patients. J Crit Care 1999;14:73–7.
25. Hallebeek JM, Beynen AC. A preliminary report on a fat-free diet formula for nasogastric enteral administration as treatment for hyperlipaemia in ponies. Vet Q 2001;23:201–5.
26. Stick JA, Slocombe RF, Derksen FJ, et al. Esophagotomy in the pony: comparison of surgical techniques and form of feed. Am J Vet Res 1983; 44(11):2123–32.
27. Sweeney RW, Hansen TO. Use of a liquid diet as the sole source of nutrition in six dysphagic horses and as a dietary supplement in seven hypophagic horses. J Am Vet Med Assoc 1990;197:1030–2.
28. MD Choice Critical Care Meals[R]. Available at: www.vetsupplements.com.
29. Naylor JM, Freeman DE, Kronfeld DS, et al. Alimentation of hypophagic horses. Comp Cont Educ Vet 1992;6:S93–9.
30. Hardy J, Stewart RH, Beard WL, et al. Complications of nasogastric intubation in horses: nine cases (1987–1989). J Am Vet Med Assoc 1992;201:483–6.
31. Lopes MAF, White NA. Parenteral nutrition for horses with gastrointestinal disease retrospective study of 79 cases. Equine Vet J 1995;34:250–7.
32. Stapleton RD, Jones N, Heyland KD, et al. Feeding critically ill patients: what is the optimal amount of energy? Crit Care Med 2007;35(9):S535–40.
33. Jeejeebhoy KN. Permissive underfeeding of the critically ill patient. Nutr Clin Pract 2004;19:477–80.
34. Marik PE. Arginine: too much of a good thing may be bad!. Crit Care Med 2006; 34:2844–7.
35. Wischmeyer PE. Glutamine: mode of action in critical illness. Crit Care Med 2007; 35(9):S541–4.
36. Routledge NB, Harris RC, Harris PA, et al. Plasma glutamine status in the equine at rest, during exercise and following viral challenge. Equine Vet J Suppl 1999;30: 612–6.
37. Singleton KD, Serkova N, Eckey V, et al. Glutamine (0.75 g/kg) attenuates lung injury and improves survival after sepsis: role of enhanced heat shock protein expression. Crit Care Med 2005;33:1206–13.
38. De-Souza DA, Greene LJ. Intestinal permeability and systemic infections in critically ill patients: effect of glutamine. Crit Care Med 2005;33:1125–35.
39. Rotting AK, Freeman DE, Constable PD, et al. Effects of phenylbutazone, indomethacin, prostaglandin E2, butyrate, and glutamine on restitution of oxidant-injured right dorsal colon of horses in vitro. Am J Vet Res 2004;65(11): 1589–95.
40. Duckworth DH, Madison JB, Calderwood-Mays M, et al. Arteriovenous differences for glutamine in the equine gastrointestinal tract. Am J Vet Res 1992; 53(10):1864–7.

41. Curi R, Lagranha CJ, Doi SQ, et al. Molecular mechanisms of glutamine action. J Cell Physiol 2005;272:G879–84.
42. Kim SH, Johnson VJ, Shin TY, et al. Selenium attenuates lipopolysaccharide-induced oxidative stress responses through modulation of p38 MAPK and NF-kappa B signaling pathways. Exp Biol Med 2004;229:203–13.
43. Van den Berghe G, Wouters P, Weekers F, et al. Intensive insulin therapy in the critically ill patients. N Engl J Med 2001;345:1359–67.
44. Van den Berghe G, Wilmer A, Hermans G, et al. Intensive insulin therapy in the medical ICU. N Engl J Med 2006;354:449–61.
45. Durham AD. Clinical application of parenteral nutrition in the treatment of five ponies and one donkey with hyperlipaemia. Vet Rec 2006;158:159–64.
46. Dunkel B, McKenzie HC. Severe hypertriglyceridaemia in clinically ill horses: diagnosis, treatment and outcome. Equine Vet J 2004;35(6):590–5.
47. Mogg TD, Palmer JE. Hyperlipidemia, hyperlipemia, and hepatic lipidosis in American miniature horses: 23 cases (1990–1994). J Am Vet Med Assoc 1995; 207:604–7.
48. Naziroglu M, Karaoglu A, Aksoy AO, et al. Selenium and high dose vitamin E administration protects cisplatin-induced oxidative damage to renal, liver and lens tissues in rats. Toxicology 2004;195(2–3):221–30.
49. Hirsch S, Bunout D, De la Maza P, et al. Controlled trial on nutrition supplementation in out-patients with symptomatic alcoholic cirrhosis. JPEN J Parenter Enteral Nutr 1993;17:119–24.

Feeding Management of Sick Neonatal Foals

Harold C. McKenzie III, DVM, MS[a,*],
Raymond J. Geor, BVSc, MVSc, PhD[b]

KEYWORDS

- Enteral and parenteral feeding • Insulin therapy
- Foal • Metabolism • Dietary support

One of the challenges faced when treating a sick foal is developing an appropriate nutritional plan to ensure that the foal has adequate energy and nutrients for basal metabolism, immune function, and growth. This should be a straightforward endeavor, where one simply calculates the number of calories required by the foal, then determines the volume of the appropriate nutrient-containing solution, and provides this nutritional source by either the enteral or parenteral route. Unfortunately, the energy requirements for sick foals are not entirely understood and may be different in each patient. As a further complication, the ability of the foal appropriately to metabolize the nutrients provided is not guaranteed, because both age and degree of illness impact the foal's ability to produce metabolic hormones and the ability of the tissues to respond to hormonal stimulation. Another difficulty arises from the fact that the energy content of mare's milk is not consistent between mares and over time, and the exact formulation of substitutes, such as artificial milk replacer, is not always known. By developing an understanding of normal foal nutrition and metabolism one can approach the sick neonate with a sound basis for developing and implementing a nutritional plan.

FOAL METABOLISM

The Healthy Foal

The foal's nutritional requirements and dietary composition change substantially during the gradual transition from neonate to weanling. Careful consideration of the foal's stage of growth is required when formulating a nutritional plan. At birth the foal must transition from a continuous supply of nutrients provided by the dam by way of the placenta to intermittent absorption of ingested nutrients. At the

[a] Marion DuPont Equine Medical Center, Virginia-Maryland Regional College of Veterinary Medicine, Virginia Polytechnic and State University, PO Box 1938, Leesburg, VA 20177, USA
[b] Department of Large Animal Clinical Sciences, D-202 Veterinary Medical Center, College of Veterinary Medicine, Michigan State University, East Lansing, MI 48824, USA
* Corresponding author. Marion DuPont Equine Medical Center, PO Box 1938, Leesburg, VA 20177.
E-mail address: hmckenzi@vt.edu (H.C. McKenzie III).

Vet Clin Equine 25 (2009) 109–119
doi:10.1016/j.cveq.2008.11.005
vetequine.theclinics.com
0749-0739/08/$ – see front matter

same time the metabolism of the neonate is no longer able to depend on the maternal glucose concentration to maintain normoglycemia, and the pancreas assumes responsibility for regulating glucose homeostasis. These dramatic alterations in energy metabolism may not always occur smoothly, and the neonatal foal possesses limited energy reserves in the form of glycogen and fat. The result is that hypoglycemia occurs frequently in even the normal neonatal foal, and the sick foal is at risk of profound hypoglycemia if deprived of energy intake for even a few hours.

The caloric requirements of the normal foal are sizable, because of the need to support not only basal metabolic needs but also to maintain a rate of growth of as much as 2.5% of bodyweight per day in the neonatal period. This means that in the neonatal period the caloric requirement is as much as 150 kcal per kilogram bodyweight per day (kcal/kg/d), but it decreases gradually to around 120 kcal/kg/d at 3 weeks of age and then to 80 to 100 kcal/kg/d by 1 to 2 months of age.[1,2] Because these measures are given in terms of foal bodyweight it is important to realize that as the energy requirement per kilogram is decreasing the foal's bodyweight is increasing, with the result that the total caloric requirement increases with age. The initial energy source for the foal is mare's milk, which has substantially greater lactose content than cow's milk, with lower milk fat content. On a dry matter basis, mare's milk averages about 64%, 22%, and 13% sugar, protein, and fat, respectively, as compared with 38%, 26%, and 30% sugar, protein, and fat, respectively, for cow's milk. As a result mare's milk derives most of its energy content from carbohydrates. Appropriate endogenous production of insulin by the pancreatic β-cells is required for the foal to metabolize and use these carbohydrates appropriately.

Maturation of pancreatic β-cell function occurs very late in gestation in the fetal foal, and is dependent on the normal rise in fetal circulating cortisol concentration, which occurs in the final days of gestation.[3] This preparturient cortisol rise is responsible for many aspects of readying the foal for birth, both in terms of endocrine function and respiratory and cardiovascular function. Following birth there is a gradual maturation of the endocrine response to ingested carbohydrates. In a recent study normal newborn pony foals demonstrated impaired glucose clearance following the administration of exogenous glucose on the first day of life, suggesting a degree of insulin resistance.[4] By day 10 after birth these foals demonstrated increased rates of glucose clearance, but this response remained lower than that which is seen in normal adult equines. This gradual maturation may be an appropriate response to changes in the composition of mares milk, because colostrum contains little lactose, and in the volume of milk ingested, which is less on the first day of life than on subsequent days.[1,4]

Starting as early as the second day of life foals begin ingesting small amounts of hay, grass, and grain while at the same time they are ingesting maternal feces, which likely provides the initial microbial flora required to support digestion of these feedstuffs. It is unlikely that grain and roughage are well digested until at least several weeks of age, at which point the foal begins the gradual transition from a milk-based diet to a forage-based diet. The amount of milk produced by the mare peaks at around 2 months of lactation and then begins a steady decline, which continues until the time of weaning, necessitating that the foal begin relying on ingestion of solid food for an increasing proportion of its nutritional requirements. At the same time, the foal's hind-gut function is increasing and is likely fully functional by around 3 to 4 months of age. By the age of 6 months the foal is receiving less than 30% of the total nutritional requirement in the form of milk, which allows for a fairly easy dietary transition when weaning occurs. As the foal's hindgut function increases there is a corollary shift in the primary energy substrate, from ingested carbohydrates absorbed in the small intestine to volatile fatty acids produced by fermentation that are absorbed from the large intestine.

The Sick Foal

When evaluating the sick neonatal foal one must always keep in mind the possibility that the disease processes at work in the foal may have had their origins in utero. Maternal illness, maternal malnutrition, maternal toxin exposure, placentitis, and placental insufficiency all have the potential profoundly to influence the development and maturation of fetal metabolism. Studies investigating the role of a restricted uterine environment on fetal development have demonstrated lifelong impairment of growth and development in affected foals.[5] Conversely, the provision of a luxurious in utero environment can lead to enhanced growth rates out to 3 years of age.[5] The influence of maternal diet is demonstrated by a study wherein the provision of a diet high in soluble carbohydrates to the mare in late gestation contributed to a decrease in insulin sensitivity of the foals at 160 days of age.[6] These studies illustrate the potential for lifelong effects on metabolic function secondary to this prenatal programming effect, potentially contributing to the development of adult metabolic disease.[7] This prenatal programming may affect the neonatal foal's ability appropriately to metabolize nutrients in the clinical setting, with foals from a compromised placental environment potentially exhibiting insulin resistance and carbohydrate intolerance.

The late gestation rise in fetal cortisol is critical in final maturation of energy metabolism, and many foals delivered prematurely fail to undergo this rise in fetal cortisol concentration and are unable to respond normally to the changes in metabolism that occur after birth. Hypoglycemia, complicated by decreased endogenous energy reserves and the impairment of nursing caused by concurrent weakness, depression, or difficulty standing, is a common problem in these foals. Following the successful delivery of nutrients by the enteral or parenteral routes these foals are likely to be intolerant of carbohydrates, because of impaired endogenous insulin productions, and may suffer profound hyperglycemia. Foals suffering from systemic inflammation, such as that associated with septicemia, may also exhibit hyperglycemia caused by insulin resistance and carbohydrate intolerance. Management of these foals may require the use of lipid-containing parenteral nutrition solutions or the administration of exogenous insulin to achieve adequate caloric input.

Attempting to determine the true caloric needs of the clinically ill foal is one of the greatest challenges in designing a nutritional strategy. Historically, it was believed that critical illness created a hypermetabolic situation, where the patient had increased energy needs caused by increased tissue energy consumption. The energy requirements of the sick foal do not seem to be as great as once was thought,[8] however, because there is a reduction in the overall metabolic rate caused by a decrease in activity level in combination with a temporary reduction in growth rate. Indirect calorimetry testing of clinically ill foals in one study revealed that the resting energy requirement was approximately 45 kcal/kg/d, which is one third of the energy requirement for growing, active, normal foals.[9]

In managing the critically ill neonatal foal it may be preferable to pursue a hypocaloric approach, wherein one endeavors to prevent the foal from entering a severely catabolic state while accepting that all of the nutritional needs of the patient may not be met.[10] This approach addresses the fact that aggressive nutritional support can result in overfeeding, the risks of which may easily outweigh the possible benefits of providing nutritional support. Excessive carbohydrate administration leads to increased generation of carbon dioxide and can worsen hypercapnia in foals with compromised respiratory function. Excessive carbohydrate delivery also causes hyperglycemia, which is considered to be a proinflammatory stimulus and has been associated with worsening of outcome in human critical illness.[11,12] Overfeeding of protein results in increased protein catabolism and can result in the potentiation or development of azotemia.[12] The excessive administration of lipids may result in hypertriglyceridemia.[13] In contrast to the risks of overfeeding there is little evidence in human patients that short-term (several days) hypocaloric nutritional support results in worsened outcomes as compared with regimens designed to meet the patient's metabolic needs.[10] Recent evidence actually indicates that this approach, especially in regards to maintaining stringent control of blood glucose levels, is associated with decreased rates of complications and improved outcomes.[11]

ENTERAL NUTRITION

The first step in the development of a nutritional plan involves selection of the route of nutrient delivery. Provision of nutritional support by the enteral route is generally preferred for two reasons.[2,14] First, this is the most natural and physiologically sound means of nutrient delivery. Second, the intestinal mucosa is partially dependent on the products of digestion for energy and nutrients. A thorough evaluation of gastrointestinal function is needed before institution of enteral nutritional support. This includes abdominal auscultation; checking for gastric reflux; and possibly, abdominal radiographs and ultrasonographic examination for evaluation of bowel dimensions and motility. Foals with evidence of gastrointestinal dysfunction, such as gastric reflux, bowel distention, increased bowel wall thickness, and ileus, are unlikely to tolerate enteral feeding. A conservative approach to enteral feeding is also indicated for premature or immature foals in which there may be incomplete development of the gastrointestinal tract. Foals with perinatal asphyxia syndrome may be intolerant of enteral feeding as a result of intestinal ischemic injury.

ENTERAL SUPPORT AND HOW TO PROVIDE IT

Mare's milk is the preferred substrate for enteral feeding. Mare's milk is highly digestible and provides the correct balance of nutrients for normal growth and development. Commercial mare's milk replacers can be used, but it should be recognized that these products are bovine in origin and have lower digestibility compared with mare's milk. This increases the risk of intestinal dysfunction associated with enteral feeding. Semi-skimmed (2% fat) cow's milk to which 20 g/L dextrose (corn sugar) is added can be used if mare's milk or mare's milk replacer is unavailable. If a mare is not available for nursing then foals may be fed using a bottle, bowl, or nasogastric feeding tube. A bottle is often used in this situation, especially if the foal is to be transitioned to a mare within a short period of time, because this most closely mimics normal nursing. Bottle feeding is very labor intensive, however, and does carry some risk of milk aspiration if the milk flow rate from the bottle is not well correlated with the foal's nursing attempts. Feeding from the bowl can be challenging initially, but is much less labor intensive once the foal is drinking consistently from the bowl. Because the foal's head is positioned with the nose down when drinking from the bowl the risk of milk aspiration is very low.

Foals that are unable to nurse the mare may be fed through a bottle, bowl, or nasogastric feeding tube. Many sick, recumbent foals have a weak or uncoordinated suck reflex, and are at risk of milk aspiration and pneumonia; therefore, milk should be administered through a feeding tube. Use of small-bore, indwelling nasogastric feeding tubes (NG1243 – 12F catheter × 108 cm [43 in], MILA International, Erlanger,

Kentucky) and feeding of small volumes at frequent intervals (eg, every 20 minutes) is preferred over repeated passage of a nasogastric tube at 1- to 2-hour intervals. Large-bolus feedings may overwhelm digestive capacity, and repeated passage of a stomach tube is an unnecessary stress on the foal. Another advantage of the small-bore, indwelling tubes is that they do not interfere with the suckle response. The tube may be left in place as the foal is transitioned to feeding from the mare. The feeding tube should be inserted with the foal in sternal recumbency, and correct placement within the esophagus should be confirmed by radiography or endoscopy. The tube should be fastened to the external nares by sutures and can also be retained in a circumferential elastic bandage around the muzzle. At each feeding, it is important to check that the tube is still in place and that there is no reflux. The foal should be in sternal recumbency or standing when it is fed. Milk should be administered by gravity flow followed by a small amount of clean water to flush the tube. The tube should be capped between feedings to prevent aspiration of air. Feeding tubes should be replaced every 1 to 2 days to reduce risk of gastrointestinal-tract infection.

A suggested initial rate of milk delivery is 2 to 3 mL/kg body weight per hour or 100 to 150 mL/h for a 50-kg foal (**Table 1**). This provides 2.4 to 3.6 L of milk to a 50-kg foal during the first 24 hours of enteral support. Dextrose-containing fluids can be administered intravenously to provide additional calories during the transition to an adequate level of enteral feeding (see later). The feeding rate can be gradually increased over the next 2 to 3 days (eg, increase to 4–5 mL/kg/h on day 2 and then to 6–8 mL/kg/h on day 3), which represents a total daily intake of 10% to 15% of body weight. Simultaneously, intravenous caloric support (dextrose) can be gradually withdrawn. This feeding level likely meets the resting energy requirements of hospitalized foals. Depending on the rate of clinical improvement and the length of hospitalization, it may be possible to increase the volume of feeding to 20% to 22% body weight per day, which approximates the milk intake of healthy neonatal foals.[1] Clinical monitoring should include frequent assessments of gastrointestinal function, including gastric reflux, intestinal sounds, abdominal distention, and quantity and quality of feces. Gastric reflux, bloating, colic, diarrhea, or constipation can indicate intolerance to enteral feeding and the need for adjustments to the feeding program. This may involve a decrease in the volume or frequency of enteral feedings. Foals fed milk replacers seem to be more likely to develop loose feces than foals fed mare's milk, and in some cases this may be associated with a syndrome of lactase deficiency. Supplementation with 6000 units of lactase (Lactaid) per 50-kg foal every 3 to 8 hours[15] either orally or mixed into the milk replacer before feeding may be of benefit in aiding milk digestion.

Table 1
Feeding recommendations for neonatal and growing foals

Foal Age (d)	Energy Requirement	Volume of Mare's Milk or Milk Replacer	Percentage of Body Weight Fed
0–1	150 kcal/kg/d	2–3 mL/kg/h	5–7
2–3	150 kcal/kg/d	4–5 mL/kg/h	10–12
4–7	150 kcal/kg/d	6–8 mL/kg/h	14–20
8–30	120 kcal/kg/d	9–10 mL/kg/h	22
30–weaning	80–100 kcal/kg/d	Gradually decreasing and replaced with solid feed	

PARENTERAL NUTRITION

It is generally preferred to support foals by way of the enteral route,[2,14] both because this is the most natural and physiologically desirable route and because the epithelial cells lining the intestine are partially dependent on the products of digestion for energy and nutrients. Unfortunately, there are a variety of situations in which a foal may be unable to receive enteral nutrition, or is unable to tolerate the volume of enteral nutrition required to support basal metabolism and growth. These range from the critically ill neonate with gastrointestinal complications to the suckling foal with severe enterocolitis. In these circumstances the provision of nutrition by intravenous infusion, a procedure termed "parenteral nutrition," aids in ensuring that the patient receives appropriate caloric and nutritional support in a controlled manner and eliminates concerns regarding intestinal absorption. The limitations of parenteral nutritional support are primarily caused by the expense of this therapy and the risk of secondary complications. These complications may include hyperglycemia, hypertriglyceridemia, thrombophlebitis, and an increased risk of bloodstream infections.[13]

The primary goal of parenteral nutrition, as with any type of nutritional support, is to ensure that the patient is supplied with adequate calories to support basal metabolism at a minimum, and ideally to provide additional support to allow for ongoing growth. If sufficient nutritional support is not provided, affected foals may develop a negative energy balance, which results in protein catabolism to use amino acids for energy production.[1,16] Failure to provide adequate nutritional support may also have a substantial negative influence on the immune response.[16–18] Short-term parenteral supplementation (less than 24 hours) does not require that the patient receive a balanced nutritional source consisting of carbohydrates, amino acids, and lipids, but if parenteral nutrition is expected to be administered for a longer period then a more complete formula should be used.

Short-Term Caloric Supplementation

Carbohydrate-containing solutions represent the simplest means of providing intravenous caloric support to foals. A solution containing 5% dextrose can be used, and there are several options available including 5% dextrose in water; lactated Ringer's solution with 5% dextrose; 0.45% saline with 5% dextrose; and hypotonic maintenance electrolyte solutions containing 5% dextrose (Normosol-M, Plasmalyte-56). Fluids containing dextrose should not be used for initial large-volume fluid resuscitation, because this almost certainly results in the delivery of excessive amounts of dextrose to a foal with any degree of dehydration, leading to profound hyperglycemia. Following initial fluid resuscitation the solutions containing electrolytes and dextrose may be used as the primary fluids for maintenance therapy in foals with minimal ongoing fluid losses. Dextrose 5% in water is not a good choice as a maintenance solution because of the absence of electrolytes, and is primarily useful in providing free water to patients suffering from hyperosmolar conditions. The caloric content of a 5% dextrose solution is 0.17 kcal/mL, so an infusion rate of 10 mL/kg/h is required to deliver approximately 40 kcal/kg/d (0.17 kcal/kg/h $\times$ 24 hours/day = 41 kcal/kg/d). This rate of infusion is over twice that which is considered to be a maintenance rate for a neonatal foal (4–5 mL/kg/h). Because an infusion rate of 5 mL/kg/h (20 kcal/kg/d) is typically the maximal limit for administering these solutions one cannot typically depend on a 5% dextrose solution as a primary form of parenteral nutrition. In addition, care must always be taken when adjusting the infusion rates of 5% dextrose–containing solutions in response to changes in the patient's fluid status, to ensure that excessive amounts of dextrose are not infused, especially in premature or very sick foals that are likely to be poorly tolerant of dextrose infusions.

Alternatively, a 50% dextrose solution can be delivered without further dilution using an infusion pump, as long as additional isotonic fluids are being administered concurrently to avoid endothelial injury caused by the hypertonic nature of this solution. Use of 50% dextrose solution should be avoided if an infusion pump is not available, because it is very easy inadvertently to administer an excessive amount of dextrose, leading to hyperglycemia. The caloric content of 50% dextrose solution is 1.7 kcal/mL, so an infusion rate of 1 mL/kg/h of this solution delivers approximately 40 kcal/kg/d (1.7 kcal/kg/h $\times$ 24 hours/day = 41 kcal/kg/d). This low rate of infusion means that the primary fluid needs of the patient can be met with a dextrose-free isotonic electrolyte-containing fluid, the infusion rate of which can be altered in response to changes in patient fluid status without concerns related to the requirements of the nutritional plan.

At the end of the first 24 hours of treatment the fluid therapy plan and nutritional plan should be revisited, to determine if the patient can begin to rely on enteral fluid and nutritional intake or if continued parenteral therapy is required. Because dextrose-containing fluids are a very incomplete nutritional source they should not be used as the primary nutritional source for more than 24 hours. Continued parenteral nutritional support requires the formulation of a more complete solution that provides amino acids and possibly lipids.

Parenteral Nutrition Formulation

One important aspect of providing parenteral nutrition to foals is the inclusion of a protein source. The metabolic response to injury and sepsis is to increase protein degradation in muscle tissue. This catabolic response can be reduced both by supplying a source of nitrogen and by increasing energy intake. The recommended ratio for nonprotein calories to nitrogen is 100 to 200 nonprotein calories per gram of nitrogen.[19] Spurlock and Donaghue[20] demonstrated that the amount of protein provided affects weight gain, because the nonprotein nitrogen calories to grams nitrogen ratio was negatively correlated with the rate of weight gain.

The inclusion of lipids in the parenteral nutrition formulation allows for the provision of a larger number of calories per unit volume compared with solutions containing only dextrose. Another advantage of lipid emulsions is that they are isotonic, thereby moderating the hypertonicity of the parenteral nutrition formulation and potentially decreasing the risk of thrombophlebitis. Unfortunately, formulating parenteral nutrition solutions with lipids increases the cost of the solution and may increase the risk of complications.[21] Hyperlipidemia can occur in association with lipid administration to foals, but does not seem to result in adverse effects.[13,21] Lipid emulsions are prone to contamination and promote bacterial growth. Because of these risks the intravenous lines through which lipid-containing solutions are administered should be changed daily, substantially increasing client costs. In a recent report the use of lipid-containing parenteral nutrition solutions allowed for the provision of 40 to 92 kcal/kg/d (mean, 63 kcal/kg/d) to foals, as opposed to only 25 to 66 kcal/kg/d (mean, 41 kcal/kg/d) with a dextrose-based solution.[13]

There are two basic approaches to the formulation of parenteral nutrition to foals. The first involves the exact determination of the anticipated metabolic needs of the patient, followed by the development of a formulation that meets all of these needs in a fairly precise manner, using a mixture of dextrose, amino acids, and lipids. This approach is fairly complex and is best performed using a computerized spreadsheet to aid in performing the various calculations. The second approach is more practical and consists of using two basic parenteral nutrition formulas (**Table 2**). One of these

Table 2
Formulation of parenteral nutrition solutions

Formulation	Composition	Caloric Density (kcal/mL)	Nonprotein Calories/g N
Formula 1	1500 mL 50% dextrose, 1500 mL 8.5% amino acids	1.02	125
Formula 2	1500 mL 50% dextrose, 500 mL 20% lipids, 2000 mL 8.5% amino acids	1.08	131

solutions is intended for short-term use and consists only of 50% dextrose and 8.5% amino acid solutions (Solution I). The second solution incorporates a lipid energy source, and is preferred for long-term administration or for administration to foals that are poorly tolerant of infused dextrose (Solution II). Solution I is formulated using equal volumes (1:1) of 50% dextrose (Dextrose 50%) and 8.5% amino acids (Travasol 8.5%), whereas Solution II is formulated with three parts of 50% dextrose, one part of 20% lipids (Intralipid 20%), and four parts of 8.5% amino acids.[13] The caloric density of these solutions is 1.02 kcal/mL for Solution I and 1.08 kcal/mL for Solution II. The ratio of nonprotein calories to nitrogen is 125 nonprotein calories per gram of nitrogen for Solution I and 131 nonprotein calories per gram of nitrogen for Solution II.

Administration of Parenteral Nutrition

An electronic infusion pump should be used when administering parenteral nutrition solutions, because the rate must be tightly controlled and adjustments to the infusion rate must be made easily and accurately. Excessive rates of administration can easily induce profound hyperglycemia, which has been shown in other species to be associated with severe complications and increased risk of death.[22] The solutions used for parenteral nutrition are all hypertonic and can cause injury to the vascular endothelium, increasing the risk of thrombophlebitis. For this reason, it is recommended that parenteral nutrition solutions be administered through a 20-cm long polyurethane long-term catheter (Arrow International, Reading, Pennsylvania) placed in the jugular vein, because this provides a central line in most foals. The use of a multiple-lumen catheter allows for one lumen to be dedicated to infusion of the parenteral nutrition solution, minimizing the risks of contamination. Catheter management is extremely important when foals are receiving parenteral nutrition and the catheter site and vein should be monitored at least twice daily for heat, swelling, or exudation. Increased resistance to fluid flow in the catheter may be an indication of thrombosis deeper within the vasculature and often necessitates the placement of a catheter in an alternative site, such as the opposite jugular vein, a cephalic vein, or a lateral thoracic vein.

All components of parenteral nutrition solutions must be mixed in a sterile manner before administration. The bag containing the final parenteral nutrition composition should be covered with a brown plastic bag during administration to protect it from light, which can degrade the amino acids within the solution. The rate of infusion (in milliliter per hour) is calculated based on the desired kilocalorie per kilogram per day to be administered. A reasonable initial goal is 40 to 60 kcal/kg/d. Although this does not fully meet the theoretic energy requirements of the neonate, it can be difficult to achieve higher rates of energy administration without encountering hyperglycemia or hyperlipidemia. The initial infusion rate of parenteral nutrition solutions should be 50% of the calculated final rate, and the rate should be gradually increased every 1 to 3 hours following monitoring of the blood glucose concentration to ensure that hyperglycemia (blood glucose >180 mg/dL) is not present. When parenteral nutrition is to be discontinued it is recommended that the infusion rate be gradually reduced by decreasing the infusion rate in 25% to 50% increments every 4 to 6 hours while gradually introducing enteral feeding. It is important that blood glucose monitoring is continued during this weaning process, to prevent the development of severe hypoglycemia.

Monitoring the Foal Receiving Parenteral Nutrition

The foal must be frequently monitored, especially during the initial phase of parenteral nutrition therapy. This monitoring should include a general physical examination, with close attention paid to neurologic status and respiratory function. Rectal temperature should also be closely monitored, because fever is a common early manifestation of systemic infection. Blood glucose concentrations should be frequently monitored, initially on an hourly basis until the patient has stabilized with the appropriate rate of parenteral nutrition infusion, followed by monitoring every 3 to 6 hours for the first day of therapy. The frequency of blood glucose monitoring is very dependent on the stability of the patient, and may need to be more frequent in the very critically ill, but may not need to be monitored beyond every 12 hours in the stable patient. Urine output should be monitored continuously, in combination with intermittent monitoring of urine glucose concentration, because of the risk of hyperglycemia-induced diuresis and glucosuria. Although the actual renal threshold for glucose is not well described in foals, glucosuria and diuresis are observed when blood glucose levels exceed 180 mg/dL in many cases. Additional clinicopathologic monitoring should consist of daily complete blood counts and serum chemistry profiles in the critical case, although these can be performed every 48 to 72 hours in more stable patients. Ideally, bodyweight should be assessed on a daily basis, to ensure that the foal is at least maintaining body weight while on parenteral nutrition.

Insulin Therapy

The critically ill foal often demonstrates a degree of insulin resistance for the reasons described previously, and this can make it very difficult to achieve even a conservative rate of administration of intravenous nutrition. This phenomenon can only be addressed by the administration of exogenous insulin. The administration of insulin to the neonatal foal is not to be undertaken lightly, however, because this therapy places additional demands on both the clinician and nursing staff to ensure that profound hypoglycemia does not occur. Intermittent dosing of subcutaneous insulin may offer some advantages in terms of simplicity of administration and moderation of effects, but this route of administration does not allow for changes in dosage over the short term. The use of continuous-rate infusion for the administration of insulin allows for a fairly rapid onset of action while also providing a simple and timely means of adjustment of the dosage. Because of the gradual saturation of the cellular insulin receptors the maximal effect of continuous-rate infusion insulin is not typically seen until approximately 90 minutes after initiation of the infusion. The response to alteration of the rate of infusion occurs over a similar time frame, so one should take care to avoid altering the rate of infusion of parenteral nutrition solutions too rapidly after changing the rate of insulin infusion.

An initial insulin infusion rate of 0.07 IU/kg/h is generally well tolerated and represents a reasonable starting point. In general, it is best to avoid simultaneous alterations in both the insulin infusion rate and the parenteral nutrition infusion rate, because this can lead to a roller-coaster ride wherein the blood glucose concentration is rising and falling wildly because of the delay in the body's response to these changes. Dramatic alterations in blood glucose concentration can be minimized by using a protocol where changes in blood glucose concentration are primarily addressed by altering the insulin infusion rate (**Fig. 1**). Blood glucose monitoring should be performed at least hourly for the first 2 to 3 hours after initiation of the insulin continuous-rate infusion, and if hyperglycemia (blood glucose >150 mg/dL) is persistent beyond the first 2 hours of insulin therapy then the insulin infusion rate may be increased by 50%, followed by hourly blood glucose monitoring for a further 2 to 3 hours. This procedure for increasing the insulin infusion rate may be repeated if hyperglycemia persists.

Conversely, if hypoglycemia (blood glucose <60 mg/dL) is noted, then a bolus of 0.25 to 0.5 mL/kg of 50% dextrose solution should be administered intravenously over 3 to 5 minutes. The blood glucose level should then be reassessed every 30 minutes for at least 90 minutes to ensure that hypoglycemia does not recur. If hypoglycemia does recur then a second bolus of dextrose is administered and the insulin infusion rate is decreased by 50%. Close monitoring then is required for a further 60 to 90 minutes to ensure that hypoglycemia does not recur and that hyperglycemia does not develop.

Further changes to the insulin infusion rate are not usually necessary once a steady state has been achieved, wherein the blood glucose level is stable and the desired rate of parenteral nutrition administration has been achieved. Patient reassessment is indicated if one finds that the foal has become even more insulin resistant (requiring additional insulin administration to avoid hyperglycemia), because this may be an early indicator of an overall deterioration in the patient's condition accompanied by increasing systemic inflammation.

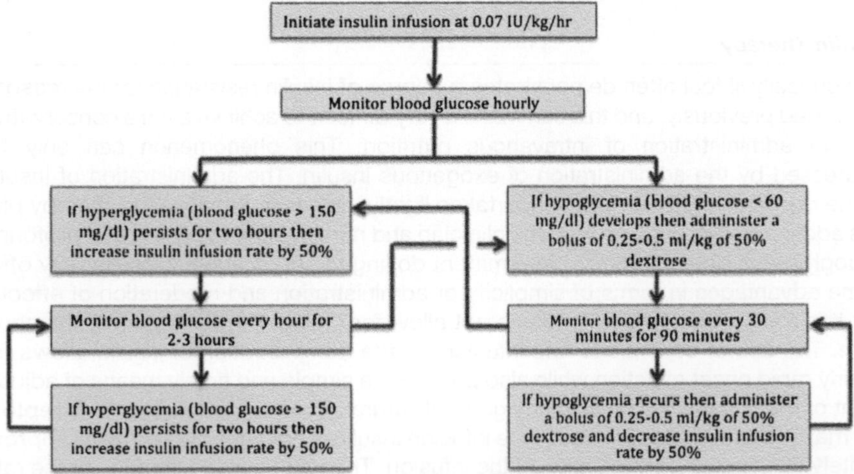

Fig. 1. A flow sheet that can be used as a guide in the administration of insulin as a continuous rate infusion to foals that develop hyperglycemia secondary to parenteral nutrition administration.

REFERENCES

1. Ousey JC, Holdstock N, Rossdale PD, et al. How much energy do sick neonatal foals require compared with healthy foals? Pferdeheilkunde 1996;12:231–7.
2. Ousey JC, Prandi S, Zimmer J, et al. Effects of various feeding regimens on the energy balance of equine neonates. Am J Vet Res 1997;58:1243–51.
3. Fowden AL, Gardner DS, Ousey JC, et al. Maturation of pancreatic beta-cell function in the fetal horse during late gestation. J Endocrinol 2005;186:467–73.
4. Holdstock NB, Allen VL, Bloomfield MR, et al. Development of insulin and proinsulin secretion in newborn pony foals. J Endocrinol 2004;181:469–76.
5. Allen WR, Wilsher S, Tiplady C, et al. The influence of maternal size on pre- and postnatal growth in the horse: III Postnatal growth. Reproduction 2004;127:67–77.
6. George LA, Staniar WB, Treiber KH, et al. Insulin sensitivity and glucose dynamics in foals following maternal dietary treatment. Proceedings of the Equine Science Society 2007;20:5–6.
7. Forhead AJ, Ousey JC, Allen WR, et al. Postnatal insulin secretion and sensitivity after manipulation of fetal growth by embryo transfer in the horse. J Endocrinol 2004;181:459–67.
8. Ousey J. Total parenteral nutrition in the young foal. Equine Veterinary Education 1994;6:316–7.
9. Paradis MR. Caloric needs of the sick foal: determined by the use of indirect calorimetry. Proceedings of the 3rd Dorothy Havemeyer Foundation Neonatal Septicemia Workshop, Talliores, France. October 2001.
10. Boitano M. Hypocaloric feeding of the critically ill. Nutr Clin Pract 2006;21: 617–22.
11. Dandona P, Mohanty P, Chaudhuri A, et al. Insulin infusion in acute illness. J Clin Invest 2005;115:2069–72.
12. Klein CJ, Stanek GS, Wiles CE III, et al. Overfeeding macronutrients to critically ill adults: metabolic complications. J Am Diet Assoc 1998;98:795–806.
13. Krause JB, McKenzie HC III, et al. Parenteral nutrition in foals: a retrospective study of 45 cases (2000–2004). Equine Vet J 2007;39:74–8.
14. Settle CS, Vaala WE. Management of the critically ill foal: initial respiratory, fluid and nutritional support. Equine Vet Educ 1991;3:49–54.
15. Magdesian KG. Neonatal foal diarrhea. Vet Clin North Am Equine Pract 2005;21: 295–312, vi.
16. Furr MO. Intravenous nutrition in horses: clinical applications. Proceedings of the 20th ACVIM Forum 2002;186–7.
17. Lopes MA, White NA II. Parenteral nutrition for horses with gastrointestinal disease: a retrospective study of 79 cases. Equine Vet J 2002;34:250–7.
18. Naylor JM, Kenyon SJ. Effect of total caloric deprivation on host defense in the horse. Res Vet Sci 1981;31:369–72.
19. Hansen TO. Nutritional support: parenteral feeding. In: Koterba AM, Drummond WH, Kosch PC, editors. Equine clinical neonatology. Philadelphia: Lea & Febiger; 1990. p. 747–62.
20. Spurlock SL, Donaghue S. Weight gains in foals on parenteral nutrition. Int Soc Vet Perinatology 2nd Sci Conf, Cambridge, England. July 1990.
21. Hansen TO. Parenteral nutrition in foals. 32nd Annu Conv AAEP 1986;153–6.
22. Hays SP, Smith EOB, Sunehag AL, et al. Hyperglycemia is a risk factor for early death and morbidity in extremely low birth-weight infants. Pediatrics 2006;118:1811–8.

Optimal Diet of Horses with Chronic Exertional Myopathies

Erica C. McKenzie, BSc, BVMS, PhD[a,*], Anna M. Firshman, BVSc, PhD[b]

KEYWORDS

- Fat • Nonstructural carbohydrate
- Exertional rhabdomyolysis • Polysaccharide
- Starch • Digestible energy

Chronic exertional rhabdomyolysis represents a syndrome of recurrent exercise-associated muscle damage in horses that arises from a variety of etiologies.[1,2] Recently, major advances have been made in the understanding of the pathophysiology of chronic exertional rhabdomyolysis, and causative genetic defects have been identified.[3,4] Dietary manipulation and environmental management comprise the most effective and convenient means of controlling clinical signs of chronic exertional rhabdomyolysis in many affected horses.[5–9]

CLINICAL SIGNS AND PATHOPHYSIOLOGY OF EXERTIONAL RHABDOMYOLYSIS

Clinical signs of exertional rhabdomyolysis typically arise soon after the onset of exercise or shortly after exercise ceases. The volume of exercise that elicits muscle necrosis and the frequency of episodes vary extensively between individuals and may be influenced by factors including the underlying cause, age, gender, fitness, exercise intensity, and the horse's temperament and diet.[1,5,10–14] Common clinical signs include excessive sweating, a stiff gait, fasciculations, and reluctance to continue exercise. Tachypnea, tachycardia, and firm painful gluteal and lumbar musculature may be appreciated, and myoglobinuria and subsequent renal failure may occur in severely affected horses.[15–18] Subclinically affected horses may have considerable elevations of serum creatine kinase (CK) and aspartate transaminase (AST) activities above normal range after exercise.[19]

Chronic exertional rhabdomyolysis in horses frequently results from underlying heritable myopathic conditions, including polysaccharide storage myopathy (PSSM) and recurrent exertional rhabdomyolysis (RER).[1,20–23] PSSM most commonly affects quarter horses, paints, warm bloods and draft horses, and their crosses and has

[a] Department of Clinical Sciences, College of Veterinary Medicine, Oregon State University, 227 Magruder Hall, Corvallis, OR 97331, USA
[b] Department of Veterinary Population Medicine, University of Minnesota, Saint Paul, MN, USA
* Corresponding author.
E-mail address: erica.mckenzie@oregonstate.edu (E.C. McKenzie).

Vet Clin Equine 25 (2009) 121–135
doi:10.1016/j.cveq.2008.12.001 vetequine.theclinics.com
0749-0739/08/$ – see front matter

also been identified in a variety of light breeds.[24–33] RER is associated with repeated episodes of muscle necrosis in exercising thoroughbreds and possibly other breeds, including standardbred and Arabian horses.[19,34,35]

PSSM is a glycogen storage disorder characterized by increased skeletal muscle glycogen concentrations and the accumulation of abnormal amylase-resistant polysaccharide in type 2A and type 2B skeletal muscle fibers.[24] The condition has a prevalence of approximately 6% to 12% in quarter horses and 36% in draft horses.[31,36] Unlike comparable glycogenoses in humans, in horses with PSSM, glycogen accumulation is not related to the inability to metabolize glycogen, and glycogenolytic and glycolytic enzyme activities are normal.[24,37] In quarter horses, PSSM is associated with a myofiber energy deficit with submaximal exercise and enhanced insulin sensitivity.[38,39] An increased rate of blood glucose clearance has been demonstrated in affected horses after a carbohydrate meal or intravenous or oral glucose tolerance tests.[40,41] Enhanced insulin sensitivity and rhabdomyolysis are apparent in affected quarter horses by 6 months of age, and subclinical rhabdomyolysis may occur as early as 4 weeks of age, although accumulation of abnormal polysaccharide in muscle biopsies may not be found until animals surpass 7 to 12 months of age.[42] Insulin sensitivity does not appear to be different between Belgian draft horses with and without PSSM, despite similarities in the histopathologic abnormalities between quarter horses and draft horses with PSSM.[25,31,32,43,44] Recently, an autosomal dominant mutation in the gene encoding the skeletal muscle glycogen synthase enzyme (*GYS1*) was identified as the primary cause of PSSM in quarter horses and draft horses and their crosses.[3]

Clinical signs associated with PSSM are variable among different breeds of horses.[33] Quarter horses tend to develop typical signs of exertional rhabdomyolysis with even mild exercise, and signs often occur in unfit horses commencing training or following a period of unaccustomed stall confinement.[25] The severity of clinical signs can vary greatly between affected individuals, possibly as a result of previous dietary and exercise management of the horse and heterozygosity or homozygosity for causative mutations.[3,5] Serum CK activity is often persistently elevated even when horses are rested for weeks.[5] Draft horses and warm blood horses with PSSM may be subclinically affected or may develop exertional rhabdomyolysis, gait abnormalities, weakness, and recumbency.[18,26,30–32,45–47] Muscle atrophy and back pain have also been reported in association with PSSM.[32,48]

In thoroughbred horses, RER is attributable to a heritable defect in intracellular calcium regulation that results in excessive muscular contraction and necrosis with exercise.[49,50] Clinically affected horses are frequently 2-year-old fillies in race training, although this apparent gender predisposition diminishes with age.[10,14] Episodes of rhabdomyolysis tend to occur during training and not racing and may become more frequent as fitness increases.[10] Stressful situations often precipitate clinical episodes, and a nervous temperament is reported to be a strong predisposing factor.[10] Subclinical episodes of muscle necrosis may be identified via intermittent elevations of serum CK and AST activity. Administration of inhalant anesthetic agents may provoke rhabdomyolysis in horses with RER or other underlying myopathic conditions.[51,52]

Sporadic exertional rhabdomyolysis may occur in otherwise healthy horses that are exerted beyond their level of conditioning, particularly after a period of rest.[13] Exhaustive exercise in well-conditioned horses can also cause rhabdomyolysis, typically observed in horses competing in endurance competition in hot weather.[53,54] Dietary electrolyte imbalances and respiratory infection with influenza virus have also been incriminated as causes of sporadic or chronic exertional rhabdomyolysis in horses.[55–57] Any horse with clinical signs of respiratory disease should be rested until signs resolve.

DIAGNOSTIC EVALUATION OF HORSES WITH SUSPECTED CHRONIC EXERTIONAL RHABDOMYOLYSIS

Horses with chronic exertional rhabdomyolysis are often presented for evaluation of a history of poor performance or muscle stiffness with exercise; however, at the time of evaluation, clinical evidence of rhabdomyolysis is frequently lacking. A thorough investigation of prior history is critical, including a description of the clinical problem, ration composition and volume, exercise routine, and the horse's temperament and behavior among other pertinent factors, to assist in establishment of the diagnosis and the development of an appropriate management plan. Diagnostic evaluation may include measurement of serum muscle enzyme activities, assessment of the horse's response to submaximal exercise, histopathologic evaluation of muscle biopsy samples, and analysis of urine samples for evidence of myoglobinuria and dietary electrolyte and mineral imbalances.[35,58] Recently, genetic testing has become available for specific mutations associated with chronic rhabdomyolysis.[3]

Demonstration of elevated serum CK activity provides evidence of muscle damage. Horses with PSSM may have persistently elevated serum CK activity at rest, particularly if they are stall confined.[59] For horses with normal serum CK activity suspected to have chronic rhabdomyolysis, serum CK activity can be measured before and 4 to 6 hours after 2 to 20 minutes of trotting exercise. Greater than a threefold to fourfold increase in serum CK activity or serum CK activity greater than 1000 U/L after exercise constitutes an abnormal response.[60–62] Because some horses, particularly those with PSSM, can develop significant rhabdomyolysis during light exercise, horses should be monitored closely for signs of stiffness, muscle fasciculation, or reluctance to continue, and an exercise test ended if such signs occur. Elevations of serum CK activity in horses with RER are often intermittent and do not occur reliably during submaximal exercise testing.

Muscle biopsy samples may be obtained to definitively confirm a diagnosis of PSSM or to investigate other causes of muscular dysfunction. Small biopsy samples can be obtained from the middle gluteal muscle using a modified Bergstrom needle. These small samples require appropriate processing for frozen sectioning; therefore, they are only performed at specific institutions.[25] A technique for open surgical biopsy of the semimembranosus muscle has been described and is recommended when samples must be shipped to a laboratory for analysis.[25] Semimembranosus samples should be wrapped in saline-moistened gauze and shipped chilled (not frozen) on ice packs within 24 hours to a specialized laboratory. Muscle sections prepared in frozen isopentane at a specialized laboratory (versus formalin fixation) allow muscle fiber typing, mitochondrial staining, and enzymatic analyses to be performed.[25]

Biopsy samples from horses with RER may display acute segmental necrosis or macrophage infiltration of a variable number of muscle fibers, a few small regenerative basophilic fibers with large central nuclei, and mature muscle fibers with centrally displaced nuclei.[62] Biopsy samples from horses with PSSM may have unstained subsarcolemmal vacuoles, variable numbers of fibers undergoing necrosis and regeneration, and a dark purple staining intensity with periodic acid–Schiff (PAS) due to elevated muscle glycogen concentrations.[24] A variable number of fibers (1%–40%) may contain cytoplasmic aggregates of amylase-resistant, PAS-positive polysaccharide, although these may not be visible in horses less than 1 year of age.[24,42,43] Increased PAS staining intensity alone should not be considered diagnostic of PSSM because it is subjective and varies extensively depending on the horse's diet, state of training, and muscle fiber composition.[43]

Recently, an arginine-to-histidine substitution in a highly conserved region of the glycogen synthase gene (*GYS1*) was found to be associated with PSSM in quarter horses and draft breeds.[3] Elevated glycogen synthase activity has been documented in affected horses, and disease associated with this mutation has been termed *type 1 PSSM*. Nevertheless, approximately 20% of quarter horses with PSSM do not have the GYS1 mutation, and it is suspected that a different type of PSSM (termed *type 2 PSSM*) may exist that is not associated with the recently identified mutation.[3] Horses with the GYS1 mutation have a variable clinical phenotype ranging from subclinical disease to exertional rhabdomyolysis to acute recumbency and death.[3] The GYS1 mutation is inherited in a dominant fashion, and homozygous individuals appear to be more severely clinically affected.[3] Variable phenotypic expression may also be attributed to environmental factors such as diet and exercise as well as modifying genes. Evidence suggests that the presence of a concurrent mutation of the skeletal muscle ryanodine receptor (RYR1) reported to cause malignant hyperthermia in quarter horses may be responsible for modifying the GYS1 phenotype, resulting in a more severe form of disease;[4,52] therefore, in quarter horses and related breeds, it may be prudent to test for both of these mutations.[4] DNA testing of whole blood or hair root samples is available through the University of Minnesota Veterinary Diagnostic Laboratory. Muscle biopsy is still recommended for horses with clinical signs of rhabdomyolysis that test negative for known causative mutations to identify the non-GYS1 (type 2) form of PSSM.

NUTRITION AND CHRONIC EXERTIONAL RHABDOMYOLYSIS

For decades, nutritional factors have been suspected to have an important role in the pathophysiology of chronic exertional rhabdomyolysis. Deficiencies of specific electrolytes, vitamins, and minerals, and the feeding of a high grain diet, particularly after a period of rest, have all been linked with the condition;[63–66] therefore, nutritional manipulation, frequently consisting of reducing or removing concentrate feed on light exercise days, has been repeatedly recommended as a management strategy. Controlled clinical trials performed recently support the assertion that reduction of dietary soluble carbohydrate can significantly improve exertional rhabdomyolysis in horses, despite differences in underlying etiologies.[5–9] Dietary management of affected horses should involve accurately establishing energy requirements and meeting vitamin and mineral requirements and providing the majority of the caloric requirement via fat and fiber sources while minimizing dietary soluble carbohydrate content.[5–7,9,58]

Estimation of Daily Digestible Energy Requirements

Energy requirements for horses are usually expressed as digestible energy (DE) in megacalories (Mcal) per day. Recommendations for DE and other nutritional requirements have recently been revised by the National Research Council.[67] Reported maintenance energy requirements (DE_m) for horses vary substantially, ranging from approximately 25 to 35 kcal/kg BW, and are influenced by individual variation, dietary composition, age, breed, environment, and body composition, among other factors.[67] Recent recommendations regarding DE_m suggest providing 30.3 kcal/kg BW for idle draft horses and 33.3 kcal/kg BW (16.7 Mcal/500 kg horse/day) for adult light breed horses with moderate voluntary activity (several hours of turnout per day or active in stall). An estimate of 36.3 kcal/kg BW (18.2 Mcal/500 kg horse/day) may apply to horses with nervous temperaments or high levels of voluntary activity. Further adjustments to DE intake to accommodate energy demands associated with growth, pregnancy, lactation, ambient environment, body condition, and other factors should be determined, and serial monitoring of body condition or weight should be performed to determine whether energy provision is adequate.[67]

Increases in energy demand related to exercise can be substantial and can be specifically calculated if factors including the exercise intensity and duration, the weight of load carried, the ambient temperature, and the breed of horse are known, and the energy intake can be adjusted accordingly. A simpler approach is to subjectively categorize exercise demands and to increase DE_m by 20%, 40%, 60%, or 90% for light, moderate, heavy (polo, race training), and very heavy exercise (racing, 3 day event), respectively.[67] Periodic body condition scoring or weighing can be used to determine whether estimated requirements are being met.

Knowledge of the energy content and composition of available feedstuffs assists in the construction of a ration of appropriate composition and volume. Ideally, proximate analysis of feedstuffs is performed to obtain this information, because the composition of individual feedstuffs can vary substantially. Manufacturer-provided information for commercial feedstuffs (**Tables 1** and **2**) or the use of appropriate literature sources to establish estimates for forage and generic feedstuffs may be more convenient methods of estimating the nutritional value of intended ration components.

Ration Composition

Traditional equine rations (forage/grain mix) have a low fat content (<3% of dry matter) and provide the majority of energy in the form of structural and nonstructural carbohydrates (NSC).[67] Structural carbohydrate refers to the fiber-related components in the diet, including cellulose, hemicellulose, and pectin. The NSC or soluble carbohydrate content of a feed encompasses simple sugars (mono- and disaccharides), oligosaccharides (fructans), and starch (amylose and amylopectin). Newer terminology identifies water soluble carbohydrates (simple sugars and fructans), ethanol soluble carbohydrates (a subset of water soluble carbohydrates), and starch. Starch can be approximately determined by subtracting the water soluble carbohydrate component from the NSC component if both are known.[67]

Rations for horses with rhabdomyolysis should provide a good quality forage (grass hay or mixed alfalfa–grass hay) preferably fed at 1.5% to 2% of bodyweight and at no less than 1% of bodyweight in horses with high DE requirements.[68] Remaining DE requirements may be met using small amounts of starch-based concentrates, soluble fibers, and fat supplements, the amount of each depending on the underlying myopathic condition and the magnitude of additional energy requirements as described later. Vitamin and mineral requirements should also be determined and appropriately addressed by additional supplementation if required.

Fat can readily replace NSC in rations for horses. Fat is extremely energy dense (each gram provides approximately 9 kcal of gross energy compared with approximately 4 kcal/g for protein and carbohydrate), and rations containing up to 15% to 20% fat (as dry matter) are well tolerated by horses providing there is a gradual introduction to fat supplementation.[69] Additionally, fat supplementation has been associated with decreased thermal stress, gut fill, and water requirement, enhanced aerobic and anaerobic performance, and calmer demeanor.[70–73] The array of commercially available fat-fortified feeds and fat supplements for horses has expanded tremendously in recent years (**Tables 1** and **2**). Vegetable sources of fat including oil and stabilized rice bran (~20% fat) based products are more digestible and palatable than animal sources of fat.[69] There is little information regarding the effect of different forms of fat on equine physiology and exertional rhabdomyolysis; however, stabilized rice bran–based feeds have been shown to significantly lower pre-exercise heart rates

Table 1
Estimate macronutrient and digestible energy content of commercially available concentrate feeds with greater than 10% crude fat by weight

Diet	Crude Fat (%)	Nonstructural Carbohydrate (%)	Starch (%)	Crude Protein (%)	Digestible Energy (kcal/kg)
Typical oats	5.0–8.5	48.0–37.0	35.0–54.0	10.5–15.0	3050–3650
Typical corn	3.0–5.5	68.0–78.0	65.0–75.0	7.7–11.0	3790–3960
Typical barley	1.5–3.7	52.0–67.0	45.0–64.0	10.0–15.0	3450–3850
Buckeye Nutrition Cadence	10.0	27.6	22.6	10.0	3630
Buckeye Nutrition Cadence Ultra	14.0	23.0	18.0	14.0	3400
Buckeye Nutrition Endurance 101	10.0	42.6	38.6	14.0	3630
Buckeye Trifecta	12.0	22.1	15.0	12.0	3850
LMF Gold	12.0	24.0	18.0	12.0	3500
Purina Mills Ultium	12.4	16.0	9.0–10.0	11.7	3800
Nutrena Equine Nutrition XTN	12.0	32.5	22.3	12.0	3650
Nutrena Equine Nutrition Vitality Ultra	10.0	27.3	21.8	12.0	3200
Re-Leve	12.5	18.0	10.0	12.5	3300
Triple Crown Nutrition 10% Performance formula	10.0	38.9	33.3	10.0	3795
Triple Crown Nutrition 14% Performance formula	10.0	38.1	31.8	14.0	3758
Triple Crown Nutrition Senior formula	10.0	11.7	6.4	14.0	3401
Triple Crown Nutrition Complete	10.0	20.6	11.8	11.0	3511
Triple Crown Nutrition Growth formula	10.0	13.9	5.6	14.0	3450

and post-exercise serum CK activity in horses with RER, supporting the use of rice bran in rations for horses with this condition.[6]

Rations for Horses with Rhabdomyolysis

Despite various underlying etiologies, horses prone to rhabdomyolysis are more likely to develop muscle necrosis when consuming high energy diets containing substantial amounts of NSC.[6,9,12] The reasons for this phenomenon have not been clearly elucidated. In horses with PSSM, it is possible that high NSC intake encourages enhanced

Table 2
Estimate macronutrient and digestible energy content of commercially available feed supplements with greater than 20% crude fat by weight

Diet	Crude Fat (%)	Nonstructural Carbohydrate (%)	Starch (%)	Crude Protein (%)	Digestible Energy (kcal/kg)
Corn oil	100	—	—	—	9000
Buckeye Nutrition Ultimate Finish	25	27.0	25.2	12	4356
Buckeye Nutrition SHINE 'N WIN	30	7.0	—	20	7260
Buckeye Nutrition Ultimate Finish Rice Bran	20	26.0	—	13	4070
Buckeye Nutrition Ultimate Finish 100	99	0	0	0	8580
Buckeye Nutrition Ultimate Finish 40	40	17.5	12.5	14	4510
Buckeye Nutrition Ultimate Finish 25	25	27.0	25.2	12	4356
Nutrena Equine Nutrition Empower	22	22.1	24.1	12	3380
Purina Mills Athlete	14	45.0–48.0	43.0	14	4182
Purina Mills Amplify	30	21.0–24.0	17.0	14	4400
Triple Crown Nutrition Rice Bran	20	23.2	16.2	13	3300–3960
Triple Crown Nutrition Rice Bran Oil Plus	98	—	—	—	8800

glucose uptake and glycogen storage in muscle. In horses with RER, high dietary NSC has been associated with excitability, a strong triggering factor for rhabdomyolysis in horses with this condition.[10]

An appropriate diet for horses with PSSM is designed to reduce glucose load and to promote the supply of fat-based substrates to exercising muscle tissue. A retrospective study in quarter horses identified a marked improvement in clinical signs associated with PSSM when a low starch, fat-supplemented diet was fed in combination with a regular exercise regimen.[5] Furthermore, a clinical trial in which horses with PSSM were fed a diet providing 4% of DE as starch and 13% of DE as fat documented normalization of 4-hour, post-exercise serum CK activity in the affected horses.[9] When the same horses were fed a diet providing 15% to 21% of DE as starch and 7% to 10% of energy as fat, a marked increase in serum CK activity was observed after exercise.[9] The beneficial effects of a low starch, fat-supplemented diet were potentially attributed to decreased glucose uptake and increased availability of free fatty acids to muscle fibers during aerobic metabolism.[9] Nevertheless, dietary manipulation alone may not successfully resolve clinical signs of rhabdomyolysis in quarter horses with PSSM, and concurrent institution of a regular exercise regimen is recommended.[5,48]

Draft horses with PSSM have been reported to display improvement in clinical signs in response to dietary fat supplementation;[8,47] however, controlled studies of dietary manipulation are needed in these breeds. Based on controlled studies of PSSM in quarter horses, the generally accepted rule is to provide a diet from which 10% or less of daily DE is provided by starch and a minimum of 13% of daily DE is supplied by fat. Some authorities anecdotally recommend that a minimum of 20% of daily DE intake be supplied as fat;[8] however, supplementation that exceeds caloric requirements may result in excessive body condition, which can be detrimental in performance horses.[74] Additionally, excessive fat supplementation may create unpalatable rations, promote digestive upsets, and potentially reduce the digestibility of other feed components. For horses with PSSM that are in good or excessive body condition, the provision of a diet with an energy content that does not exceed calculated or estimated DE requirements and that is high in fiber and low in starch, with additional moderate fat supplementation (~13% DE), may be the best compromise to avoid excessive weight gain.

In contrast to horses with PSSM, horses with RER appear to benefit from dietary fat supplementation only when the total DE intake is high, exceeding 21 Mcal DE/day. Rations with a high energy content based on starch can promote increased excitability and rhabdomyolysis in predisposed horses.[6,12,14] Horses with RER fed a high energy diet (28.8 Mcal DE/day) based on starch had significantly greater serum CK activity after exercise than when they consumed a lower energy diet (21.4 Mcal DE/day) in which additional calories were provided as either starch or fat.[12] Furthermore, horses with RER consuming two isocaloric high energy diets (28.8 Mcal DE/day) were shown to have post-exercise serum CK activity that was substantially lower and within normal range when 20% of DE was supplied as fat. In contrast, serum CK activity after exercise was significantly elevated above the normal range in the same horses when fat calories were substituted by starch.[6] Additionally, horses consuming the fat-supplemented diets had lower resting heart rates and packed cell volumes and were subjectively more tractable.[6,12] Given the close connection between a nervous temperament and tying-up in RER horses, modulating anxiety and nervousness by reducing dietary starch and increasing dietary fat may decrease the predisposition to episodes of rhabdomyolysis by making these horses calmer before exercise.[6,10] Current recommendations are to feed horses with RER requiring high energy intakes less than 20% of daily DE from starch sources and 15% to 25% of DE from fat sources, depending on daily energy requirements.[58]

Impact of Fat Supplementation

Studies indicate that horses can be fed a fat-supplemented ration for long periods of time with no negative effects;[75] however, the time required to elicit improvement in horses with exertional rhabdomyolysis has not been clearly elucidated. It has been suggested that dietary control of exertional rhabdomyolysis may require several months in horses with PSSM.[76] Nevertheless, clinical impressions suggest a beneficial effect may occur in some horses within weeks. Furthermore, establishing a structured exercise regimen may result in improvement within several weeks regardless of dietary fat supplementation.[5] PSSM horses that are stall confined and that consume a forage-based diet may still have persistent increases in serum CK activity; therefore, the success of dietary intervention and the avoidance of unnecessary weight gain in horses with PSSM requires limited periods of confinement (less than 12 hours at a time) with turnout or forced exercise.[5,48]

Horses with RER fed a diet providing 20% of DE as fat and 9% of DE as starch displayed significant reductions in, or normalization of, post-exercise serum CK activity within 1 week of commencing the fat-supplemented diet, with no alterations in muscle lactate and glycogen concentrations.[6] Rhabdomyolysis did not abate when these horses consumed an isocaloric diet providing 40% of DE as starch. It was suggested that the rapid improvement might relate to neurohormonal changes reducing anxiety and decreasing the occurrence of stress-induced rhabdomyolysis in the predisposed horses.[6] While the horses were consuming the fat-supplemented diet, post-exercise serum CK activity was significantly higher when exercise occurred after 2 consecutive days of stall rest when compared with the values obtained after the horses performed consecutive days of the same amount of submaximal exercise; therefore, dietary manipulation should be accompanied by management strategies that minimize stall rest. It is possible that exercise exerts beneficial effects on horses with chronic exertional rhabdomyolysis that are separate from the impact of dietary intervention, and the failure to implement an appropriate exercise routine may compromise attempts to control rhabdomyolysis in predisposed horses.

Vitamins, Electrolytes, Minerals, and Dietary Additives

A wide variety of dietary supplements and additives have been recommended for the management of horses with chronic rhabdomyolysis, particularly sodium bicarbonate.[77] To date, no specific dietary additives have proven to be efficacious. Deficiencies of vitamin E and selenium have not been identified in affected horses, and further supplementation with these substances has not been beneficial.[78] For mature horses, the ration should likely provide 1 IU/kg BW per day of vitamin E and 1 to 3 mg (total) of selenium per day.[67] Additional vitamin E (100–200 IU/100 g of added oil) is recommended for prophylaxis against oxidant stress when oil is directly added to the ration.[79]

Chronic rhabdomyolysis has previously been attributed to dietary electrolyte and mineral imbalances, specifically deficiencies of sodium, potassium, and calcium.[55,56] Dietary deficiencies of these substances can be determined via ration analysis or by determining the fractional excretion (FE) of these individual substances in urine. Such procedures should be considered wherever it is possible that dietary electrolyte or mineral composition may be initiating or exacerbating episodes of rhabdomyolysis. FE values can be determined via measurement of the specific substance in question in simultaneously obtained urine and serum samples using the following equation:

$$FE\%(x) = \frac{[Cr]serum}{[Cr]urine} \times \frac{[X]urine}{[X]serum} \times 100$$

where *Cr* and *X* are creatinine and electrolyte or mineral concentrations, respectively, in urine or serum.[80] Confidence intervals (95%) for urine FE values based on noncentrifuged and acidified urine samples are as follows: sodium, 0.1%–0.55%; potassium, 18.0%–51.5%; chloride, 0.1%–1.4%; calcium, 6.0%–15.0%; phosphorus, 0%–5.0%; and magnesium, 7.8%–22.5%.[81] Serum and urine samples for analysis of FE values should be obtained once a day for 3 days and preferably at the same stage of the horse's daily routine because considerable within day variation in urinary electrolyte and mineral excretion can occur. Samples can be pooled or the results of the three analyses averaged. Urine should be analyzed by flame photometry or emission spectrophotometry techniques because high potassium concentrations may interfere with ion-specific electrode measurement of urine sodium concentrations. Additionally, urine samples should not be obtained following administration of alpha-2 agonist sedatives or diuretics, and samples should be acidified and not centrifuged before analysis of calcium, phosphorus, and magnesium to dissolve mineral-containing urine crystals.[81] FE values below the reported ranges are suggestive of conservation and possibly inadequate dietary intake that may require supplementation.[55]

Heavily exercised horses should be supplemented appropriately for electrolytes and minerals through the addition of sodium-, potassium-, and chloride-containing salts to the ration at a ratio approximating 2:1:4, respectively.[82] Supplementation should be regulated according to the ambient temperature and duration of exercise, but horses working in moderate-to-hot conditions can lose 50 to 100 g of electrolytes per hour of intense exercise (primarily sodium and chloride).[82,83] Provision of a salt block to exercising horses does not constitute adequate supplementation due to inconsistent voluntary intake.

Additional Management Strategies

Instituting a daily exercise routine, commencing with exercise of a duration and intensity that can be tolerated without clinical signs of muscle pain, will greatly assist control of exertional rhabdomyolysis, especially in horses with PSSM.[5,48] Stall confinement should be minimized, preferably not exceeding 12 hours per day, and pasture turnout is ideal. In horses with RER, management strategies to reduce stress and anxiety may help reduce the frequency of episodes of rhabdomyolysis. Maximizing turnout time, exercising or feeding affected horses before other horses, and providing compatible equine company may be beneficial. Low dose tranquillization may also be of benefit for anxious horses during training.[84]

Supplemental feeds should be reduced in amount on days when energy demands decline, particularly if the horse is at risk of weight gain. Dietary strategies that decrease the intensity of the postprandial glycemic response may be particularly important in horses with PSSM and include feeding small meals, providing at least 1.5% to 2.0% of body weight per day in forage, and feeding forage or a fat source concurrently with any grain.[85,86] High starch supplements such as molasses should be avoided. Additionally, it may be beneficial to avoid feeding grain in the 2 to 3 hours preceding exercise, because carbohydrate feeding may inhibit lipid oxidation in the muscle cell, possibly contributing to the occurrence of rhabdomyolysis in horses with PSSM.[87]

SUMMARY

The optimum diet for horses with chronic exertional rhabdomyolysis should consist of a good quality forage source, a fat supplement, and adequate vitamins and minerals. For horses with PSSM, starch should be decreased to less than 10% of daily DE intake by eliminating high starch concentrates and molasses. Rice bran, fat-fortified concentrates, fat supplements, or oil can be gradually introduced to supply at least 13% of daily DE intake as fat. Horses with RER consuming a high caloric intake will benefit from a diet providing no more than 20% of daily DE intake as starch and 20% to 25% of DE as fat. Although some grain concentrates may be added to the diet to achieve high caloric intakes, horses with RER should not receive more than 5 pounds of grain per day. Additionally, optimum success of dietary manipulation, particularly in horses with PSSM, requires institution of a regular daily exercise regimen.

REFERENCES

1. Valberg SJ, Mickelson JR, Gallant EM, et al. Exertional rhabdomyolysis in quarter horses and thoroughbreds: one syndrome, multiple aetiologies. Equine Vet J 1999;30:533–8.
2. Aleman M. A review of equine muscle disorders. Neuromuscul Disord 2008;18(4): 277–87.
3. McCue ME, Valberg SJ, Miller MB, et al. Glycogen synthase (GYS1) mutation causes a novel skeletal muscle glycogenosis. Genomics 2008;91(5):458–66.

4. McCue ME, Valberg SJ, Jackson M, et al. The polysaccharide storage myopathy phenotype in quarter horse–related breeds is modified by an RYR1 mutation [abstract no. 172]. In: Proceedings of the ACVIM Forum, San Antonio, 2008.
5. Firshman AM, Valberg SJ, Bender JB, et al. Epidemiologic characteristics and management of polysaccharide storage myopathy in quarter horses. Am J Vet Res 2003;64(10):1319–27.
6. McKenzie EC, Valberg SJ, Godden SM, et al. Effect of dietary starch, fat and bicarbonate content on exercise responses and serum creatine kinase activity in equine recurrent exertional rhabdomyolysis. J Vet Intern Med 2003;17(5): 693–701.
7. De La Corte FD, Valberg SJ, MacLeay JM, et al. The effect of feeding a fat supplement to horses with polysaccharide storage myopathy. World Equine Veterinary Review 1999;4:12–9.
8. Valentine BA, Van Saun RJ, Thompson KN, et al. Role of dietary carbohydrate and fat in horses with equine polysaccharide storage myopathy. J Am Vet Med Assoc 2001;219(11):1537–44.
9. Ribeiro W, Valberg SJ, Pagan JD, et al. The effect of varying dietary starch and fat content on creatine kinase activity and substrate availability in equine polysaccharide storage myopathy. J Vet Intern Med 2004;18(6):887–94.
10. MacLeay JM, Sorum SA, Valberg SJ, et al. Epidemiologic analysis of factors influencing exertional rhabdomyolysis in thoroughbreds. Am J Vet Res 1999;60(12): 1562–6.
11. MacLeay JM, Valberg SJ, Pagan JD, et al. Effect of diet on thoroughbred horses with recurrent exertional rhabdomyolysis performing a standardised exercise test. Equine Vet J 1999;30:458–62.
12. MacLeay JM, Valberg SJ, Pagan JD, et al. Effect of ration and exercise on plasma creatine kinase activity and lactate concentration in thoroughbred horses with recurrent exertional rhabdomyolysis. Am J Vet Res 2000;61(11):1390–5.
13. McGowan CM, Posner RE, Christley RM, et al. Incidence of exertional rhabdomyolysis in polo horses in the USA and the United Kingdom in the 1999/2000 season. Vet Rec 2002;150:535–7.
14. McGowan CM, Fordham T, Christley RM, et al. Incidence and risk factors for exertional rhabdomyolysis in thoroughbred racehorses in the United Kingdom. Vet Rec 2002;151:623–6.
15. Beech J. Chronic exertional rhabdomyolysis. Vet Clin North Am Equine Pract 1997;13(1):145–68.
16. Harris PA. The equine rhabdomyolysis syndrome in the United Kingdom: epidemiological and clinical descriptive information. Br Vet J 1991;147(4):373–84.
17. Schmitz DG. Toxic nephropathy in horses. Compendium on Continuing Education for the Practicing Veterinarian 1988;10(1):104–10.
18. Sprayberry KA, Madigan J, LeCouteur RA, et al. Renal failure, laminitis and colitis following severe rhabdomyolysis in a draft horse cross with polysaccharide storage myopathy. Can Vet J 1998;39(8):500–3.
19. Valberg S, Haggendal J, Lindholm A, et al. Blood chemistry and skeletal muscle metabolic responses to exercise in horses with recurrent exertional rhabdomyolysis. Equine Vet J 1993;25(1):17–22.
20. Valberg SJ, Geyer C, Sorum SA, et al. Familial basis of exertional rhabdomyolysis in quarter horse–related breeds. Am J Vet Res 1996;57(3):286–90.
21. MacLeay JM, Valberg SJ, Sorum SA, et al. Heritability of recurrent exertional rhabdomyolysis in thoroughbred racehorses. Am J Vet Res 1999;60(2): 250–6.

22. Collinder E, Lindholm A, Rasmuson M, et al. Genetic markers in standardbred trotters susceptible to the rhabdomyolysis syndrome. Equine Vet J 1997;29(2): 117–20.
23. Dranchak PK, Valberg SJ, Onan GW, et al. Inheritance of recurrent exertional rhabdomyolysis in thoroughbreds. J Am Vet Med Assoc 2005;227(5):762–7.
24. Valberg SJ, Cardinet GH, Carlson GP, et al. Polysaccharide storage myopathy associated with recurrent exertional rhabdomyolysis in horses. Neuromuscul Disord 1992;2(5-6):351–9.
25. Valberg SJ, MacLeay JM, Mickelson JR, et al. Exertional rhabdomyolysis and polysaccharide storage myopathy in horses. Compendium on Continuing Education for the Practicing Veterinarian 1997;19:1077–86.
26. Valentine BA, Credille KM, Lavoie JP, et al. Severe polysaccharide storage myopathy in Belgian and Percheron draught horses. Equine Vet J 1997;29(3):220–5.
27. Valentine BA. Polysaccharide storage myopathy in draft and draft-related horses and ponies. Equine Pract 1999;21:16–9.
28. Valentine BA, McDonough SP, Chang YF, et al. Polysaccharide storage myopathy in Morgan, Arabian, and Standardbred related horses and Welsh-cross ponies. Vet Pathol 2000;37(2):193–6.
29. Valentine BA, Habecker PL, Patterson JS, et al. Incidence of polysaccharide storage myopathy in draft horse–related breeds: a necropsy study of 37 horses and a mule. J Vet Diagn Invest 2001;13(1):63–8.
30. Bloom BA, Valentine BA, Gleed RD, et al. Postanaesthetic recumbency in a Belgian filly with polysaccharide storage myopathy. Vet Rec 1999;144: 73–5.
31. Firshman AM, Baird JD, Valberg SJ, et al. Prevalences and clinical signs of polysaccharide storage myopathy and shivers in Belgian draft horses. J Am Vet Med Assoc 2005;227(12):1958–64.
32. Quiroz-Rothe E, Novales M, Guilera-Tejero E, et al. Polysaccharide storage myopathy in the M. longissimus lumborum of show jumpers and dressage horses with back pain. Equine Vet J 2002;34(2):171–6.
33. McCue ME, Ribeiro WP, Valberg SJ, et al. Prevalence of polysaccharide storage myopathy in horses with neuromuscular disorders. Equine Vet J 2006;36:340–4.
34. Lindholm A, Johansson HE, Kjaersgaard P, et al. Acute rhabdomyolysis ("tying-up") in standardbred horses: a morphological and biochemical study. Acta Vet Scand 1974;15:325–39.
35. Valberg SJ. Diseases of muscles. In: Smith BP, editor. Large animal internal medicine. Fourth edition. St. Louis (MO): Mosby Elsevier; 2008. p. 1388–418.
36. McCue ME, Valberg SJ. Estimated prevalence of polysaccharide storage myopathy among overtly healthy quarter horses in the United States. J Am Vet Med Assoc 2007;231(5):746–50.
37. Valberg SJ, Townsend D, Mickelson JR, et al. Skeletal muscle glycolytic capacity and phosphofructokinase regulation in horses with polysaccharide storage myopathy. Am J Vet Res 1998;59(6):782–5.
38. Annandale EJ, Valberg SJ, Essen-Gustavsson B, et al. Effects of submaximal exercise on adenine nucleotide concentrations in skeletal muscle fibers of horses with polysaccharide storage myopathy. Am J Vet Res 2005;66(5):839–45.
39. Annandale EJ, Valberg SJ, Mickelson JR, et al. Insulin sensitivity and skeletal muscle glucose transport in horses with equine polysaccharide storage myopathy. Neuromuscul Disord 2004;14(10):666–74.
40. De La Corte FD, Valberg SJ, MacLeay JM, et al. Glucose uptake in horses with polysaccharide storage myopathy. Am J Vet Res 1999;60(4):458–62.

41. De La Corte FD, Valberg SJ, Mickelson JR, et al. Blood glucose clearance after feeding and exercise in polysaccharide storage myopathy. Equine Vet J 1999;30: 324–8.
42. De La Corte FD, Valberg SJ, MacLeay JM, et al. Developmental onset of polysaccharide storage myopathy in 4 Quarter Horse foals. J Vet Intern Med 2002;16(5): 581–7.
43. Firshman AM, Valberg SJ, Bender JB, et al. Comparison of histopathologic criteria and skeletal muscle fixation techniques for the diagnosis of polysaccharide storage myopathy in horses. Vet Pathol 2006;43:257–69.
44. Firshman AM, Valberg SJ, Baird JD, et al. Insulin sensitivity in Belgian horses with polysaccharide storage myopathy. Am J Vet Res 2008;69(6):818–23.
45. Valentine BA. Diagnosis and treatment of equine polysaccharide storage myopathy. Journal of Equine Veterinary Science 2005;25:52–61.
46. Valentine BA, de Lahunta A, Divers TJ, et al. Clinical and pathologic findings in two draft horses with progressive muscle atrophy, neuromuscular weakness, and abnormal gait characteristic of shivers syndrome. J Am Vet Med Assoc 1999;215:1661–5.
47. Valentine BA. Equine polysaccharide storage myopathy. Equine Veterinary Education 2003;11:326–34.
48. Hunt LM, Valberg SJ, Steffenhagen K, et al. An epidemiological study of myopathies in warm blood horses. Equine Vet J 2008;40(2):171–7.
49. Lentz LR, Valberg SJ, Balog EM, et al. Abnormal regulation of muscle contraction in horses with recurrent exertional rhabdomyolysis. Am J Vet Res 1999;60(8):992–9.
50. Lentz LR, Valberg SJ, Herold LV, et al. Myoplasmic calcium regulation in myotubes from horses with recurrent exertional rhabdomyolysis. Am J Vet Res 2002;63(12):1724–31.
51. Waldron-Mease E. Correlation of postoperative and exercise-induced equine myopathy with the defect malignant hyperthermia. Proceedings of the American Association of Equine Practitioners 1978;24:95–9.
52. Aleman M, Riehl J, Aldridge BM, et al. Association of a mutation in the ryanodine receptor 1 gene with equine malignant hyperthermia. Muscle Nerve 2004;30: 356–65.
53. Carlson GP. Medical problems associated with protracted heat and work stress in horses. Compendium on Continuing Education for the Practicing Veterinarian 1985;7:S542–50.
54. Geor RJ, McCutcheon LJ. Thermoregulation and clinical disorders associated with exercise and heat stress. Comp Contin Educ Pract Vet 1996;18:18436–44.
55. Harris P, Colles C. The use of creatinine clearance ratios in the prevention of equine rhabdomyolysis: a report of four cases. Equine Vet J 1988;20(6):459–63.
56. Harris PA, Snow DH. Role of electrolyte imbalances in the pathophysiology of the equine rhabdomyolysis syndrome. In: Persson SGB, editor. Equine exercise physiology 3. Davis (CA): ICEEP Publications; 1991. p. 435–42.
57. Harris PA. An outbreak of the equine rhabdomyolysis syndrome in a racing yard. Vet Rec 1990;127:468–70.
58. McKenzie EC, Valberg SJ, Pagan JD. Nutritional management of exertional rhabdomyolysis. In: Robinson NE, editor. Current therapy in equine medicine 5. St. Louis (MO): Saunders; 2003. p. 727–34.
59. Finno CJ, Spier SJ, Valberg SJ, et al. Equine diseases caused by known genetic mutations. Vet J 2008; May 8 [Epub ahead of print].
60. De La Corte F, Valberg SJ. Treatment of polysaccharide storage myopathy. Compend Cont Educ Pract Vet 2000;22:782–8.

61. Valberg SJ, MacLeay JM, Billstrom JA, et al. Skeletal muscle metabolic response to exercise in horses with "tying-up" due to polysaccharide storage myopathy. Equine Vet J 1999;31(1):43–7.
62. Valberg S, Jonsson L, Lindholm A, et al. Muscle histopathology and plasma aspartate aminotransferase, creatine kinase and myoglobin changes with exercise in horses with recurrent exertional rhabdomyolysis. Equine Vet J 1993; 25(1):11–6.
63. Farrow FA, Roloff DH, Westman CW, et al. Treatment for azoturia and tying-up. Mod Vet Pract 1976;57(1):413–6.
64. Harris PA. Equine rhabdomyolysis syndrome. In: Robinson NE, editor. Current therapy in equine medicine 4. Philadelphia: WB Saunders; 1987. p. 115–21.
65. Carlstrom B. The etiology and pathogenesis in horses with haemoglobinaemia paralytica. Acta Physiologica Scandinavica 1932;63:164–212.
66. Wilson TM, Morrison HA, Palmer NC, et al. Myodegeneration and suspected selenium/vitamin E deficiency in horses. J Am Vet Med Assoc 1976;169(2):213–7.
67. National Research Council. Nutrient requirements of horses. Sixth revised edition. Washington, DC: National Academies Press; 2007.
68. Hintz HF. Nutrition and equine performance. J Nutr 1994;124:2723S–9S.
69. Rich GA, Fontenot JP, Meacham TN, et al. Digestibility of animal, vegetable and blended fats by the equine. In: Proceedings of the 7th Equine Nutrition and Physiology Symposium. Warrenton; 1981;7:30.
70. Harkins JD, Morris GS, Tulley RT, et al. Effect of added dietary fat on racing performance in thoroughbred horses. J Equine Vet Sci 1992;12:123–9.
71. Scott BD, Potter GD, Greene LW, et al. Efficacy of a fat-supplemented diet to reduce thermal stress in exercising thoroughbred horses. In: Proceedings of the 13th Equine Nutrition and Physiology Symposium. 1993;66–9.
72. Kronfeld DS. Dietary fat affects heat production and other variables of equine performance under hot and humid conditions. Equine Vet J 1996; 22:24–34.
73. Holland JL, Kronfeld DS, Meacham TN. Behavior of horses is affected by soy lecithin and corn oil in the diet. J Anim Sci 1996;74:1252–5.
74. Lawrence L, Jackson S, Kline K, et al. Observations on body weight and condition of horses in a 150 mile endurance ride. J Equine Vet Sci 1992;12:320–4.
75. Pagan JD, Burger I, Jackson SG, et al. The long term effects of feeding fat to 2-year-old thoroughbreds in training. Equine Vet J 1995;18:343–8.
76. Valentine BA, Hintz HF, Freels KM, et al. Dietary control of exertional rhabdomyolysis in horses. J Am Vet Med Assoc 1998;212(10):1588–93.
77. Robb EJ, Kronfeld DS. Dietary sodium bicarbonate as a treatment for exertional rhabdomyolysis in a horse. J Am Vet Med Assoc 1986;188(6):602–7.
78. Roneus B, Hakkarainen J. Vitamin E in serum and skeletal muscle tissue and blood glutathione peroxidase activity from horses with the azoturia tying-up syndrome. Acta Vet Scand 1985;26:425–7.
79. Siciliano PD, Wood CH. The effect of added dietary soybean oil on vitamin E status of the horse. J Anim Sci 1993;71:3399–402.
80. Morris DD, Divers TJ, Whitlock RH, et al. Renal clearance and fractional excretion of electrolytes over a 24-hour period in horses. Am J Vet Res 1984;45:2431–5.
81. McKenzie EC, Valberg SJ, Godden SM, et al. Comparison of volumetric urine collection versus single sample urine collection in horses consuming diets varying in cation-anion balance. J Vet Intern Med 2002;16(3):336.
82. McCutcheon LJ, Geor RJ. Sweating: fluid and ion losses and replacement. Vet Clin North Am Equine Pract 1998;14(1):75–95.

83. McCutcheon LJ, Geor RJ. Sweat fluid and ion losses in horses during training and competition in cool vs. hot ambient conditions: implications for ion supplementation. Equine Vet J 1996;22:54–62.
84. Freestone JF, Kamerling SG, Church G, et al. Exercise induced changes in creatine kinase and aspartate aminotransferase activities in the horse: effects of conditioning, exercise tests and acepromazine. J Equine Vet Sci 1989;9:275–80.
85. Pagan JD, Harris PA. The effects of timing and amount of forage and grain on exercise response in thoroughbred horses. Equine Vet J 1999;30:451–7.
86. Stull CL, Rodiek AV. Responses of blood glucose, insulin and cortisol concentrations to common equine diets. J Nutr 1988;118:206–13.
87. Jose-Cunilleras E, Hinchcliff KW, Sams RA, et al. Glycemic index of a meal fed before exercise alters substrate use and glucose flux in exercising horses. J Appl Phys 2002;92(1):117–28.

Feeding Management of Elite Endurance Horses

Patricia Harris, MA, PhD, VetMB, MRCVS

KEYWORDS

- Endurance racing • Electrolytes • Forage
- Oil supplementation • Antioxidants

The sport of endurance racing is probably the most demanding of the equine athletic disciplines, with horses required to complete distances of up to 160 km in a single day (and longer distances during multiday races). Furthermore, particularly at the international level, the recent trend has been for very high racing speeds. The winner of the 2005 World Equine Endurance Championship race in Dubai covered the 160 km distance at an average speed of 22.5 km per hour (~14 mph). These high work rates pose several challenges for the endurance horse. First, high energy demands may result in the depletion of substrate stores, particularly muscle and liver glycogen, resulting in poor performance. Second, because the evaporation of sweat is the major mechanism for heat dissipation during exercise, there is a substantial loss of body water and electrolytes (especially sodium and chloride). Failure to mitigate the resultant dehydration and electrolyte disturbances via replacement strategies is another potential reason for poor performance and elimination from the race. Additionally, dehydration and electrolyte imbalances increase the risk for metabolic problems, including heat stress, synchronous diaphragmatic flutter, and rhabdomyolysis. In a recent survey of horses that participated in 16 Concours de Raid d'Endurance International or Concours de Raid d'Endurance National events in France, 48% of the horses were disqualified during the races: 51.8% because of lameness, 29.3% for metabolic reasons (with 12.5% of the starters requiring veterinary care), and 12.7% for other causes.[1] It can be argued that appropriate nutritional management may help reduce the incidence of metabolic problems that result in race disqualification or the need for veterinary intervention.

Because several factors influence the choice of feeding program for an individual endurance horse (eg, temperament, housing [pasture versus confinement], the level of training and competition, and owner/rider preference), there is no single correct

WALTHAM Centre for Pet Nutrition, Freeby Lane, Waltham-on-the-Wolds, Melton Mowbray, Leicestershire LE14 4RT, United Kingdom
E-mail address: pat.harris@eu.effem.com

Vet Clin Equine 25 (2009) 137–153
doi:10.1016/j.cveq.2009.01.005

way to feed an endurance horse. Nonetheless, a few general principles should guide the development of a diet and feeding plan. This article reviews guidelines for the feeding management of endurance horses.

ENERGY METABOLISM

For athletic horses, the supply of energy from the diet is crucial for maintenance of body weight plus condition for storage and availability of the substrates needed to fuel muscular work. An increase in energy (ie, caloric) intake is required for avoidance of weight loss and probably loss of performance in the face of the increased energy demands of training and competition. In addition, some evidence suggests that the source of dietary energy can affect the storage and use of the primary substrates used to fuel muscular work, namely, glycogen (liver, skeletal muscle) and fat.

The body condition score (BCS) and body fat content may influence performance during endurance rides. In one study of horses that competed in a 150-mile ride, the average BCS (scale of 1–9) was 4.67, and the percentage of body fat estimated from ultrasound assessment of rump fat thickness was 7.8%.[2] Among the top finishers, the estimated total fat was approximately 6.5% of body mass, whereas the fat content of nonfinishers averaged approximately 11%. In another study, the mean BCS of horses that completed the 100-mile Tevis Cup ride was 4.5 (measurement taken pre-ride); all horses with a BCS of less than 3 failed to complete.[3] Horses eliminated for metabolic reasons had a mean pre-ride BCS of 2.9 compared with a BCS of 4.5 for those disqualified for nonmetabolic problems such as lameness. It was suggested that, at least in more difficult rides such as the Tevis Cup, thin horses (ie, BCS <3) might be at a disadvantage because of lower energy reserves (and potentially lower muscle mass) when compared with horses with a higher body condition. Overconditioned horses (BCS >6) also could have problems due to the extra weight carried plus the insulating effect (impairment to heat dissipation) of the additional subcutaneous adipose tissue.[1,3] In general, feeding programs for endurance horses should target a BCS of approximately 4 to 4.5 on the 9-point scale.

The capacity for endurance exercise is dependent on the availability of substrate for the synthesis of ATP, the cell's energy "currency." Stored energy in the form of muscle and liver glycogen, intramuscular and adipose triglycerides, along with glucose and fatty acids derived from the feed ingested during longer rides are used for synthesis in working tissues. It has been estimated that a 450-kg horse has around 1400 to 2800 g of muscle triglyceride, 40,000 g of adipose triglyceride, 3000 to 4000 g of muscle glycogen (1%–2% skeletal muscle weight), and 100 to 200 g of liver glycogen.[4] Fat stores are therefore comparatively large, and it is currently thought that fatigue during endurance racing in horses is due to depletion of muscle and liver glycogen stores[5,6] combined with fluid and electrolyte disturbances.[7]

At low-to-moderate work intensities, oxidative phosphorylation (aerobic metabolism) of glucose and fatty acids is an efficient mechanism for regeneration of ATP. At higher workloads (eg, canter and gallop), ATP demand cannot be met by oxidative metabolism alone, and nonoxidative breakdown (anaerobic metabolism) of glycogen and glucose (fatty acids cannot be metabolized by anaerobic mechanisms) contributes to ATP resynthesis. Anaerobic glycogenolysis is far less efficient in terms of ATP yield per gram of glucose metabolized and results in lactic acid accumulation within skeletal muscle, which contributes to the development of fatigue.[7] Historically, aerobic metabolism of fatty acids has been thought to predominate during endurance rides undertaken at an average speed of 12 to 14 km per hour (8–9 mph), with a shift to anaerobic metabolism for only brief periods of time (eg, during controlled sprints that some riders use at the beginning or the end of the ride or when hill climbing). This assumption may not apply to contemporary elite level endurance racing wherein the more sustained periods of high-speed running invoke a larger contribution from anaerobic metabolism and greater demands for use of the more limited body glycogen stores. Even with the low rate of glycogen use during submaximal exercise (<10 mph), if such exercise is sufficiently long term, muscle glycogen stores may be depleted by more than 50% to 75%.[8] There is increasing interest in the application of strategies (eg, diet, training, racing strategy) that might reduce the speed or extent of this glycogen depletion.

ENERGY REQUIREMENTS

Energy requirements for horses are most commonly expressed as megacalories (Mcal) or megajoules (MJ) of digestible energy (DE), where 1 Mcal = 4.184 MJ. For an endurance horse, energy needs depend not only on work duration and intensity but also on factors such as the environmental conditions, terrain, weight of the rider and tack, ability of the rider, and fitness of the horse.[4,9] In general terms, the requirement is the sum of maintenance requirements plus an allowance for the work being undertaken. Maintenance DE requirements for a 450-kg endurance horse[9] are around 13.6 to 16.3 Mcal per day (~57–68 MJ per day). Training or competition requirements depend on the weight of the horse plus rider and tack as well as the speed of work[5,8,9] as illustrated in **Table 1**.[10] A 450-kg horse (plus 75 kg for the rider and tack) given a 3-hour training ride at a medium trot (~250 m/min) would have an estimated additional DE requirement of 15 Mcal (63 MJ), giving a total requirement of approximately 29 to 31 Mcal (~120–130 MJ) for that day. The most recent National Research Council (NRC) publication on nutrient requirements for horses[9] includes elite endurance horses in the very heavy work category, for which the energy requirement is estimated as follows: DE (Mcal/d) = (0.0363 × BW) × 1.9, giving a value of ~31Mcal/d (130 MJ) for a 450-kg horse. In a US survey of aspiring international level competitors,[11] the average estimated daily DE intake (from forage and supplementary feeds) during training was 24 Mcal (~100 MJ); however, many of the horses surveyed were kept at pasture, and the estimate did not account for DE intake from pasture forage.

Horses are individuals; therefore, actual DE requirements may deviate from calculated estimates and vary widely among horses of similar body weight undertaking

Table 1
A guide to potential digestible energy requirements above maintenance at various speeds

Gait	Speed (m/min)	DE Mcal/kg BW (of Horse Plus Rider Plus Tack)/h	DE MJ/kg BW (of Horse Plus Rider Plus Tack)/h
Slow walk	59	0.0017	0.0071
Fast walk	95	0.0025	0.0105
Slow trot	200	0.0065	0.0272
Medium trot	250	0.0095	0.03975
Fast trot/slow canter	300	0.0137	0.0573
Medium canter	350	0.0195	0.0816

DE (kJ per kilogram of horse, rider, and tack) = $4.184 \times \{[e^{(3.02 + 0.0065Y)} - 13.92] \times 0.06\}/0.57$ where Y is the speed (meters per minute) and 0.57 accounts for the efficiency of utilization of DE.

Abbreviation: BW, body weight.

Data from Pagan JD, Hintz HF. Equine energetics. II. Energy expenditure in horses during submaximal exercise. J Anim Sci 1986;63: 822–30.

the same amount and type of work. From a practical aspect, weekly or biweekly monitoring and assessment of body weight or BCS[12] will enable the feeding program to be individually tailored.

MEETING ENERGY REQUIREMENTS

The four main sources of energy[4] in horse feeds are as follows:

Hydrolysable carbohydrates (eg, simple sugars and starches): These substances can be digested by mammalian enzymes to hexoses which are absorbed from the small intestine. If they escape digestion in the small intestine, they are rapidly fermented in the hindgut (ie, cecum and colon).

Fermentable fiber (cellulose, hemicelluloses, and pectins): These components are not digestible by mammalian enzymes but can be fermented by the microorganisms predominantly located in the hindgut. The speed of fermentation and site likely influence the energy value to the horse.

Oils/fats: Although horses evolved on diets with low concentrations of oils and fats, they are able to digest and use up to 20% of the diet (dry matter basis) as oil if suitably introduced (see further comments below).

Protein: Protein is not primarily fed as an energy source because the metabolism of amino acids to useable energy is inefficient relative to that of carbohydrates and fats.

Different feeds and feedstuffs contain differing amounts of gross energy. The efficiency of conversion from gross to useable or net energy also differs widely[13] between feedstuffs and between individual animals. Vegetable oils provide proportionally more net energy than cereal grains (approximately two and one half times as much DE as maize/corn and three times as much as oats). Cereal grains, in turn, provide more net energy than hay, whereas the net energy from hay is twofold higher than that available from straw.[13]

Forage Should be the Foundation

Forage should be the foundation of the diet for all horses. In the aforementioned US survey of feeding practices,[11] about 80% of the horses had 24-hour pasture turnout (with additional preserved forage provided some of the year). On average, 78% of the ration was forage, which is much higher in comparison with the diet of other types of sports horses (eg, the ration of racehorses may be no more than 30% forage). Although there is no agreement on the recommended amount of dietary fiber, the inclusion of some long-stem roughage in the diet is thought to be important for the maintenance of hindgut function and health and for a reduction in the risk of gastric ulceration and abnormal behaviors.[14,15] Fiber may provide energy during an endurance ride as fermentation of fiber and absorption of volatile fatty acids (acetate, propionate) continues long after the fiber has been ingested. Propionic acid from the hindgut fermentation of fiber is an important precursor for gluconeogenesis.[16]

Some fiber sources (eg, beet pulp, soya hulls) may augment the size of the large intestinal fluid reservoir, which may represent as much as 8% to 10% of body weight and 10% to 20% of total body Na, K, and Cl.[17,18] This increase in intestinal fluid may assist in the maintenance of hydration during exercise by acting as a reservoir for water and electrolytes.[17] Extrapolating from studies in ponies[17] during low intensity exercise, approximately 10 L of water, 19 g of Na, and 10 g of Cl may be absorbed from the gastrointestinal tract of horses during 2 to 3 hours of exercise, potentially offsetting some of the sweat fluid losses that occur during endurance rides.[19] Recent work has suggested that differences in fiber type, which affect total body water, might influence core temperature during endurance type exercise;[20] however, the potential benefits of a high-fiber diet with respect to improved water and electrolyte balance must be weighed against possible energetic disadvantages associated with an increase in hindgut weight (bowel ballast). For example, in a 450-kg horse, an extra 4 kg in hay intake can be estimated to increase bowel ballast by between 10 and 24 kg.[21] The optimal mix of dietary fibers is not known, but it is common for endurance horses to consume a variety of fiber sources, including long-stem hay, beet pulp, and soya hulls.[22] Practical recommendations include the following:

- Feed at least 1.0 kg of forage (hay or equivalent—if haylage/silage is fed, the minimal amount needs to increase to ensure adequate fiber [and potassium] provision) per 100 kg of body weight and preferably 1.5 to 2.0 kg per 100 kg of body weight.
- Avoid very mature forages (due to reduced digestibility and possibly available water reservoir capacity).
- Select hay with a low-to-moderate protein content (ie, grass hay with crude protein of 8%–14%) rather than a legume hay (often with crude protein >20%) because of concerns regarding high protein intake. Select good quality grass hay or a grass/alfalfa mix in which alfalfa is no more than 30% of the mix.
- Avoid high intakes of calcium-rich forages (ie, alfalfa) due to the perceived increased risk of synchronous diaphragmatic flutter ("thumps") during endurance rides when horses are fed a high calcium ration.

Supplemental Energy Sources

Cereal grains

Many endurance horses are Arabian, at least in part, and tend to be "easy" keepers; however, even good quality pasture/preserved forage may not be sufficient to maintain body weight and condition. Some cereals are commonly required; the average amount in the aforementioned survey[11] was 2.27 kg per day. Higher quantities are likely to be required by horses engaged in heavier training and higher level racing.

Starch, a hydrolyzable carbohydrate, is the principal component of cereal grains (~50% of oats and 70% of corn). Large cereal-based meals may overwhelm the small intestine's relatively low capacity for starch hydrolysis, resulting in rapid fermentation of the starch reaching the hindgut with potential adverse clinical consequences.[23] In one study, providing around 400 g of oat starch per 100 kg of body weight in a single feeding/meal was suggested to saturate the small intestine's digestive capacity for starch.[24] Consequently, it has been recommended to feed no more than 300 g of starch per100 kg of body weight per meal.[25] More caution is required when feeding unprocessed corn or barley starch, which has substantially lower pre-cecal digestibility when compared with oat starch.[26] The pre-cecal starch digestibility of corn or barley starch is improved by heat treatment (cooking or micronization).[25,27] Regardless of the starch source, it is advisable to limit the size of individual grain-based meals to no more than 1.5 kg (for a 450-kg horse). Some nutritionists also advocate providing grain-based meals separately from a large meal of long fibrous hay due to concerns of lower pre-cecal starch digestibility when these feeds are ingested together.[28]

Highly digestible fiber sources

The feeding of sugar beet pulp and soya hulls to horses has gained popularity recently.[29] When compared with more traditional fiber sources such as hay, these highly digestible or "super fibers" contain lower indigestible material (eg, lignin) and higher amounts of nonstarch polysaccharides, pectins, and gums which can be digested to a large extent within the time period that they remain within the gastrointestinal tract. This digestibility translates to a higher energy yield.

Vegetable oils

Energy rich vegetable oils contain no starch or sugar and potentially may provide other advantages, including reduced heat production (important in conditions of high heat and humidity), a reduced amount of feed needed to achieve desired energy intake, and possible behavioral advantages.[4,9,23,30,31] Reduced bowel ballast due to the substitution of some cereals by oil helps to balance to a certain extent the recommendation for a high-fiber intake (which creates more bowel ballast) in endurance horses.

Of more interest is the potential for oil-supplemented diets to provide a more direct performance advantage. More than 30 years ago, it was reported that horses fed a diet containing 12% fat (9% added corn oil) and ridden 67 km over mountainous terrain for 8 to10 hours performed better and had higher blood glucose concentrations at the end of the ride than horses fed a control diet (3% fat).[32] Subsequent studies have demonstrated that oil supplementation is characterized by a dose-dependent increase in the activity of lipoprotein lipase and, in some reports, an increase in the activity of skeletal muscle citrate synthase and beta-hydroxy acyl-CoA dehydrogenase.[3,33] These alterations in enzyme activities may result in increased uptake and oxidation of free fatty acids in skeletal muscle.[34] Horses fed a diet providing 25% to 30% of DE from oil had a lower respiratory exchange ratio[33,34] and decreased glucose use[34] during low intensity exercise (~25%–35% VO_{2max}) than horses fed a control (nonsupplemented) ration. Another study that used compartmental modeling techniques to evaluate glucose kinetics observed that horses adapted to a fat and fiber supplement used less glucose during exercise (4 m/s on a treadmill) when compared with horses fed a starch-rich supplement.[35] Theoretically, this enhancement of lipid oxidation and sparing of plasma glucose use should result in muscle glycogen sparing and perhaps an increase in endurance performance. Preliminary work also suggests that adaptation to fat and fiber-rich feeds lowers serum insulin concentration during endurance rides in association with improved performance;[36] however, overall, the effect of diet composition on performance during endurance races remains equivocal.[4,9]

The ideal type (including the fatty acid profile) and the amount of vegetable oil for supplementation of horse diets have not been determined. Corn oil tends to be one of the most palatable,[37] but several other vegetable oils also show acceptable palatability providing they are fresh, not rancid, and of a good quality, preferably human grade. Any supplemental oil should be introduced slowly (over 14–21 days) to avoid intestinal disturbances, because the capacity to hydrolyze lipids appears to occur over time.[38] The equine pancreas has high lipase activity,[39] which might explain why horses are able to digest and use up to 20% or more of the diet as oil.[38] There is conflicting evidence regarding the effect of soya oil on fiber digestibility, with several studies[38] suggesting no effect and others[40] reporting depressed digestibility when soya oil represents 15% of dry matter intake. Practical recommendations are that vegetable oil should be 5% to 8% of the total diet (with 10% as an upper limit) if this level of energy is required. An alternative recommendation is to feed up to 100 g of oil per 100 kg of body weight per day. For reference, 450 mL of oil (~420 g) provides about 3.4 Mcal (14 MJ) of DE. This daily amount should be divided into two to three meals and introduced gradually (eg, starting at 50 mL/d). To obtain metabolic benefits of dietaryoil, it has been recommended that the oil be fed for several weeks if not months.[4,34]

With the exception of vitamin E (variable amounts), vegetable oils do not provide other nutrients. Indeed, adding oil to an existing ration has the potential to create multiple imbalances; therefore, it is recommended to feed a diet in which the oil has been balanced in relation to all of the essential nutrients in the feed. Alternatively, a vitamin/mineral supplement may be needed to achieve the desired balance and ensure that nutrient requirements are met. Although oil supplementation may enhance vitamin E absorption in horses,[41] studies in humans suggest that the requirement for vitamin E increases with increasing dietary polyunsaturated fatty acid content.[42] The increased fat oxidation that occurs during submaximal exercise following fat supplementation[33] is likely to increase the production of peroxyl free radicals and the need for additional dietary antioxidants. Based on studies in other species, it has been estimated that the vitamin E requirement is 0.6 mg of alpha-tocopherol per gram of linoleic acid and around 3 mg of alpha-tocopherol per gram of omega-3 polyunsaturated fatty acid.[43] Currently, the author recommends an additional 100 to 150 iu of vitamin E per 100 mL of added vegetable oil.

Muscle Glycogen Storage

During exercise, horses appear to rely more heavily on carbohydrate for energy transduction from muscle glycogen and blood glucose than humans.[44] Suboptimal liver and muscle glycogen content at the onset of exercise may reduce performance.[6,45] The carbohydrate-based nutritional strategies employed by human marathon runners to raise muscle glycogen levels (exercise-linked depletion followed by a high carbohydrate diet) do not appear to be of any value in the horse. Several studies have shown that diet has minimal impact on the slow rate of muscle glycogen restoration in the horse following glycogen-depleting exercise.[6,7,44,46] One study concluded that "after substantial exercise-induced muscle glycogen depletion (~55% of initial values) feeding status only minimally affects net muscle glycogen concentrations after exercise at 24 hours post" (the diets were no feed, high cereal grain, or a hay only diet fed 15 minutes and 4 hours post exercise).[46] Another study demonstrated that feeding large starch-rich meals at 8-hour intervals after glycogen-depleting exercise resulted in a modest increase in glycogen storage at 48 and 72 hours when compared with no feeding or a hay diet;[47] however, the risk-benefit of this aggressive grain-feeding practice is questionable.

A recent study reported that oral administration of a hypotonic electrolyte solution after prolonged moderate intensity exercise enhanced the rate of muscle glycogen storage when compared with no fluid treatment.[48] The investigators suggested that post exercise dehydration may be one factor that contributes to the slow muscle glycogen replenishment in horses.

TIMING OF FEEDING RELATIVE TO EXERCISE

Evidence from several studies suggests that the timing and composition of a meal consumed before exercise can influence the metabolic response in horses.[49,50] In particular, the hyperglycemia and insulinemia associated with the digestion and absorption of grain meals affects the mix of substrates used during a bout of exercise. Insulin is a potent inhibitor of lipolysis and fatty acid oxidation in skeletal muscle and also promotes glucose uptake into muscle via recruitment of the glucose transporter protein GLUT4 to the sarcolemma. Hyperinsulinemia at exercise onset will suppress free fatty acid availability and lipid oxidation and increase reliance on carbohydrate stores (including plasma glucose) for energy transduction. The decrease in plasma glucose that occurs when horses are exercised 2 to 3 hours after a grain meal tends to be relatively short term;[28] however, plasma free fatty acids and lipid oxidation may remain lower in fed animals when compared with the fasted state throughout certain types of exercise.[50] The impact of pre-exercise feeding may be more complex in endurance horses because they are fed at rest stops during rides. In this circumstance, exercise-associated alterations in hormones (eg, increased catecholamines, decreased insulin) may counterbalance the effect of hormonal changes induced by feeding.

Large meals (hay or grain/concentrate or mixtures) may result in a decrease in plasma volume as a result of fluid shifts into the gastrointestinal tract[28] and should be avoided. Although the effects of pre-exercise grain feeding on endurance exercise performance in the field have not been reported, the potential acceleration in carbohydrate oxidation and suppression of fat oxidation lead to the recommendation that grain or concentrate-based meals should not be fed within 3 hours of a race.

PROTEIN NUTRITION

Additional protein over maintenance amounts may be needed with exercise and training because of the accompanying muscular development, the need for muscle repair, and the need to replenish the nitrogen lost in sweat (~20–25 g/kg sweat loss). The precise protein requirements for exercise are unknown. The current NRC recommendations[9] are an average of 1.26 g of crude protein per kilogram of body weight per day for maintenance plus between 0.089 and 0.354 g of crude protein per kilogram of body weight per day depending on the exercise level to allow for muscle gain and then an allowance for nitrogen loss in the sweat. The author's current recommendations are to allow around 2.0 to 2.5 g of crude protein per kilogram of body weight per day. Some evidence suggests that the dietary protein level alters urea metabolism in the horse. It has been estimated that a change in dietary crude protein from 10% to 15% of dry matter intake would increase water requirements by approximately 5% because of an obligate increase in urine production for clearance of endogenous urea.[51] Higher protein diets may also be undesirable because of the effects of excess dietary protein on heat production, acid-base balance (especially as speeds increase), and possibly respiratory health (due to ammonia accumulation in confinement housing).[52] It has been recommended[53] that endurance horses should not be fed more than 2 g of digestible protein/kg BW/day (around 3–4 g CP depending on the feedstuffs), and some potential advantages[52] have been demonstrated with a restricted protein diet (7.5% CP with added lysine and threonine), but this has not been proven in the field to date.

The quality and nature of the protein fed is important, especially in growing horses and those in hard or repetitive work.[9] The lysine and possibly threonine content of the diet of actively exercising horses should be considered. A recommended allowance for lysine is 0.08 to 0.1 g per kilogram of body weight per day. Soya bean meal or flakes are a good source of lysine. The amount of additional lysine needed will depend on the hay and pasture being fed; alfalfa and other legumes have a higher lysine content than many meadow hays and grasses.

Branch Chain Amino Acids

Supplementation with branch chain amino acids (BCAA) (valine, leucine, and isoleucine) has been advocated as a strategy to improve performance. One theory suggests that BCAA supplementation increases the concentration of trichloroacetate intermediates (anaplerosis) available for condensation with acetyl-CoA, enabling an increase in the turnover rate of the cycle. A second theory is that BCAA can influence fatigue during exercise by preventing the rise of free, unbound plasma tryptophan, which results in elevated brain serotonin and the development of central fatigue; however, this theory has been disputed,[54] and recent research in the horse has failed to show any effect of BCAA supplementation.[55,56] Certainly, changes in plasma BCAA concentrations have been observed in horses during simulated[57] and actual endurance competitions,[58] but further studies are needed before recommendations can be given regarding BCAA supplementation.

ANTIOXIDANTS

Free radical reactions are responsible for many key biochemical events, and, under controlled circumstances, they are essential for life. Free radicals can also cause irreversible denaturation of essential cellular components and result in several degenerative disease processes.[59] During exercise, there is a marked increase in free radical production in the horse due to increased activity of xanthine oxidase during anaerobic exercise, degradation of purine nucleotides, and the partial reduction of oxygen during oxidative phosphorylation within the mitochondria. It is believed that free radical production may have a role in muscle damage and the fatigue of exercise if the production exceeds the capacity of natural defense mechanisms.[60] A system of natural antioxidant defenses is present in the body to help counteract such free radical–induced damage, including vitamins E and C and the selenium-containing enzyme glutathione peroxidase. Glutathione peroxidase reduces the production of hydroxyl radicals, vitamin E scavenges free radicals, and vitamin C assists by reducing the tocopheroxyl radicals formed during this scavenging process. In addition, vitamin E helps to block lipid peroxidation and may also form an important part of membrane structure. All horses, but especially those in hard work such as the endurance horse, need vitamin E and selenium. The levels of plasma antioxidants throughout an endurance race may depend to some extent on the difficulty of the race and the environmental conditions. Additional antioxidant supplementation above the levels recommended by the NRC[5] may be of value before and during the race.[61–63] The author recommends providing vitamin E at approximately 2000 IU per day and selenium at approximately 2 mg per day (for a 450-kg horse). In the total ration, selenium should not exceed 1 mg per100 kg of body weight per day. Additional vitamin E is required if the horse is fed a vegetable oil–supplemented diet (see above).

ELECTROLYTES

The evaporation of sweat is one of the major mechanisms for the removal of excess heat produced during energy use. The onset of substrate depletion, hyperthermia, and disturbances to fluid, electrolyte, and acid-base homeostasis may result in elimination of the horse from the ride (so-called "metabolic failure"). The amount of sweat produced depends on the environmental conditions, the nature of the work performed (which, in turn, will depend on the rider's ability and the terrain), and the animal's fitness.[64] Body weight losses during an endurance ride reflect a balance among changes in gastrointestinal tract weight, sweat loss, plus water and feed intake. Net losses of 3% to 7% of body weight commonly occur during endurance rides, and some horses may lose up to 10% of body weight.[64,65] These losses are only partially compensated for during overnight stops, perhaps owing to persistent loss in the intestinal content which takes longer than an overnight period to recover to pre-race levels.[66]

Sweat production seems to decrease only after extreme water loss. Although there may be some changes in sweat composition over time, sweat fluid production results in an obligate loss of electrolytes.[64] Sweat contains relatively low levels of calcium (~0.12 g/L), magnesium (~0.05 g/L), and phosphate (<0.01 g/L), and small amounts of various trace elements (eg, iron ~4.3 mg/L, zinc ~11.4 mg/L), but relatively high levels of sodium (~3.1 g/L), potassium (~1.6 g/L), and chloride (~5.3 g/L).[9,53,67] Water and electrolyte replacement is vitally important for mitigating the risk of thermoregulatory failure and other metabolic problems associated with dehydration and electrolyte disturbances.[64]

Currently, considerable confusion exists regarding the optimal amounts and types of electrolytes that should be given to endurance horses, as well as how they should be supplied. Options for provision include the administration of hypertonic electrolyte pastes before and during the race, the addition of electrolytes to meals offered at rest stops, and the provision of hypotonic electrolyte solutions for voluntary consumption.[64] Using a straightforward factorial approach to replenishment seems to overestimate the daily requirements of horses, especially those that lose large quantities of sweat fluid. Several factors may contribute to this overestimation. First, sweat electrolyte losses may be offset by the absorption of ions in the large intestinal fluid reservoir. Second, respiratory water loss (devoid of electrolytes) is included in estimates derived from body weight loss. Third, the electrolyte content of sweat fluid may be lower in some animals when compared with the values derived from research studies. It is possible that not all losses need to be replenished immediately.

As an example, on a factorial basis, the sodium requirement for a horse at rest has been estimated to be 20 mg per kilogram of body weight per day.[5,68] Sodium requirements for exercise would then take into consideration the sodium content of sweat (allow for replacement ~3.45g/L [ie, 3.1g/L loss with sodium having a 90% availability]) and the volume of sweat fluid lost (for light, moderate, hard, and very heavy exercise, respectively, around 0.5–1 L, 1–2 L, 2–5 L, and 7–8 L per 100 kg of body weight).[67] Horses under more extreme environmental conditions may lose up to 10 to 15 L of sweat per hour of exercise. On a factorial basis, a 500-kg horse that loses 8 kg of sweat per day should receive 10 g + 28 g = 38 g of Na or approximately 100 g of salt per day. This calculation assumes that the sodium sources are 90% available, which may be an overestimate.[68] In addition, this high level of supplementation has been demonstrated to affect acid-base balance, at least in the short-term.[68] The author recommends no more than 50 to 60 g of salt per day under the circumstances described previously.

The forage-based diet should provide an adequate reserve for potassium; therefore, the main concern should be for salt replenishment during training. Recently, it has been suggested that because moderate-to-fast exercise can result in hyperkalemia, the provision of potassium-containing electrolyte formulations during fast loops of an endurance ride may increase the risk of cardiac arrhythmia and muscle cramping.[69,70] More research in the field is required before recommendations can be made.

One study has suggested that the repeated oral administration of hypertonic electrolyte pastes may increase the risk of gastric ulceration.[71] As a consequence, some riders add antacid medications to electrolyte mixtures administered to horses during endurance rides. The efficacy of this treatment is not known; however, the coadministration of antacid medications with electrolytes may not be advisable due to potential effects on electrolyte availability.

Most commercial feeds, and home mixed rations, do not provide adequate Na and Cl for horses that lose substantial sweat during training. For horses performing little or no work, the provision of a salt block or free choice salt may be adequate (sited so that its use by that individual horse can be monitored). When a commercial feed or a vitamin-mineral supplement is being fed, the block should be pure salt rather than a salt-mineral type. Owners should be advised to not use blocks formulated for other species. Because adequate salt intake from a block cannot be guaranteed,[64,72–74] it is generally recommended to provide loose salt to horses in hard training, either added to feed or provided in a separate vessel. Salt should be introduced or removed from a feed gradually.

The optimal level of salt supplementation most likely varies between horses. In practice, riders will establish the most appropriate replacement strategy for their horse by a process of trial and error, ideally through the evaluation of different approaches during training rides.

SUGGESTED FEEDING AND MANAGEMENT STRATEGIES AROUND RACE DAYS

Pre-Ride

An endurance horse should start the competition fully hydrated with optimal amounts of liver and muscle glycogen and, after appropriate physical conditioning, with metabolic processes primed for efficient energy use. Exercise training increases the amount of glycogen in muscle and to some extent influences the metabolic characteristics of muscle, both of which help to increase the workload/running speed before onset of substantial anaerobic metabolism (ie, delays the onset of the lactate threshold). Recommendations include the following:

- Training should be light for the 4 to 5 days before a race, which combined with regular feeding will help to ensure that the glycogen stores are "topped" up.
- Forage intake should be high before a ride, and good quality forage should be used during the ride.
- Ensure adequate antioxidant and micronutrient provision.
- A high glycemic meal (in a grain-adapted horse) the night before may be helpful to top up liver glycogen stores; however, it is important not to overload the digestive capacity of the small intestine.
- Avoid changes in the ration in the period leading up to the race.
- The practice of "electrolyte loading" during the 2- to 3-day period leading up to a race is not recommended (most of the administered electrolyte will be quickly excreted).
- The horse should be allowed to ingest small amounts (1–2 kg as fed) of hay or other forage in the 1- to 3-hour period before the race. Given the recent work suggesting some advantage with respect to gastric buffering of feeding alfalfa hay,[74,75] the inclusion of alfalfa in the forage may be helpful; however, more work is needed in this area before firm conclusions can be drawn.
- Grain-based concentrates should not be fed within 3 hours of the ride. Short chopped fiber (eg, hay chop) and oil-based feeds may be advantageous (in horses adapted to oil feeding).
- Electrolytes given a few hours before prolonged exercise may be of value if adequate water is also provided and the horse is adequately hydrated.[76] Do not give excessive amounts.

During the Ride

- Water should be provided at frequent intervals during a ride (eg, every 30–40 minutes), especially in hot weather. Ideally, horses should be trained to take any opportunity to drink either plain water or appropriate salt/electrolyte solutions.
- Glycerol administration does not seem to be of value and may increase water electrolyte loss.[77]
- Anecdotally and unlike in humans, there have been reports of a detrimental effect (eg, poor heart rate recovery at veterinary checks) in horses receiving certain carbohydrate supplements during rides (eg, as glucose polymers). Fructose is absorbed in the horse and at low levels may be used as an alternative or partial substitute for glucose if required during exercise.[78,79]
- Small amounts of calcium and magnesium can be provided during the ride, but predominantly sodium and chloride are required.

Some recommend adding some electrolytes to the feed if this does not discourage eating. Alternatively, electrolyte pastes may be given after the horse has consumed feed and water. Pastes can be a convenient way to administer electrolytes providing the horse has adequate access to and drinks water.[80] The administration of hypertonic electrolyte pastes is contraindicated in horses with a poor drinking response or those with or prone to gastric ulceration.

There are no hard and fast rules on what to feed during a race. It depends to a large extent on what the horse will eat. Certainly, the horse should be offered high quality feedstuffs and plenty of water. Typically, a "smorgasbord" of feeds is provided because the primary goal is to encourage feed consumption. Appetite is an indicator of overall health, and feed intake may assist in the maintenance of normal gastrointestinal motility. Consumed feed also helps to support work performance by providing a source of energy and perhaps water plus electrolytes. Mash or slurry mixtures are popular; ingredients often used include alfalfa meal, cereals, wheat bran, stabilized rice bran, and some molasses. Most riders will also provide plain forage (often soaked). It has been suggested, but not proven, that forage-based pellets or cubes may be advantageous because they may be consumed faster and reach the cecum more quickly where they can be fermented to produce volatile fatty acids, resulting in enhanced energy availability.

Post Ride

Provide water immediately. It may be beneficial in horses adapted to the consumption of saline solutions to offer salt water (0.9% NaCl, 9 g in 1 L of water) immediately after exercise and then plain water free choice.[65,81] The temperature of the water may also be of importance for some horses.[81]

If the horse exhibits an appropriate drinking response, a further dose of an electrolyte supplement may be given.

Provide free choice hay followed by some cereal or mash (as per the ride) and then maintain the horse on a normal diet for the next few days. Do not attempt to replenish all of the lost energy in the immediate (12–24 hour) post ride period. Most endurance horses are only given light exercise (eg, walking, pasture turnout) for a few days post race combined with a return to a normal feeding pattern.

Provide supplementary electrolytes over the 24-hour post race period. It is essential to include potassium in this supplement.

SUMMARY

If one considers the perfect endurance horse as one that "stays healthy and sound" and "wins," many factors are involved, the most obvious being genetics (intrinsic ability), conformation, training, and veterinary and paraprofessional support. Nutrition and management have both enabling and supporting roles. Appropriate nutrition during the training period and the race can help to minimize metabolic problems; therefore, it is very important for all persons involved in this complex sport to have a good understanding of nutritional practices. Sound nutrition will only help a horse to be able to compete optimally. It will not improve the intrinsic ability of the horse. Poor or inappropriate nutrition, on the other hand, may impose limits on the animal's ability to perform.

REFERENCES

1. Langlois C, Robert C. Epidemiology of metabolic disorders in endurance racing horses. Pratique Veterinaire Equine Editions du Point Veterinarire 2008;157. 51–60.

2. Lawrence LM, Jackson S, Kline K, et al. Observations on body weight and condition of horses in a 150 mile endurance ride. J Equine Vet Sci 1992;12:320–4.
3. Garlinghouse SE, Burrill MJ. Relationship of body condition score to completion rate during 160 km endurance races. Equine Vet J 1999;Suppl 30:591–5.
4. Harris PA. Energy sources and requirements of the exercising horse. Annu Rev Nutr 1997;17:185–210.
5. Farris J, Hinchcliff KW, McKeever KH, et al. Effect of tryptophan and of glucose on exercise capacity of horses. J Appl Phys 1998;85:807–16.
6. Lacombe V, Hinchcliff KW, Geor RJ, et al. Muscle glycogen depletion and subsequent replenishment affect anaerobic capacity of horses. J Appl Phys 2001;91: 1782–90.
7. Pösö AR, Hyyppa S, Geor R. Metabolic responses to exercise and training. In: Hinchcliff KW, Kaneps AJ, Geor RJ, editors. Equine sports medicine and surgery. London: WB Saunders; 2004. p. 771–92.
8. Snow DH, Kerr MG, Nimmo MA, et al. Alterations in blood, sweat, urine and muscle composition during prolonged exercise in the horse. Vet Rec 1982;110: 377–84.
9. Anon. National Research Council nutrient requirements of horses. 6th edition. Washington (DC): National Academy Press; 2007.
10. Pagan JD, Hintz HF. Equine energetics. II. Energy expenditure in horses during submaximal exercise. J Anim Sci 1986;63:822–30.
11. Crandell K. Trends in feeding the American endurance horse. In: Proceedings of the Kentucky Equine Research Nutrition Conference, Lexington (KY), 2002. p. 135–9.
12. Gee H, Harris PA. Condition scoring and weight estimation: practical tools. In: Harris PA, Mair TS, Slater JD, et al (editors). Equine nutrition for all. Proceedings of the 1st British Equine Veterinary Association & WALTHAM Nutrition Symposia, 2005. Harrogate (UK). 15–24.
13. Martin Rosset W, Vermorel M, Doreau M, et al. The French horse feed evaluation systems and recommended allowances for energy and protein. Livestock Production Science 1994;40:37–56.
14. Goodwin D, Davidson HPB, Harris P. Foraging enrichment for stabled horses: effects on behaviour and selection. Equine Vet J 2002;34:686–91.
15. Shirazi-Beechey SP. Molecular insights into dietary induced colic in the horse. Equine Vet J 2008;40:414–21.
16. Ford EJH, Simmons HA. Gluconeogenesis from caecal propionate in the horse. Br J Nutr 1985;53:55–60.
17. Meyer H, Coenen M. Influence of exercise on the water and electrolyte content of the alimentary tract. In: Proceedings of the 11th Conference of the Equine Nutrition and Physiology Society; 1989. p. 3–7.
18. Warren L, Lawrence LM, Roberts A. The effect of dietary fiber on gastrointestinal fluid volume and the response to dehydration and exercise. In: Proceedings of the 17th Conference of the Equine Nutrition and Physiology Society; 2001. p. 148–9.
19. Geor R, Harris PA. Nutritional management of endurance horses. In: Harris PA, Mair TS, Slater JD, et al, editors. Equine nutrition for all. Proceedings of the 1st British Equine Veterinary Association & WALTHAM Nutrition Symposia, 2005. Harrogate (UK). 71–8.
20. Spooner HS, Nielsen BD, Harris PA, et al. Hydration status of horses during endurance exercise as affected by dietary fiber type. Maryland. In: Proceedings of the 20th Equine Science Symposium; 2007. p. 24–5.
21. Kronfeld D. Body fluids and exercise: influences of nutrition and feeding management. J Equine Vet Sci 2001;21:417–28.

22. Kronfeld D. Body fluids and exercise: replacement strategies. J Equine Vet Sci 2001;21:368–75.
23. Harris PA, Kronfeld DS. Influence of dietary energy sources on health and performance. In: Robinson NE, editor. Current therapy in equine medicine 5. Philadelphia: WB Saunders; 2003. p. 698–704.
24. Potter G, Arnold F, Householder D, et al. Digestion of starch in the small or large intestine of the equine. Pferdeheilkunde 1992;1:109–11.
25. Kienzle E. Small intestinal digestion of starch in the horse. Revue de Medecine Veterinaire 1994;145:199–204.
26. De Fombelle A, Frumholtz P, Poillion D, et al. Effect of botanical origin of starch on its prececal digestibility measured with the mobile bag technique. In: Proceedings of the 17th Equine Nutrition & Physiology Society Symposium; 2001. p. 153–5.
27. McLean BML, Hyslop JJ, Longland AC, et al. Physical processing of barley and its effects on intracaecal fermentation parameters in ponies. Animal Feed Science Technology 2000;85:79–87.
28. Pagan JD, Harris PA. The effects of timing and amount of forage and grain on exercise response in thoroughbred horses. Equine Vet J 1999;Suppl 30:451–8.
29. Palmgren Karlsson C, Jansson A, Essen-Gustavsson B, et al. Effect of molassed sugar beet pulp on nutrient utilisation and metabolic parameters during exercise. Equine Vet J 2002;Suppl 34:44–9.
30. Harris PA, Harris R. Nutritional ergogenic aids in the horse: uses and abuses. In: Lindner A, editor. Proceedings of the Conference on Equine Sports Medicine and Science. The Netherlands: Wageningen Press; 1998. p. 203–18.
31. Holland J, Kronfeld DS, Meacham TN. Behavior of horses is affected by soy lecithin and corn oil in the diet. J Anim Sci 1996;74:1252–5.
32. Slade LM, Lewis LD, Quinn CR, et al. Nutritional adaptations of horses for endurance performance. Pomona (CA). In: Proceedings of the Equine Nutrition & Physiology Society Symposium; 1975. p. 114–28.
33. Dunnett C, Marlin DJ, Harris RC. Effect of dietary lipid on response to exercise: relationship to metabolic adaptation. Equine Vet J 2002;Suppl 34:75–80.
34. Pagan JD, Geor RJ, Harris PA, et al. Effects of fat adaptation on glucose kinetics and substrate oxidation during low intensity exercise. Equine Vet J 2002;Suppl 34:33–8.
35. Treiber KH, Geor RJ, Boston RC, et al. Dietary energy source impacts glucose kinetics in trained Arabian geldings at rest and during endurance exercise. J Nutr 2008;138:964–70.
36. Hess TM, Kronfeld DS, Treiber KH, et al. Fat adaptation affects insulin sensitivity and elimination of horses during an 80 km endurance ride. Pferdeheilkunde 2007; 23:241–6.
37. Holland J, Kronfeld DS, Rich GA, et al. Acceptance of fat and lecithin containing diets by horses. Appl Anim Behav Sci 1998;56:91–6.
38. Kronfeld DS, Holland JL, Rich G, et al. Fat digestibility in *Equus caballus* follows increasing first order kinetics. J Anim Sci 2004;82:1773–80.
39. Lorenzo-Figueras M, Morisset SM, Morisset J, et al. Digestive enzyme concentrations and activities in healthy pancreatic tissue of horses. Am J Vet Res 2007;68: 1070–2.
40. Jansen WL, Sloet van Oldruitenborgh-oosterbaan MM, Cone JW. Studies on the mechanism by which a high intake of soybean oil depresses the apparent digestibility of fibre in horses. Animal Feed Science Technology 2007;138:298–308.
41. Siciliano PD, Wood CH. The effect of added dietary soybean oil on vitamin E status of the horse. J Anim Sci 1993;71:3399–402.

42. Wardlaw GM. Perspectives in nutrition. 4th edition. New York: WBC McGraw-Hill; 1999.
43. Anon. Omega-3 fatty acids. Roche Report 1987;A5:1–5.
44. Jose-Cunilleras E, Hinchcliff KW, Lacombe VA, et al. Ingestion of starch-rich meals after exercise increases glucose kinetics but fails to enhance muscle glycogen replenishment in horses. Vet J 2006;171:468–77.
45. Lacombe VA, Hinchcliff KW, Geor RJ, et al. Exercise that induces substantial muscle glycogen depletion impairs subsequent anaerobic capacity. Equine Vet J 1999;Suppl 30:293–7.
46. Essen Gustavsson B, Blomstrand E, Karlstroom K, et al. Influence of diet on substrate metabolism during exercise. In: Persson SGB, Lindholm A, Jeffcott LB, editors. Equine exercise physiology 3. Davis (CA): ICEEP Publications; 1991. p. 288–98.
47. Lacombe VA, Hinchcliff KW, Kohn CW, et al. Effects of feeding meals with various soluble carbohydrate content on muscle glycogen synthesis after exercise in horses. Am J Vet Res 2004;65:916–23.
48. Waller A, Heigenhauser GJF, Geor RJ, et al. Fluid and electrolyte supplementation after moderate intensity exercise enhances muscle glycogen resynthesis in standardbred horses. J Appl Phys 2009;106:91–100.
49. Harris PA, Graham-Thiers P. To evaluate the influence that “feeding” state may exert on metabolic and physiological responses to exercise. Equine Vet J 1999;Suppl 30:633–6.
50. Jose-Cunilleras E, Hinchcliff KW, Sams RA, et al. Glycemic index of a meal fed before exercise alters substrate use and glucose flux in exercising horses. J Appl Phys 2002;92:117–28.
51. Kronfeld DS. Dietary fat affects heat production and other variables of equine performance under hot and humid conditions. Equine Vet J 1996;Suppl 22: 24–35.
52. Graham-Thiers PM, Kronfeld DS, Kline KA, et al. Dietary protein level and protein status in Arabian horses during interval training and repeated sprints. J Equine Vet Sci 2000;20:516–21.
53. Meyer H. Nutrition of the equine athlete. In: Robinson NE, editor. Equine exercise physiology 2. Davis (CA): ICEEP Publications; 1987. p. 644–73.
54. Grimmett A, Sillence MN. Calmatives for the excitable horse: a review of L-tryptophan. Vet J 2005;170:24–32.
55. Casini L, Gatta L, Magni B, et al. Effect of prolonged branch chain amino acid supplementation on metabolic responses to anaerobic exercise in standardbreds. J Equine Vet Sci 2000;20:120–3.
56. Steffanon B, Bettini C, Guggia P. Administration of branched chain amino acids to standardbred horses in training. J Equine Vet Sci 2000;20:115–9.
57. Trottier NL, Nielsen BD, Lang KL, et al. Equine endurance exercise alters serum branched chain amino acid and alanine concentrations. Equine Vet J 2002;Suppl 34:168–72.
58. Nery J, Assenza A, Pinna W, et al. A study of horse’s blood constituents and weight variations during endurance competitions. Pferdeheilkunde 2005;21:103–4.
59. Halliwell B. Free radicals and antioxidants: a personal view. Nutr Rev 1994;52: 253–65.
60. Marlin DJ, Dunnett CE, Deaton CM. The role of antioxidants. In: Harris PA, Mair TS, Slater JD, et al, editors. Equine nutrition for all. Proceedings of the 1st British Equine Veterinary Association & WALTHAM Nutrition Symposia, 2005. Harrogate (UK): Equine Veterinary Journal; 2005. p. 39–48.

61. Hargreaves BH, Kronfeld DS, Waldron JE, et al. Antioxidant status and muscle cell leakage during endurance exercise. Equine Vet J 2002;Suppl 34:116–21.
62. Marlin DJ, Fenn K, Smith N, et al. Changes in circulatory antioxidant status in horses during prolonged exercise. J Nutr 2002;132:1622S–7S.
63. Williams CA, Kronfeld DS, Hess TM, et al. Antioxidant supplementation and subsequent oxidative stress of horses during an 80-km endurance race. J Anim Sci 2004;82:588–94.
64. Jose-Cunilleras E. Abnormalities of body fluids and electrolytes in athletic horses. In: Hinchcliff KW, Kaneps AJ, Geor RJ, editors. Equine sports medicine and surgery. London: Elsevier; 2004. p. 898–917.
65. Butudom P, Schott HC II, Davis MW, et al. Drinking salt water enhances rehydration in horses dehydrated by frusemide administration and endurance exercise. Equine Vet J 2002;Suppl 34:513–8.
66. Schott HC, McGlade KS, Hines MT, et al. Body weight, fluid and electrolyte, and hormonal changes in horses that successfully completed a five day, 424 kilometre endurance competition. Equine Athlete 1997;40–4.
67. Harris PA, Coenen M, Frape D, et al. Equine nutrition and metabolic disease. In: Higgins A, Snyder J, editors. Equine manual. London: Elsevier; 2006. p. 151–222.
68. Zeyner A, Romanowski K, Müller A-M, et al. Effects of different doses of sodium chloride on the acid-base balance of horses. Proceedings of the European Society of Veterinary Comparative Nutrition 10(1):40–4.
69. Hess TM, Kronfeld DS, Carter RA, et al. Does usefulness of potassium supplementation depend on speed? Equine Vet J 2006;Suppl 36:74–82.
70. Hess TM, Greiwe-Crandell KM, Waldron JE, et al. Potassium-free electrolytes and calcium supplementation in an endurance race. Comparative Exercise Physiology 2008;5:33–41.
71. Holbrook TC, Simmons RD, Payton ME, et al. Effect of repeated oral administration of hypertonic electrolyte solution on equine gastric mucosa. Equine Vet J 2005;37:501–4.
72. Jansson A, Dahlborn K. Effects of feeding frequency and voluntary salt intake on fluid and electrolyte regulation in athletic horses. J Appl Phys 1999;86:1610–6.
73. Jansson A, Rytthammar Å, Lindberg JE, et al. Voluntary salt (NaCl) intake in standardbred horses. Pferdeheilkunde 1996;12:443–5.
74. Kennedy MAP, Entrekin P, Harris PA, et al. Voluntary intake of loose vs. block salt and its effect on water intake in mature idle thoroughbreds. In: Proceedings of the Kentucky Equine Research Equine Nutrition Conference for Feed Manufacturers. Lexington (KY): Kentucky Equine Research, Inc.; 1998. p. 73–5.
75. Lybbert T, Gibbs P, Cohen N, et al. Gastric ulcer syndrome in exercising horses fed different types of hay. In: Proceedings of the 20th Equine Science Society Symposium; 2007. p. 128–9.
76. Coenen M, Meyer H, Steinbrenner B. Effects of NaCl supplementation before exercise on metabolism of water and electrolytes. Equine Vet J 1995;Suppl 18: 270–3.
77. Schott HC II, Dusterdieck KJ, Eberhart SW, et al. Effects of electrolyte and glycerol supplementation on recovery from endurance exercise. Equine Vet J 1999; Suppl 30:384–93.
78. Bullimore SR, Pagan JD, Harris PA, et al. Carbohydrate supplementation of horses during endurance exercise: comparison of fructose and glucose. J Nutr 2000;120:1760–5.

79. Vervuert I, Coenen M, Bichmann M. Comparison of the effects of fructose and glucose supplementation on metabolic responses in resting and exercising horses. Journal of the American Veterinary Medical Association 2004;51:171–7.
80. Düsterdieck KF, Schott HC II, Eberhart SW, et al. Electrolyte and glycerol supplementation improve water intake by horses performing a simulated 60 km endurance ride. Equine Vet J 1999;Suppl 18:418–24.
81. Schott HC II, Butudom P, Nielsen BD, et al. Strategies to increase voluntary drinking after exercise. In: Proceedings of the 49th American Association of Equine Practitioners Meeting; 2003. p. 132–9.

Nutrition of the Aged Horse

Nicola G. Jarvis, BVetMed, MRCVS

KEYWORDS

• Nutrition • Horse • Aged • Geriatric • Management

Ageing is defined as the "accumulation of changes in an organism or object over time."[1] As a horse ages, the body undergoes changes with respect to failing dentition, degenerative disease, and alteration in gut absorption, which all provide challenges when formulating an individual's diet.[2]

Although it is difficult to state an exact time when a horse moves from being "mature" to being "aged," a survey in Massachusetts found that owners perceived their horses as being old at approximately 22 years of age.[3] The survey compared two groups of horses according to age, in which horses aged 20 years or older were considered old and those younger than the age of 20 years were considered young. The results highlighted the popularity of using commercial "senior" feeds (51%), long-term medication (25%), and feed supplements in the older horse group. A further report showed that although only 2.2% of total admissions to a large animal hospital in 1989 were older than 20 years of age, this figure rose sharply to 12.5% in 1999.[4] This perhaps demonstrates improved longevity in horses and owner's expectations for increased levels of veterinary treatment and care.

The terms *aged* and *geriatric* are often used interchangeably in the literature. Strictly speaking, however, in human medicine, the term *geriatrics* refers to a branch of medicine dedicated to the diseases associated with old age,[1] and perhaps should not therefore be applied to a "healthy" older horse. A postal survey of horse owners in Australia revealed an increased prevalence of disease in the aged horse: 42.9% of horses aged older than 20 years were considered have disease compared with 33.3% in the 6- to 10-year-old age group.[5] This article aims to bring together the current thoughts on nutrition of the older horse in health and disease.

MANAGEMENT TO MAXIMIZE FOOD INTAKE

Weight loss or difficulty in maintaining adequate body condition is one of the most common problems encountered in the older horse. Although there are several potential causes for inability to maintain body condition (eg, dental abnormalities, renal and hepatic disease, pituitary pars intermedia dysfunction [PPID, equine Cushing's

Redwings Horse Sanctuary, Hapton, Norwich, Norfolk, England NR15 1SP, UK
E-mail address: njarvis@redwings.co.uk

Vet Clin Equine 25 (2009) 155–166
doi:10.1016/j.cveq.2009.01.003
vetequine.theclinics.com

disease]), an important first step in diagnostic workup is evaluation of diet and feeding management. In many cases, changes in the quantity or quality of feed or in the method of feeding can result in improvement in feed intake and body condition. A young horse kept in a group situation may be at the top of the pecking order, but as ageing progresses, the horse may eventually drop to the bottom of the order, especially when new horses are introduced to the herd. Loss of a companion horse also can change herd social dynamics and contribute to reduced appetite and feed intake. Feed intake may be improved by feeding the older horse in a separate enclosure (corral) within the pasture. This approach is useful for horses that are "slow eaters" because of poor dentition.

When standing normally, the center of gravity of a horse lies just behind the withers, but when the horse lowers the head to graze, the center of gravity moves forward, concentrating over the forelimbs (**Fig. 1**).[6] A horse that has osteoarthritis (OA), especially of the forelimbs, may experience increased pain when grazing or eating from the floor. In this author's experience, a simple raised manger on a gate or fence bracket can markedly improve feed intake in the arthritic horse (**Fig. 2**). If the arthritis is generalized, the horse is likely to be reluctant to move around the field to graze and a change in housing may be warranted (eg, provision of a flat paddock in which the water tank is located close to the gate and shelter, housing in a small drylot rather than at pasture). OA of the neck may hinder grazing and make "pulling" hay from a net difficult. In these cases, feeding loose hay in a raised hay bin or using hay nets with larger holes may resolve the problem.

In this author's experience, some older horses with poor appetite show improved appetite and feed intake if fed with companion horses. This has certainly been

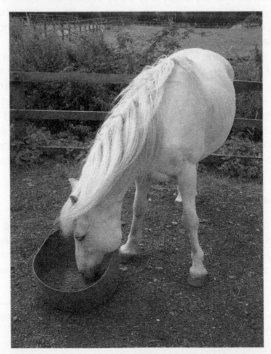

Fig.1. Feeding from the floor can prove difficult for a horse with osteoarthritis of the neck or forelimbs.

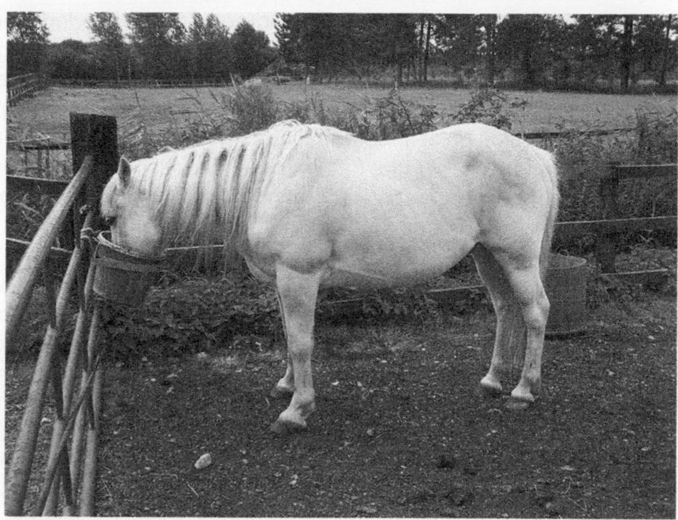

Fig. 2. Feeding from a raised bucket improves comfort and can lead to increased feed intake and weight gain.

demonstrated in human beings, in whom it was found that elderly patients consumed more if they ate in a communal dining room than alone by their beds.[7,8] Warming food, especially if soaked, and the addition of molasses, pureed apple, or flavoring (eg, crushed ginger cookies) to feed seem to increase intake in the aged horse (author's observations in stall-kept horses).

AGE-RELATED CHANGES IN DIGESTIVE FUNCTION

A article frequently cited regarding digestive function in the older horse is that by Ralston and colleagues[8] In that study, the apparent digestibility of a commercial alfalfa pellet diet was compared in groups of aged horses (>20 years old) and young horses (<10 years old). The main findings included statistically significant decreases in digestibility of crude protein (CP) and phosphorus and a trend for reduced fiber digestibility. This research group subsequently demonstrated similar reductions in CP and phosphorus digestibility in a group of young horses after resection of 90% of the large colon.[8,9] It was concluded that the decrease in CP, phosphorus, and fiber digestion observed in the old horses was attributable to changes in large colon function, perhaps secondary to chronic parasitic damage. A subsequent study failed to demonstrate an effect of old age on feed digestibility, however.[10] The investigators speculated that damage to the large colon associated with chronic parasitism or poor dentition may have explained the reduction in digestion observed in the old horses of their original study. Therefore, it is reasonable to assume that a healthy older horse with good dentition that has received regular anthelmintic treatment over the years has digestive capacity similar to that of younger horses and can be fed as per normal adult horse guidelines.[11]

Dietary modifications are indicated in older horses with poor dentition that are struggling to maintain weight, however. Almost all feed companies now sell products designed for nutritional support of old or geriatric horses. These senior feeds are often formulated with higher CP (12%–16%) than feeds formulated for mature horses (10%–12%), with inclusion of high-quality protein sources, such as soybean meal. Grain or grain byproducts are mechanically (ground) or thermally (popped or heat-extruded) treated to improve prececal starch digestibility. Some of these products are entirely extruded, with the rationale that this treatment improves digestibility. Vegetable oil (eg, corn) may be added, with many feeds containing 4% to 7% crude fat (ether extract). Senior feeds are usually designed to be fed as the sole component of the diet (a "complete feed") with inclusion of substantial fiber (usually at least 12% crude fiber) from soya hulls, alfalfa meal, or beet pulp, for example. The recommended feeding rate for these feeds is generally approximately 2.0% of body weight (ie, ~9 kg/d for a 450-kg horse). This daily ration should be provided in a minimum of four feedings.

The calcium-to-phosphorus ratio should be maintained at between 1.5:1 and 2:1. Excessive calcium intake should be avoided (eg, feeding legumes) because calcium can adversely affect phosphorus digestibility in any adult horse[12] and is of concern in the older horse, in which digestion of phosphorus may be reduced. Diets containing approximately 1% calcium and 0.45% to 0.6% phosphorus are recommended.[13]

It has been reported that aged horses have lower plasma ascorbic acid concentrations than younger healthy horses.[14] For this reason, vitamin C supplementation has been recommended; one reference suggests supplementation at 10 g given twice daily,[13] and another suggests 25 g given twice daily.[15] Ralston[13] described an increased antibody response to vaccination in old horses receiving vitamin C supplementation, especially those that had PPID, and suggested that supplementation may be useful in horses with chronic infections. One hypothesis is that the reduced plasma ascorbic acid in older horses that have PPID is attributable to elevated cortisol, which may result in decreased ascorbate production. Ascorbyl palmitate is absorbed more easily than ascorbic acid and is preferred when supplemental vitamin C is indicated.[15] Supplemental vitamin E (4000 IU/d) also may be of value in supporting immune function in old horses.

DENTAL CONSIDERATIONS IN THE OLDER HORSE

Horses evolved to cope with a predominantly fibrous diet, the digestion of which highly depends on thorough mastication to provide sufficient surface area. In the adult horse, the cheek teeth form solid arcades of enamel ridges that provide an abrasive surface for grinding forage.[16] Horses possess hypsodont (long-crowned) teeth, which erupt throughout life and are gradually worn away at the occlusal surface. The average rate of eruption is 2 to 3 mm/y, and, ideally, this would be matched by the rate of attrition at the occlusal surface. The teeth continue to erupt until approximately 20 years of age, when the reserve crown has shortened to the extent that the teeth are shed.[17]

A multitude of dental problems can occur with the normal ageing process. As the reserve crown erupts, the circumference of the tooth narrows, such that, over time, spaces appear between the teeth known as diastema (plural diastemata). These gaps allow food to be trapped, leading to recession of the gum line, periodontal disease, and infection. In addition, the narrowing of the teeth reduces the available surface area for grinding. Normal attrition of the first molar and fourth premolar (the first teeth to erupt), along with tooth fractures and shedding, can lead to development of "wave mouth," which can result in difficulty in chewing feed. A "step mouth" can develop from the loss of one tooth and subsequent overgrowth of the opposing cheek tooth. Again, this can lead to difficulty with mastication.[18] In extremely old horses, as the teeth approach shedding, there is a natural loss of the enamel ridges responsible for efficient grinding, a condition known as "smooth mouth."

Dietary management has an impact on changes in dentition. When grains and concentrate feeds are added to the ration, there is a usually a decrease in forage intake. When compared with forage ingestion, there is less time spent chewing and less lateral excursion of the jaw during mastication when grain is consumed.[16,19] Over time, sharp enamel ridges develop, especially on the buccal surface of the upper arcades, which can lead to oral erosions and pain. This problem may be exacerbated in older horses when the diet is switched to predominantly concentrate feed to compensate for the decreased ability to cope with forage.

Clinical signs of a dental problem may include weight loss, quidding of partially chewed feed, choke, halitosis, feed packing in cheeks, and diarrhea. Periodontal disease can be quite painful, as can loose or infected teeth, and the horse may be slow to finish feed or exhibit complete anorexia.[20] In one study, the incidence of periodontal disease in horses older than 15 years of age was 60%, whereas another study reported a similar incidence in horses older than 20 years of age.[21,22] A review of equine skulls examined at an abattoir, most of which were from old horses, showed a high prevalence of step or wave mouth and concluded that 72% would have benefited from dental work.[23] Indeed, there is a strong association between dental pathologic conditions and poor body condition score in horses.[24]

Examination of the feces can provide clues regarding the impact of dental pathologic conditions on digestion. The average length of fibrous material in equine feces is typically 3.7 mm.[25] Excessive fiber length is suggestive of dental problems.

All old horses should receive a regular (annual or biannual) oral examination, with correction of problems when indicated. Horses that have oral cavity disease often require diet modification to improve feed intake and body condition, the extent of which depends on the severity of dental problems. A decision must be made regarding the type of fiber provided in the diet. Long-stem hay can be fed to horses with only mild dental problems, with preference for high-quality forages (high leaf-to-stem ratio) that are softer and easier to chew. When available, pasture turnout is desirable, because grass is soft, easy to digest, and requires less mastication than other forage. Provided that the grass is reasonably long, most equids seem to thrive regardless of incisor status.[11,26] If there is a history of choke, chopped hay can be fed as an alterative to long-stem hay; again, a soft grass forage should be used for preparation of the hay chop. A report has suggested that feeding of coarse or chopped fiber may contribute to interdental feed packing and development of periodontal disease.[27] The risk for these complications may be higher in horses with many diastemata.

More severe dental problems may make it necessary to provide a "no long-fiber" diet. This can be achieved using one of the many commercial senior feeds, which, as previously mentioned, are often marketed as complete feeds. These feeds can be blended with other fiber sources (eg, alfalfa cubes, hay pellets, soaked sugar beet pulp) to ensure adequate fiber intake. Vegetable oil can be added to augment the caloric density of the ration (oils are easy to digest and, compared with the equivalent quantity of cereal grain, provided ~2.25-fold higher digestible energy). Although vegetable oil is often added to commercial feeds designed for old horses, it is safe to add an additional 1 to 2 cups (200-400 mL) per day.[28] Vitamin E (~100 IU per 100 mL of added oil) should be added to the ration, because studies in human beings and laboratory animals suggest an increased requirement for vitamin E when dietary polyunsaturated fat levels are increased. Corn, linseed, and soya oils are popular choices, but any vegetable oil is suitable provided that it is not rancid and is introduced slowly to avoid potential gastrointestinal disturbances (colic and greasy loose feces). Some horses may be slow to adapt to the taste and texture of oils; thus, gradual introduction helps to avoid refusal of food. Stabilized rice bran (~20% fat) can be used if the oil supplement proves unpalatable.

Horses with few teeth or periodontal disease may require any ration to be soaked before feeding to make it easier to chew. It is important to remember that soaking the feed results in the volume of the feed increasing, often to double the original size. This may result in reduced intake of calories over the course of a day. Warm water should be used to soak feed, particularly on cold days, because chilled wet feed is likely to be refused. A horse with a painful mouth also may appreciate the choice of warmed drinking water, especially in winter.

If a no long-fiber diet is fed, mimicking the natural trickle feeding pattern of the horse can increase overall daily intake and reduce the risk for colic or diarrhea. Ideally, the ration should be divided into at least four or five feedings. This strategy also helps to prevent boredom in the stabled horse.

OSTEOARTHRITIS AND NUTRITION

OA is a common condition of the older horse. One report that surveyed the clinical conditions of 467 geriatric horses found that 24% (n = 111) had musculoskeletal problems, of which OA accounted for 40% of the diagnoses.[4] OA is a chronic degenerative process characterized by the progressive deterioration and erosion of articular hyaline cartilage occurring as a consequence of enzymatic degradation and the release of inflammatory mediators. Clinical signs of joint effusion, lameness, and decreased range of movement can range from mild to severe and often deteriorate over time.[29,30]

Several oral supplements ("nutraceuticals") have been advocated for use in older horses, with speculation that these agents can slow the development of OA. Glucosamine and chondroitin sulfate are the most common ingredients in oral supplements marketed for use in horses, and one or both are sometimes incorporated into feeds designed for old horses. Glucosamine is a precursor of glycosaminoglycans, such as keratin sulfate and hyaluronan, which form the extracellular matrix of cartilage. Hence, supplementation with glucosamine is thought to provide the building blocks for cartilage repair. Chondroitin sulfate is a normal constituent of the cartilage matrix. In addition, glucosamine and chondroitin sulfate reduce the degree of proteoglycan degradation and suppress production of inflammatory mediators.[31–33] In vitro studies have shown a synergistic effect with the combination of glucosamine and chondroitin sulfate.[31]

The oral bioavailability and clinical efficacy of these oral chondroprotective agents are, however, controversial. Studies to date suggest that oral bioavailability of glucosamine and chondroitin sulfate is much lower in horses than in human beings, dogs, and rats,[31,34,35] suggesting the need for higher doses to achieve a therapeutic concentration at the site of action (ie, joints). Evidence-based dosage recommendations are not available for horses, however. A further concern is the huge variation in quality and purity of supplements containing glucosamine and chondroitin sulfate. A study of human products found that more than 84% did not meet their label claims for actual content even when marked "guaranteed analysis,"[31] and similar problems were found on analysis of products marketed for use in horses.[36] Although there are reports of improved gait and decreased lameness in horses with OA after supplementation with glucosamine or chondroitin sulfate,[31,37] there remains a lack of valid blind studies. Use of these supplements may be justified in horses that have mild or early OA (provided that a high-quality product is administered), but they are unlikely to be of value in horses that have more severe or chronic OA lesions, in which there is extensive cartilage erosion and exposure of subchondral bone.[34]

Antioxidant nutrients (eg, vitamin C, manganese, zinc) also may play a role in mitigating the progression of OA.[13] Many of the oral chondroprotective supplements contain these and other antioxidant nutrients. A recent study examined the efficacy of avocado and soybean unsaponifiable (ASU) extracts for treatment of horses with experimentally induced OA, based on positive results from clinical trials in human beings.[38] After 70 days of treatment, there was no reduction in the level of lameness and pain; however, there was a significant reduction in the severity of articular cartilage erosion, and an increase in glycosaminoglycan synthesis within the joint was observed. The value of ASU extracts for management of OA in old horses warrants investigation.

NUTRITION AND HEPATIC DISEASE

It has been suggested that between 60% and 70% of liver function may have been lost before signs of liver failure become apparent.[39] Although liver "failure" is relatively uncommon in horses, underlying liver "disease" may be far more prevalent.[40] Certainly, chronic weight loss in the older horse should be investigated further, once dentition and feeding management have been evaluated, to rule out the possibility of liver disease. In some locations, the cumulative effects of years of exposure to ragwort (*Senecio jacobeae*), found on badly managed pasture and in poor-quality hay, can lead to pyrrolizidine alkaloid hepatotoxicosis, and clinical signs of disease may not develop until the horse is aged.

Nutritional support of chronic hepatic disease involves reducing the workload of the liver in energy metabolism and the processing of metabolic wastes. Because the liver's capacity for gluconeogenesis is reduced, it is important to provide a steady supply of glycemic carbohydrate (eg, sweet feeds, corn, molassed beet pulp).[40–42] A suggested feeding rate of grain or sweet feed is 0.5 to 0.6 kg per 100 kg of body weight (BW) per day, divided into four to six meals.[39] Lower protein diets (<10% CP) with a high branched chain (BCAA)-to-aromatic amino acid (AAA) ratio are frequently advocated in the management of liver disease to decrease gastrointestinal ammonia production and accumulation of aromatic amines. Higher protein intake may be needed in horses with chronic hepatic disease and poor body condition for avoidance of further muscle wasting, however. Corn, beet pulp, milo (sorghum), and wheat bran have reasonably high levels of BCAA and are suitable for horses that have hepatic disease. Wheat and oats should be avoided because of their low BCAA/AAA ratio.[39,41,43] Grass, rather then legume, hay should be offered. Supplementation with vegetable oil may be inadvisable, given the liver's role in fat metabolism,[40] but the effect of dietary fat in horses with liver disease has not been determined.

Supplementation with a multivitamin preparation is recommended, because synthesis of some of the B-vitamins may be impaired, although absorption of fat-soluble vitamins (A, D, E, and K) may be decreased because of reduced bile salt production. The supplement should be devoid of iron because of concern that horses that have hepatic disease may be susceptible to iron overload of the liver.[39] Supplementation with antioxidant nutrients (eg, vitamin E, selenium) has been advocated because of the increased rate of oxidation stress found in liver disease.[39]

NUTRITION AND RENAL DISEASE

Chronic renal disease is uncommon in the horse. In one retrospective study of horses admitted to a veterinary teaching hospital, the prevalence of chronic renal failure (CRF) was only 0.12%. The prevalence of CRF was 0.23% in horses older than 15 years of age, however.[44] Typical signs of CRF include weight loss, polyuria or polydipsia, ventral edema, and a decrease in appetite because of uremia. The disease is usually progressive and irreversible, although some horses can survive for months or years if given appropriate nutritional support.[44]

Good-quality pasture and grass hay can help to encourage intake in horses with a poor appetite. Fresh water should be available at all times, and the horse should have access to a salt block or loose salt. Excess dietary protein exacerbates azotemia; therefore, grass, rather than legume, forage should be provided. The total diet should be 10% to 12% CP; extremely low-protein diets may aggravate muscle wasting and debilitation. Sweet feeds, grains, or vegetable oil can be used to boost digestive energy intake and combat weight loss. Use of omega-3–enriched oils (eg, flax, linseed, fish) may be of benefit, because studies in dogs and cats have demonstrated that supplementation with fish oil (rich in omega-3 fatty acids) slowed the progression of CRF.[45] Provision of an antioxidant supplement has also been advocated; as mentioned previously, supplemental vitamin E should be given when oil is added to the ration.

High dietary phosphorus decreases survival time in dogs with CRF; thus, avoidance of feedstuffs high in phosphorus (eg, wheat bran) is recommended. Avoidance of sugar beet pulp and alfalfa hay is also advocated. Both contain high levels of calcium and are thought to increase the risk for renal calculi in the older horse. In addition alfalfa, although highly palatable, is typically high in CP.[46]

ANTIOXIDANT SUPPLEMENTATION

In human beings, there is evidence that free radicals and reactive oxygen species (ROS), such as superoxide and peroxyl radicals, play a role in the ageing process and the development of chronic diseases (eg, arthritis, cancer, asthma, renal and hepatic disease).[47] Furthermore, studies in laboratory animals have demonstrated associations between the production of free radicals from cellular metabolism, tissue concentrations of specific antioxidants, and life span. Free radicals and ROS are by-products of normal cellular metabolism and can damage DNA, lipids, proteins, and carbohydrates. Antioxidants work to reduce this potential damage by stabilization of free radicals by means of electron donation, direct suppression of production, or chelation of certain metals that would otherwise promote production of these pro-oxidant species.[48] The body's balance between pro-oxidants and antioxidants is known as the antioxidant status. Disease and infection cause oxidative stress, and the associated increase in the production of free radicals and ROS contributes to progression of the disease.[47,48] Therefore, there may be a rationale for antioxidant supplementation in old horses that have chronic diseases, such as OA and recurrent airway obstruction (RAO). Several trace minerals are constituents of enzymatic and nonenzymatic antioxidants, including copper, manganese, selenium, and zinc. Vitamins A, C, and E and lipoic acid are antioxidants. Supplementation of vitamin C and lipoic acid in the healthy adult horse should be unnecessary because they are synthesized endogenously. As discussed previously, however, the synthesis of vitamin C may be impaired in older horses, especially if they are affected by PPID. It should be borne in mind that oversupplementation is a potential risk, particularly with the fat-soluble vitamins and trace metals.[48,49]

In a cross-sectional study of 80 clinically healthy horses, age did not contribute to variation in blood markers of antioxidant status, including superoxide dismutase, and concentrations of zinc and selenium.[50] The oldest horse in the group was 17 years of age, however, and studies of a wider age range are needed to determine whether antioxidant status is affected by age. RAO is more prevalent in the older horse,[51] and recent studies have evaluated the effect of antioxidant supplementation in horses with this condition. Lower plasma and bronchoalveolar lavage fluid ascorbic acid concentrations were observed in RAO-affected horses when compared with healthy controls,[52] suggesting that horses that have RAO may be more susceptible to oxidant challenges. Because exercise increases oxidative stress, exercise protocols have been incorporated into the design of trials to assess the effect of antioxidant supplementation. One study demonstrated enhanced exercise tolerance and a reduction in endoscopic score for pulmonary inflammation in horses that had RAO and were provided a mixed antioxidant supplement.[53] Although other studies have shown conflicting results,[54] dietary antioxidant supplementation may be beneficial in horses that have RAO.

SUMMARY

Older horses (>20 years of age) in good health and body condition do not require alterations in diet. Older horses in poor body condition require a complete clinical examination and evaluation of diet and feeding management to determine the cause of weight loss and the need for a dietary change, however. Common causes of weight loss and poor body condition in old horses include dental or oral cavity abnormalities (eg, tooth loss, periodontal disease), PPID, and reduced feed intake attributable to competition from herd mates or pain associated with OA. Feed intake and body condition may improve after institution of management changes (eg, separation from herd mates during feeding). Thin but otherwise healthy old horses can benefit from a diet that provides 12% to 16% CP and includes highly digestible feedstuffs (eg, sugar beet pulp, alfalfa meal, heat-treated grains or grain byproducts, vegetable oils). In horses with severe irreversible dental problems, long-stem fiber (hay) should be replaced by soaked hay cubes, short chopped hay, or heavily soaked sugar beet pulp. Evidence of chronic endocrine, hepatic, or renal disease dictates dietary modifications.

REFERENCES

1. Wikipedia. Available at: http://www.wikipedia.me.uk.
2. Jarvis NG, Harris PA, Lockyer C. Nutrition and the older horse. In: Harris PA, Mair TS, Slater JD, et al, editors. Proceedings of the First BEVA and Waltham Nutrition Symposia. Suffolk: England: EVJ Ltd.; 2005. p. 49–54.
3. Brosnahan MM, Paradis MR. Assessment of clinical characteristics, management practices and activities of geriatric horses. J Am Vet Med Assoc 2003;223(1): 99–103.
4. Brosnahan MM, Paradis MR. Demographic and clinical characteristics of geriatric horses: 467 cases (1989–1999). J Am Vet Med Assoc 2003;223(1):93–8.
5. Cole FL, Hodgson DR, Reid SWJ, et al. Owner reported equine health disorders: results of an Australia-wide postal survey. Aust Vet J 2005;83(8):490–5.
6. Skerrit GC, McLelland J. Mammalian locomotion. In: Skerritt GC, McLelland J, editors. Functional anatomy of the limbs of the domestic animals. Julish: Germany: CESMAS; 1984. p. 224–35.
7. Wright L, Hickson M, Frost G. Eating together is important: using a dining room in an acute elderly medical ward increases energy intake. J Hum Nutr Diet 2006; 19(1):23–6.
8. Ralston SL, Squires EL, Nockels CF. Digestion in the aged horse. J Equine Vet Sci 1989;9:203–5.
9. Bertone AL, Ralston SL, Stashak TS. Fibre digestion and voluntary intake in horses after adaption to extensive large colon resection. Am J Vet Res 1989; 50(9):1628–32.

10. Ralston SL, Malinowski K, Christensen R, et al. Digestion in aged horses—revisited. Veterinary review. J Equine Vet Sci 2001;21(7):310–1.
11. Siciliano PD. Nutrition and feeding of the geriatric horse. Vet Clin North Am Equine Pract 2002;18:491–508.
12. Van Doorn DA, Van Der Spek ME, Everts H, et al. The influence of calcium intake on phosphorus digestibility in mature ponies. J Anim Physiol Anim Nutr (Berl) 2004;88:412–8.
13. Ralston SL. Management of geriatric horses. In: Pagan JD, Geor RJ, editors. Advances in equine nutrition II. Nottingham: Nottingham Press; 2001. p. 393–6.
14. Ralston SL, Nockels CF, Squires EL. Differences in diagnostic test results and haematological data between young and aged horses. Am J Vet Res 1988; 49(8):1387–92.
15. Vervuert I, Coenen M, Nutritional management in horses: selected aspects to gastrointestinal disturbances and geriatric horses. In: Proceedings of the Second European Nutrition and Health Congress. Lelystad, Netherlands: 2004. p. 20–30.
16. Dacre I. The impact of nutrition on dental health and management of equine teeth for optimal nutrition. In: Lindner A, editor. Applied equine nutrition. Equine Nutrition Conference ENUCO; 2005. p. 27–41.
17. Dixon PM. Dental anatomy. In: Baker GJ, Easley J, editors. Equine dentistry. WB Saunders; 2003. p. 3–28.
18. Lowder MQ, Mueller E. Dental disease in geriatric horses. Vet Clin North Am Equine 1998;14(2):365–80.
19. Graham BP. Dental care in the older horse. Vet Clin North Am Equine 2002;18: 509–23.
20. Knottenbelt DC. The systemic effects of dental disease. In: Baker GJ, Easley J, editors. Equine dentistry. Philadelphia: WB Saunders; 2003. p. 127–38.
21. Baker GJ. Some aspects of dental disease. Equine Vet J 1970;2:105–10.
22. Wafa NS. A study of dental disease in the horse. National University of Ireland. Faculty of Veterinary Medicine. Dublin, Ireland: University College Dublin. p. 1–205.
23. Brigham EJ, Duncanson GR. An equine post-mortem dental study: 50 cases. Equine Vet Edu 2000;12(2):59–62.
24. Roy C. Dental problems in debilitated equines in Delhi. In: Proceedings of the Fourth International Colloquium on Working Equines. Hama, Syria. 20th April 2002.
25. Easley KJ. Dental and oral examination. In: Baker GJ, Easley J, editors. Equine dentistry. Philadelphia: WB Saunders; 2003. p. 107–26.
26. Pugh DG. Feeding the geriatric horse. Current concepts in equine nutrition. Proceedings of the American Association of Equine Practitioners 2002;48:21–3.
27. Miles AEW, Grigson C. Colyer's variations and diseases of the teeth of animals. Cambridge: Cambridge University Press; 1990.
28. Geor RJ. Cushing's disease and other problems of the older horse. In: Pagan JD, editor. Advances in equine nutrition III. Nottingham, UK: Nottingham University Press; 2007. p. 447–52.
29. Cary J, Turner T. Geriatric musculoskeletal disorders of the horse. In: Bertone J, editor. Equine geriatric medicine and surgery. Saunders: Elsevier; 2006. p. 135–45.
30. Payne R. Osteoarthritis—management in the older horse. Lecture from BEVA geriatric horse course. Newmarket: British racing school; 23rd May 2008.
31. Neil KM, Caron JP, Orth MW. The role of glucosamine and chondroitin sulphate in treatment and prevention of osteoarthritis in animals. Reference point. J Am Vet Med Assoc 2005;226(7):1079–88.

32. Neil KM, Orth MW, Coussens PM, et al. Effects of glucosamine and chondroitin sulphate on mediators of osteoarthritis in cultured equine chondrocytes stimulated by use of recombinant equine interleukin-1b. Am J Vet Res 2005;66(11):1861–9.
33. Dechant JE, Baxter GM, Frisbie DD, et al. Effects of glucosamine hydrochloride and chondroitin sulphate, alone and in combination, on normal and interleukin-1 conditioned equine articular cartilage explant metabolism. Equine Vet J 2005;37(3):227–31.
34. Malone ED. Managing chronic arthritis. Vet Clin North Am Equine 2002;18:439–52.
35. Platt D. The role of oral disease modifying agents glucosamine and chondroitin sulphate in the management of equine degenerative joint disease. Equine Vet J 2001;13:206–15.
36. Oke S, Aghazadeh-Habashi A, Weese JS, et al. Evaluation of glucosamine levels in commercial equine oral supplements for joints. Equine Vet J 2006;38:93–5.
37. Forsyth RK, Bridgen CV, Northrop AJ. Double blind investigation of the effects of oral supplementation of combined glucosamine hydrochloride (GHCL) and chondroitin sulphate (CS) on stride characteristics of veteran horses. Equine Vet J Suppl 2006;36:622–5.
38. Kawcak CE, Frisbie DD, McIlwraith CW, et al. Evaluation of avocado and soybean unsaponifiable extracts for treatment of horses with experimentally induced osteoarthritis. Am J Vet Res 2007;68(6):598–604.
39. Bergero D, Nery J. Hepatic diseases in horses. J Anim Physiol Anim Nutr 2008;92(3):345–55.
40. Durham AE, Newton JR, Smith KC, et al. Retrospective analysis of historical, clinical, ultrasonographic, serum biochemical and haematological data in prognostic evaluation of liver disease. Equine Vet J 2003;35(6):542–7.
41. Pearson EG. Liver disease in the mature horse. Equine Vet Edu 1999;11(2):87–96.
42. Menzies-Gow NJ. Liver disease in the geriatric horse. In: Bertone J, editor. Equine geriatric medicine and surgery. Missouri: WB Saunders; 2006. p. 209–16.
43. Stratton-Phelps M, Fascetti AJ, Geor RJ. Nutritional support in selected metabolic, hepatic, urinary and musculoskeletal conditions. In: Robinson NE, editor. Current therapy in equine medicine 5. Philadelphia: WB Saunders; 2003. p. 718–20.
44. Schott HC, Kristi SP, Fitzgerald SD, et al. Chronic renal failure in 99 horses. Proceedings of the Annual Convention of the American Association of Equine Practitioners 1997;43:345–7.
45. Schott HC. Chronic renal failure in horses. Vet Clin North Am Equine Pract 2007;23(3):593–612.
46. Ralston SL. Evidence-based equine nutrition. Vet Clin North Am Equine Pract 2007;23:365–84.
47. Blumberg JB, Halpner AD. Antioxidant status and function: relationships to ageing and exercise. In: Papas AM, editor. Antioxidant status, diet, nutrition and health. Florida: CRC Press LLC; 1999. p. 251–75.
48. Marlin DJ, Dunnett CG, Deaton CM. The role of antioxidants. In: Proceedings of First BEVA and Waltham Nutrition Symposia. Harrogate, England. 17–18th September 2005. p. 39–48.
49. National Research Council (NRC). Nutrient requirements of horses. 6th revised edition. Washington (DC): National Academies Press; 2007. p. 183–201.

50. Gorecka R, Sitarska E, Klucinski W. Antioxidant parameters of horses according to age, sex, breed and environment. Pol J Vet Sci 2002;5(4):209–16.
51. Dixon PM, Railton DI, McGorum BC. Equine pulmonary disease: a case control study of 300 referred cases. Part 2: details of animals and of history and clinical findings. Equine Vet J 1995;27(6):422–7.
52. Denton CM, Marlin DJ, Smith NC, et al. Pulmonary epithelial lining fluid and plasma ascorbic acid concentrations in horses affected by recurrent airway obstruction. Am J Vet Res 2004;65:80–7.
53. Kirschvink N, Fievez L, Bougnet V, et al. Effect of nutritional antioxidant supplementation on systemic and pulmonary antioxidant status, airway inflammation and lung function in heaves-affected horses. Equine Vet J 2002;34(7):705–12.
54. Deaton CM, Marlin DJ, Smith NC, et al. Antioxidant supplementation in horses affected by recurrent airway obstruction. J Nutr 2004;134:2065S–7S.

Role of Diet and Feeding in Normal and Stereotypic Behaviors in Horses

Becky Hothersall, PhD*, Christine Nicol, MA, DPhil

KEYWORDS

• Equine behavior • Diet • Crib-biting • Stereotypy • Weaning
• Tryptophan • Insulin

In this article, the authors review the effects of diet on equine feeding behavior and feeding patterns, before considering the evidence that diet affects reactivity in horses. A growing body of work suggests that fat- and fiber-based diets may result in calmer patterns of behavior, and possible mechanisms that may underpin these effects are discussed.

In contrast, the authors highlight the current lack of evidence that herbal- or tryptophan-containing supplements influence equine behavior in any measurable way. The role of diet in the development of abnormal oral behaviors, particularly the oral stereotypy crib-biting, is discussed, and suggestions for future work are presented.

NORMAL BEHAVIOR

Modern Husbandry and Feeding Patterns

Surprisingly few studies have directly examined the effects of diet and feeding on behavior. Relative to the natural grazing state, modern nutritional management is associated with substantial changes in the nature, quantity, and frequency of feed consumption in horses, and it can be hard to separate diet from other aspects of management. For example, horses receiving a substantial proportion of their energy requirements as discrete meals of concentrate feeds are likely to be those that are regularly stabled. Stabling reduces opportunities not only for foraging but for various other behaviors in the horse's normal repertoire, such as locomotion and social contact. Behavioral changes associated with diet are likely to be confounded by frustration, excess energy reserves, or lack of stimulation. Experiments comparing groups of horses kept under similar conditions or examining the behavior of the same individuals over time can help to illustrate how diet and feeding patterns might alter behavior.

School of Veterinary Science, University of Bristol, Langford, North Somerset, BS40 5DU, UK
* Corresponding author.
E-mail address: b.hothersall@bris.ac.uk (B. Hothersall).

Vet Clin Equine 25 (2009) 167–181
doi:10.1016/j.cveq.2009.01.002
vetequine.theclinics.com

Many of these suggest that even if the provision of concentrate feeds removes the physiologic need to forage throughout the day, the motivation may remain. Through a series of experimental manipulations using fistulae and injection of nutrients, Ralston[1] concluded that oropharyngeal stimuli (taste, chewing, and smell), nutrient feedback, and changes in energy availability (measured as glucose and insulin levels) all exert some degree of control over feeding behavior in horses. Horses given ad libitum access to concentrate feed ate around 10 meals per day and engaged in multiple "nibbling" bouts (<150 g) between meals, which were rarely separated by more than 3 hours.[2] Behaviors like coprophagy (ingestion of feces), wood-chewing, and bed-eating are often considered to be aberrant but may simply reflect motivation to feed outside of mealtimes because of cues from gut fill, time since the last meal, or a drop in blood glucose. These behaviors may specifically represent attempts to ingest fiber because they are often ameliorated by greater provision of roughage. Bed-eating is most common in horses bedded on straw and those lacking access to fibrous feed.[3] Horses fed an all-concentrate diet spent significantly more time engaged in wood-chewing and coprophagy than horses fed only hay.[4] When Zeyner and colleagues[5] varied the amount of hay provided in addition to oats, they observed restless and nervous behavior in the horses with the lowest intake. Behavior was "quieter" and aggressive behavior at feeding time and coprophagy were eliminated when the diet contained more hay. In this particular study, total caloric intake was lower in horses fed less hay; thus, hunger may also have been an important determinant of behavior.

The common perception that excess energy from concentrate feeds causes "fizzy" or unwanted excitable behavior[6] may have a basis in digestive processes. Large high-starch meals result in marked fluctuations in plasma glucose and insulin after feeding,[7–9] which are likely to cause peaks and troughs of energy. Low-fiber high-starch diets are also associated with several digestive and metabolic disorders.[10] Many problems seem to stem from the horse being unable to regulate gut acidity during digestion and absorption.[11] After ingesting large cereal-based meals, the higher proportion of dry matter in the stomach contents slows the mixing of feed and gastric juice, leading to the potential for dysfermentation in the stomach.[12] The vastly decreased time spent chewing (compared with a grazing lifestyle) exacerbates matters by reducing opportunities to moisten food with alkaline saliva. As a consequence, large starchy meals can result in discomfort and even gastric colic[13] and are associated with gastric ulceration.[14] Large meals can overwhelm the capacity of the stomach and small intestine and increase transit rates of digesta; this leads to intense episodes of hydrolysable carbohydrate fermentation in the hindgut and a drop in pH.[4,15,16] Discomfort caused by the overflow of undigested carbohydrates into the hindgut has been linked with increased anxiety and aggression in rats[17] and with abnormal oral behaviors in horses. The latter was reduced by dietary supplementation with virginiamycin, an antibiotic that altered fecal pH.[18] Presumably, selective bacterial proliferation was halted, preventing rapid fermentation of sugar and starch.

Effects of Dietary Carbohydrate, Fiber, and Oil on Behavior

Although mimicking the natural eating patterns of the ancestral horse by providing prolonged access to a low-nutrient diet of hay or pasture seems to be desirable, horses in heavy work may not be able to sustain requirements for energy or specific nutrients through forage alone. Another approach to easing problems caused by meal feeding, limited roughage, and high starch levels is the replacement of some carbohydrates with fiber and oil as an energy source. This may be beneficial in minimizing glycemic and insulinemic fluctuations,[19] with more energy coming from gradual and sustained hindgut digestion of fermentable carbohydrates from fiber.[12] In human children, breakfast foods with a lower glycemic index are associated with improved performance in attention tasks;[20,21] a comparable response in horses might result in calmer or less distractible behavior. The slowing of feed intake and gastric emptying rates caused by the addition of fiber and oil[13,22] may decrease the behavioral need to forage by extending satiety and potentially reducing fermentation- or acidosis-related discomfort. Although the mechanisms have rarely been pinpointed, several small-scale studies have produced preliminary results indicating that behavior can indeed be influenced by oil or fiber supplementation (although Ralston[14] notes the confounding influence of a simple reduction in dietary starch in most studies). Coprophagy and aggressive behavior observed by Zeyner and colleagues[5] in horses fed a high-starch diet (despite high hay intake) was not seen if starch was partially replaced by fat. Holland and colleagues[23] reported reduced spontaneous locomotion and reactivity to sudden visual stimuli when horses were fed test diets containing additional fats; similar trends were seen in reactivity toward acoustic and pressure stimuli. Holland and colleagues[24] found that foals given access to a fat and fiber (FF) dietary supplement performed more grazing behavior and seemed to be less stressed than foals provided with a starch and sugar (SS)-based supplement in at least some of the weaning groups observed. The foals in the FF group also had lower cortisol levels before and after weaning, and it was suggested that this diet help foals to cope with the stress of weaning. In a pair of related trials, foals given an FF supplement fed more[25] and tended to be more relaxed[26] during a feed preference test than foals fed an SS supplement. Nicol and colleagues[27] examined behavior in a larger sample of 17 foals fed an FF or SS diet at weaning and during validated behavioral tests[28] administered after weaning. Weaning is widely accepted to be a stressful time for foals, and heart rates recorded by Visser and colleagues[29] indicated that the selected novel object and handling tests used were likely to have induced a state of mild fear. Under these conditions, foals in the FF diet group demonstrated consistently reduced reactivity and increased investigation. Behavior at weaning depended somewhat on whether foals were barn- or paddock-weaned; however, in both cases, locomotion was reduced in foals in the FF diet group. In behavioral tests at 9 to 10 months, foals fed an FF diet spent more time investigating and less time looking at a novel object (a slowly twirling golf umbrella). They also spent less time walking away from a novel person and completed a handling test in a shorter time than foals fed an SS diet. A related study by researchers at the University of Bristol recently found complementary results in 17 unweaned 3-month-old foals born to mares fed an FF or SS diet in the last trimester of pregnancy. In a similar novel object test, foals fed an FF diet spent a greater proportion of time walking toward the umbrella and investigating the environment than foals fed an SS diet; foals fed the SS diet spent longer looking at the umbrella without approaching (**Fig. 1**). Latency to approach the umbrella was shorter in foals fed the FF diet, and only individuals from this group touched it.[30] It is notable that although fearfulness and investigative behavior seemed to be affected in challenging situations, few differences were observed in the normal behavioral profiles of the groups at pasture in either of these studies.

Evidence for Diet-Mediated Physiologic Changes

In a companion study to that of Nicol and colleagues,[27] Wilson and colleagues[31] examined the effects of the two diets on various physiologic variables in the study foals. Fecal pH was not altered by diet, and gastric mucosa was healthy in both groups. When tested at 40 weeks of age, blood glucose rose more sharply after a meal in foals fed an SS diet, which had significantly higher total blood glucose

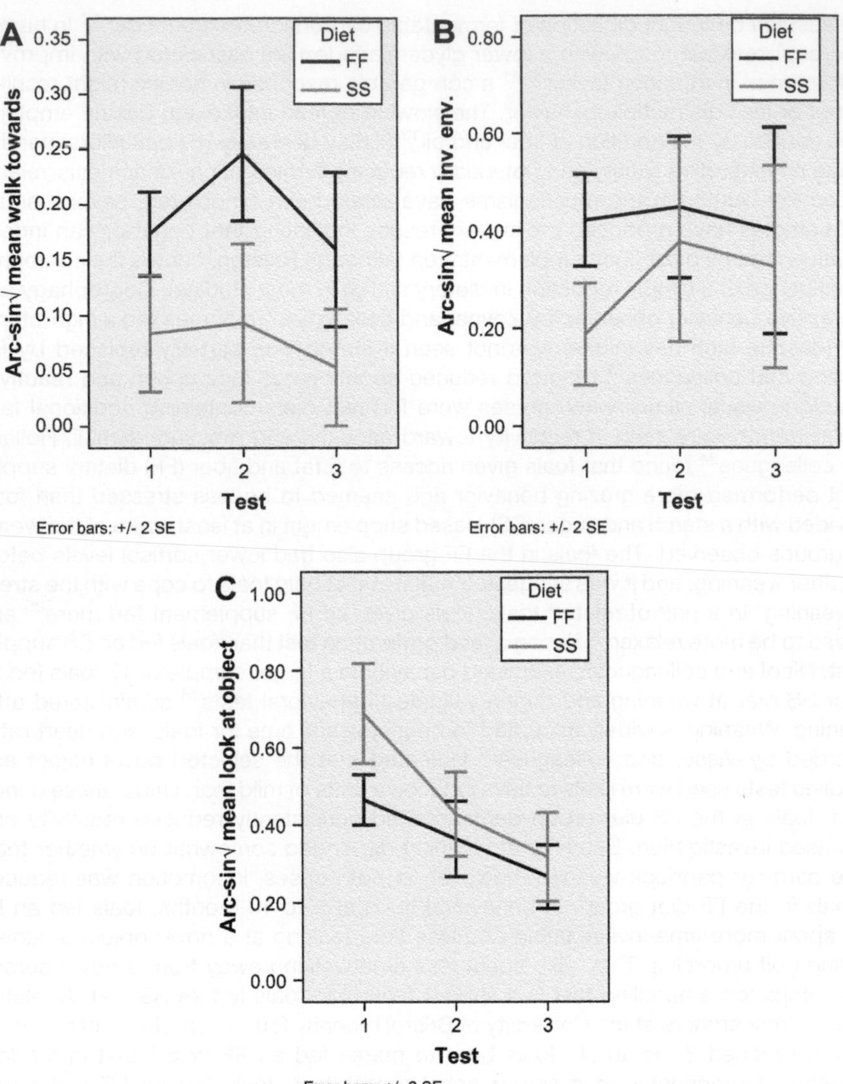

Fig. 1. Mean durations for foals fed a starch and sugar (SS) or fat and fiber (FF) diet for walking toward novel object (*A*), investigating the environment (inv. env.) (*B*), and looking at novel object across three novel object tests (*C*).

and lower total blood gastrin than foals fed an FF diet during the 6-hour period after a meal. Insulin levels also seemed to increase faster in foals fed an SS diet, but the difference did not reach significance. Because gastrin stimulates the secretion of gastric acid, the lack of difference in gastric mucosa condition despite increased gastrin production in foals fed an FF diet was slightly unexpected. Additional gastrin production may have been balanced by increased eating time, and therefore saliva production, in the foals fed an FF diet, however, increasing the water content of the swallowed bolus. This and the slower gastric emptying of the oily fibrous food would buffer the stomach from acid secretion and enhance mixing with gastric juices, reducing the risk for dysfermentation by stomach flora. Foals in the study of Nicol and colleagues[27] were not fed a standardized time before tests, however, and the 3-month-old foals[30] ate extremely small quantities of feed in proportion to their body weight. This makes it unlikely that the findings can be explained by glycemic response or digestive processes. Because gastric conditions also did not differ between the groups studied by Nicol and colleagues[27] and Wilson and colleagues,[31] the authors next consider some longer term mechanisms that may underlie the behavioral differences observed.

Glucoregulation and the Serotonergic System

Recent studies on insulin resistance[32] suggest that over a period of many months, FF diets may facilitate better glucoregulatory patterns, which could have consequent effects on brain function. The serotonergic system modulates mood and emotion, and low levels of serotonin are reliably associated with depression in laboratory animals and human beings.[33] Serotonin synthesis depends on the availability of its precursor amino acid tryptophan in the brain.[34] Increased insulin decreases plasma concentrations of most amino acids but raises levels of tryptophan. This also influences the extent to which free tryptophan is taken up by a transporter protein by reducing the availability of competing large neutral amino acids (LNAAs). The best proxy measure of central nervous system serotonin level is therefore the ratio of tryptophan to LNAA.[35,36] Although the groups did not differ overall in tryptophan/LNAA ratios, changes over the testing period suggest that foals fed the FF diet in the study of Wilson and colleagues[31] may have had a higher baseline tryptophan/LNAA ratio. It is also possible that glucoregulation may be further influenced by mare diet in gestation. Mares in late pregnancy undergo changes in insulin sensitivity that function to reserve glucose for fetal requirements,[10] and these were more evident in mares fed an FF diet than in mares fed an SS diet.[37] There is also preliminary evidence that mare diet in pregnancy can affect insulin sensitivity in foals: up to the age of 80 days, basal plasma glucose concentrations were higher, and insulin tended to be higher, in foals born to mares fed an SS diet compared with an FF diet during the last trimester. Foals of mares fed an SS diet also tended to have lower insulin sensitivity at 160 days. Notably, these results were seen despite all mares being fed the FF diet postpartum.[38]

Behavior Modification by Calmative Supplements

There is evidence that tryptophan depletion causes anxious and depressive behavior in rats[39] and enhanced tryptophan/LNAA ratios increase alertness and attention in human beings.[36] On the basis of such results, tryptophan is sold commercially as a calmative for horses, alone or in a mixture of vitamins, minerals (eg, magnesium), or herbs. A recent review concluded that although calming effects of supplementation have been demonstrated in some species, there is currently no scientific evidence for tryptophan's efficacy in horses; indeed, some studies indicate that at low doses, it may cause excitability.[40] Two studies subsequently confirmed that a commercial dose of tryptophan did not affect any behavioral parameters in response to social isolation, a novel person or object, or a handling test,[41,42] even though plasma tryptophan levels were raised.[42] Evidence from other species suggests that effects may be more apparent on aggression rather than on fear or reactivity,[40] however, and comparable tests have not yet been applied to the horse.

Other than tryptophan, calming supplements commonly include magnesium, complexes of B-vitamins, including thiamine, lecithins, essential amino acids, probiotics, and herbs or herbal extracts. The basis for including many of these ingredients seems to be that deficiencies can cause clinical problems; for example, severe thiamine deficiency can cause convulsions.[43] There is an absence of controlled trials indicating that high intake levels, conversely, have a calming effect, in addition to which commercial concentrate feed formulations mean that a horse's normal diet is, in many cases, likely to provide adequate levels of such nutrients. The inclusion of lecithins, probiotics, and, in some cases, "gastric herbs" indicates a growing recognition that digestive processes may contribute to excitable behavior. No studies have examined the effects of probiotic or lecithin supplements on behavior, but it is plausible that supplements improving digestive comfort might result in changes similar to those seen in FF versus SS feeds. Indeed, many high-starch cereal feeds now include a live yeast supplement, with the purpose of limiting undesirable changes within the intestinal environment associated with grain feeding. A supplement of *Saccharomyces cerevisiae* increased the concentration of viable yeast cells in the cecum and colon (with minimal effect on microbial counts) and modified pH, lactic acid, ammonia, acetate, and butyrate concentrations in horses fed a diet causing a starch overload.[44] Conversely, in a recent study of thoroughbred geldings, direct-fed lactic acid bacteria supplements had limited effects in preventing acidosis induced by increased starch intake.[45] A trend was noted toward an increase in fecal pH in horses fed a *Lactobacillus acidophilus* (but not a mixed *Lactobacillus*) supplement, however, and the researchers suggest that significant effects might be observed under more severely acidotic conditions.

Ralston[14] outlined the paucity of evidence for health benefits of equine herbal supplements. The capacity for herbal ingredients to modify behavior in horses has been subject to even less validation, and claims for calming effects are, at best, likely to be extrapolations from human beings or other species. Common ingredients include valerian, vervain, withania somnifera (Indian ginseng), passion flower, hops, chamomile, lemon balm, and peppermint. Although the calming effect of some of these ingredients is probably limited to their pleasant aroma, others may have potent effects and should be considered as medicines rather than food additives. For example, valerian is used as a sedative in human beings and contains several active compounds, including valerenic acid 5a, whose properties are similar to those of phenobarbitol.[46] Its effects on horses have not been studied adequately, but owners should be aware that valerian is banned during competition under International Federation for Equine Sport (FEI) rules.[14] A valerian-based supplement significantly diminished increases in heart rate variables in response to vibration stress[47] in pigs. Bioactive glycowithanolides, isolated from the roots of *Withania somnifera*, produced anxiolytic and antidepressant effects in rats similar to the benzodiazepine lorazepam and the tricyclic antidepressant imipramine, respectively.[48] Unlike synthetic drugs, the active ingredients of herbs are affected by unpredictable parameters, including growing conditions, harvesting and storage procedures, and contamination.[49] Whole plants may contain a range of active compounds. Given the chemical evidence for their pharmaceutic properties, there is a great deal of scope for herbal preparations to modify behavior; the concern is that it may be impossible to assess the dosage or even to identify what active ingredients are responsible for any behavioral changes observed. This obviously creates difficulties in predicting their effects and assessing their safety.

Overall, well-designed and peer-reviewed clinical trials are needed to assess clinical evidence of efficacy, side effects, and interactions with drugs before any calming supplements can be recommended for behavioral modification. Even if they prove effective, supplements many simply treat the symptoms and not the cause. To ensure good welfare, attempts to relieve behavioral problems should begin by examining whether aspects of management, such as diet, exercise, and the social environment, could be improved. Most evidence seems to suggest that mimicking the horse's natural eating patterns by lowering starch, increasing roughage, and feeding little and often is beneficial. Many owners have limited opportunities to implement such changes, however; access to pasture may be limited, particularly in the winter months, and, for a lot of people, work routines prohibit repeated feeding every few hours.

Foraging Enrichment

There is some evidence that implementing simple techniques of foraging enrichment may provide an alternative method for beneficially altering patterns of behavior in stabled horses. Horses provided with a feed-dispensing foraging device filled with high-fiber pelleted feed spent around 14% of their time engaged in using it. When the device was present, they spent significantly less time moving, ingesting concentrates, standing, and nosing their bedding.[50] Concerns have been voiced, however, that frustration behavior may be directed toward such devices when they become empty.[51,52] Horses fed more frequently and for longer in total during trials in which multiple rather than single types of feed were available. Similar patterns were seen whether concentrates or forages were used,[53–55] and with concentrates, provision of multiple feeds also resulted in horses spending less time standing.[54] Horses offered a choice between stables containing multiple or single forages generally entered the closest stable but then moved to the one offering multiple forages.[56] Overall, there seems to be promise in using foraging enrichments to replicate patterns of more natural patch foraging behavior. Particularly when these result in prolonged roughage intake, they are likely to promote good welfare by combining digestive benefits with provision of stimulation and opportunities for activity. Studies examining how well these effects persist over longer periods would be helpful.

ABNORMAL ORAL BEHAVIOR

In comparison to the surprisingly limited literature regarding diet and normal behavior in horses, there is now a substantial body of research implicating diet and feeding in the etiology of abnormal oral behavior. Crib-biting and wood-chewing are considered abnormal because they appear, at first sight, to serve no function. Crib-biting occurs when a fixed object is grasped by the incisor teeth, the lower neck muscles contract to retract the larynx caudally, and air is drawn into the cranial esophagus, producing a characteristic grunt.[57] Wind-sucking involves the same suite of movements, except that the horse does not actually grasp a fixed object. Frequently, the terms are used interchangeably, but the authors use the term *crib-biting* to cover both. Once developed by an individual horse, crib-biting tends to become increasingly fixed and rigid in form and orientation over time. It is also a behavior that is performed repetitively, sometimes excessively so. Nicol and colleagues[58] reported on one foal that performed crib-biting for nearly 50% of the time. Clegg and colleagues[59] observed crib-biting for 30 seconds in every 5-minute period for 22 hours per day and, by extrapolation, estimated that the horses in their study performed an average of 1470 crib-bites during each 22-hour stabled period. It is clear that crib-biting meets the key criteria of repetitiveness, invariance, and apparent lack of function used to define behaviors as stereotypic.[60] Wood-chewing is a more varied and flexible behavior pattern that is sometimes wrongly called crib-biting by horse owners. Scientists would argue that it lacks the invariant movements of a true stereotypy, and it is perhaps best described as a redirected behavior. Wood-chewing is a behavior worthy of study, however, because it often precedes or is associated with crib-biting.[61] Waters and colleagues[61] found that some 30.3% of young horses showed wood-chewing; however, of the horses that developed crib-biting, some 74% had previously shown wood-chewing.

Prevalence of Abnormal Oral Behavior

Many cross-sectional surveys have estimated the prevalences of these oral behaviors. Nicol[62] summarized the results of some early surveys performed in the United Kingdom,[63] Italy,[64] Sweden,[65] and Canada.[66] Overall mean prevalence for crib-biting was 4.13%, and for wood-chewing, it was 11.78%.[62] Subsequent reports have indicated an owner-declared prevalence of approximately 2.5% for wind-sucking in UK thoroughbreds,[67] 2.9% for crib-biting, and 1.1% for wood-chewing in 25 Italian riding centers;[68] a prevalence of 3% for aerophagia (wind-sucking), 2.2% for crib-biting, and 1.3% for wood-chewing in 690 horses observed at a veterinary school in Iran;[69] and an owner-declared prevalence of 3.8% for crib-biting and 3.8% for wood-chewing in a survey of 312 nonracing horses in Prince Edward Island.[70] By far the lowest prevalence was reported by Bachmann and colleagues,[71] who found that just 3.5% of a Swiss population of horses showed either oral or locomotor stereotypy.

Even the higher estimates obtained in these cross-sectional surveys are substantially lower than those observed in a 4-year longitudinal study of 225 foals, in which crib-biting was initiated by 10.5% of horses at a median age of 20 weeks and wood-chewing by 30.3% of horses at a median age of 30 weeks.[61] The higher figures observed in this study compared with the cross-sectional surveys of adult populations suggest that some young horses cease wood-chewing and crib-biting as they mature or that these individuals are differentially lost to the adult population.

Diet and Feeding Practices as Risk Factors

Crib-biting has not been reported in studies of feral or free-living domestic horses, but it has been observed when Przewalski horses are kept in captivity,[72] suggesting that domestic management practices are a necessary cause of the behavior. Increasing evidence suggests that it is the interaction between feeding practices and digestive function that has a primary influence on the development of crib-biting. The evidence for this comes from multiple sources. First, crib-biting is temporally associated with the delivery of concentrated feed. The rate of crib-biting in horses fed concentrates once daily rose dramatically in the period immediately after feeding, peaking some 4 to 8 hours after meal delivery.[59] This was in stark contrast to the diurnal pattern of the locomotor stereotypy weaving, which exhibited a peak frequency just before feeding.[59,73] Weaving occurs when confined horses anticipate an exciting or stressful event but are frustrated by their inability to leave the confined area. Weaving is therefore stimulated by events like the sight or sound of feed preparation or the departure of companions. Correspondingly, dividing the daily concentrate ration into smaller more frequent meals has been shown to reduce the overall incidence of crib-biting but to increase the incidence of weaving.[74] Factors that reduce the general aversiveness of the confined environment, particularly providing increased visual access to other horses, can significantly reduce the incidence of weaving.[75,76]

In contrast, general enrichment of the stabled environment seems to have little effect on the incidence of crib-biting.[62] Rather, the risk for crib-biting is increased by a low-forage or high-grain diet [57,61,65,71] and is decreased by the use of straw bedding, possibly because this may function as an additional source of dietary fiber.[57,70] Crib-biting is also associated with some forms of colic,[77–79] gastric ulceration,[58] and altered gut-transit time.[80,81] Most of these studies have been cross-sectional in nature; thus, conclusions about cause and effect have to be drawn with great care. A longitudinal study has also shown that feeding practices have a significant effect on the relative rate of development of oral stereotypies, however. Waters and colleagues[61] found that feeding grain-based feeds immediately after weaning resulted in a fourfold increase in risk.

Causation of Crib-Biting

Because horses secrete acid into the stomach continuously, it has been suggested that wood-chewing and crib-biting may be adaptive attempts by the horse to reduce excessive acidity. When horses are kept at pasture, stomach acidity is naturally buffered by a regular and continual throughput of forage and by the release of alkaline saliva. In contrast, when horses are kept under conditions in which most of their daily intake is supplied by means of concentrated grain-based rations, problems with foregut irritation can arise. The horse has a limited capacity to digest starch in the small intestine, and large grain-based meals, which contain rapidly fermentable material and a high dry matter content, can result in dysfermentation in the stomach.[13] Additionally, such meals require less biting and chewing; as a result, overall food consumption time is much less than for a horse with ad libitum forage. Horses produce saliva only when biting or chewing;[82] thus, horses fed restricted forage also produce lower amounts of neutralizing saliva. It has been proposed that horses that have foregut acidity problems may wood-chew or crib-bite in an attempt to stimulate additional saliva production.[83] This hypothesis has not been tested directly, but there is some indirect evidence in support. First, the stomachs of crib-biting foals show significantly greater evidence of inflammation and early ulceration than those of normal foals.[58] Second, feeding antacids reduces these clinical signs and also tends to result in a reduction in crib-biting behavior.[58,84] Third, crib-biting results in the production of small amounts of saliva from the submandibular gland.[85] It is important to note that even if crib-biting is an adaptive attempt by the horse to produce saliva, it may not be entirely successful in solving the underlying problem. The repetitive nature of stereotypies results from the fact that they are attempts to solve problems rather than solutions in themselves. If a recently captured tiger paced once around its enclosure and then found an escape route, its pacing would never develop into the stereotypic route-tracing commonly seen in captive large carnivores. It is the fact that no solution exists that leads an initially adaptive behavior to become fixed, invariant, and increasingly functionless.[86]

The Role of Stress

Previous studies have examined possible links between stress and stereotypy in horses. These have generally been inconclusive, with no differences in plasma cortisol concentrations or average heart rates between crib-biting, weaving, and control horses detected[59] and with inconsistent effects when comparing concentrations of plasma beta-endorphin.[80,87,88] The difficulty with these studies is the lack of information about the physiologic status of the control horses and the stereotypic horses in the period before the onset of stereotypy. Horses with a predisposition to develop stereotypy may be more reactive, or have different digestive physiology, than horses with no such predisposition. The onset and performance of stereotypy may alter the physiology of stereotypic horses to varying degrees, perhaps to levels that no longer differ significantly from those of normal horses. Therefore, longitudinal studies of individual horses, initiated before the onset of stereotypy, are needed to understand causality, but there are precious few of these. Waters and colleagues[61] noted that stressful weaning methods, particularly methods that involved the isolation of foals at weaning, significantly increased the risk for abnormal behavior. This strongly suggests that stress may play a role, but the authors suggest that this could be primarily by means of a modulation of normal feeding behavior. The newly isolated young foal, suddenly deprived of its milk-based nutrients and severely stressed by the absence of its mother, is unlikely to chew its forage rations calmly. The isolated foal is therefore particularly at risk for the gut-related problems outlined previously. Even short periods of not eating can lead to stomach acidity, early onset of ulceration,[89] and an increased risk for some types of colic.[79]

Individual Predisposition

Not all foals exposed to the same combinations of risk factors develop abnormal behavior, suggesting that biologic predisposition interacts with environmental risk. Differences in suckling motivation are a potential source, or consequence, of varying predisposition, which could interact with all the major identified environmental risk factors for abnormal oral behavior: feeding, weaning, and mare rank. Suckling influences the acidity of the stomach and the digestive physiology of the foal in complex ways,[90–92] and foals with different suckling patterns may vary in their tolerance to concentrate or grain-based feeds. In a prospective study of the foal behavior, Nicol and Badnell-Waters[93] found that 42 of 186 foals developed abnormal oral behavior (wood-chewing, crib-biting, or both) after weaning. These 42 foals had, before weaning, spent more time suckling and twice as much time teat nuzzling as other foals. It is possible that foals with the greatest suckling motivation may be most affected by sudden weaning methods that instantly prevent suckling.

SUMMARY

The start of a coherent body of work examining links between diet and equine behavior is long overdue, but the mechanisms underlying some of the effects of diet on reactivity would be easier to understand if future studies examined the role of different dietary components separately. There is also a need for a greater understanding of the mechanisms whereby diet may influence the development of abnormal oral behavior. Understanding causality is important, and further longitudinal studies are needed to fill in current gaps in knowledge.

REFERENCES

1. Ralston SL. Controls of feeding in horses. J Anim Sci 1984;59:1354–61.
2. Ralston SL, Vandenbroek G, Baile CA. Feed-intake patterns and associated blood-glucose, free fatty-acid and insulin changes in ponies. J Anim Sci 1979; 49:838–45.
3. Mills DS, Eckley S, Cooper JJ. Thoroughbred bedding preferences, associated behaviour differences and their implications for equine welfare. J Anim Sci 2000;70:95–106.
4. Willard JG, Willard JC, Wolfram SA, et al. Effects of diet on cecal pH and feeding behavior of horses. J Anim Sci 1977;45:87–93.
5. Zeyner AC, Geißler C, Dittrich A. Effects of hay intake and feeding sequence on variables in faeces and faecal water (dry matter, pH value, organic acids, ammonia, buffering capacity) of horses. J Anim Physiol Anim Nutr 2004;88:7–19.
6. Jansson A, Nyman S, Lindholm A, et al. Effects of dietary starch and sugar on exercise metabolism. Equine Vet J 2002;(Suppl 34):17–21.
7. Harris PA. Hints on nutrition for optimal growth. In: Proceedings of the First BEVA and Waltham Nutrition Symposia "Equine Nutrition for All." Harrogate (UK); 2005. p. 63.

8. Stull CL, Rodiek AV. Responses of blood glucose, insulin and cortisol concentrations to common equine diets. J Nutr 1988;118:206–13.
9. Pagan JD, Harris PA, Kennedy MAP, et al. Feed type and intake affects glycaemic response in Thoroughbred horses. In: Proceedings of the Equine Nutrition and Physiology Symposium. Raleigh (NC); 1999. p. 149.
10. Hoffman RM. Carbohydrate metabolism in horses. Available at: In: Ralston SL, Hintz HF, editors. Recent advances in equine nutrition, Vol 1. Ithaca (NY): International Veterinary Information Service; 2003 www.ivis.org; 2003. Accessed June 30, 2008.
11. Mills DS, Clarke A. Housing, management and welfare. In: Waran N, editor. The welfare of horses, Vol 1. Dordrecht: Klewer Academic Publishers; 2002. p. 77–97.
12. Harris PA, Coenen M, Frape DL, et al. Nutrition and metabolic disease. In: Higgins A, Synder J, editors. Equine manual. London: Elsevier Saunders; 2006. p. 151–222.
13. Harris PA, Arkell K. How understanding the digestive process can help minimise digestive disturbances due to diet and feeding practices. In: Proceedings of the First BEVA and Waltham Nutrition Symposia "Equine Nutrition for All." Harrogate (UK); 2005. p. 9.
14. Ralston SL. Evidence-based equine nutrition. Vet Clin North Am Equine Pract 2007;23:365–84.
15. Clarke LL, Roberts MC, Argenzio RA. Feeding and digestive problems in horses: physiologic responses to a concentrated meal. Vet Clin North Am Equine Pract 1990;6:433–50.
16. Rowe JB, Lees MJ, Pethick DW. Prevention of acidosis and laminitis associated with grain feeding in horses. J Nutr 1994;124(Suppl 12):2742S–4S.
17. Hanstock TL, Clayton EL, Li KM, et al. Anxiety and aggression associated with the fermentation of carbohydrates in the hindgut of rats. Physiol Behav 2004;82: 357–68.
18. Johnson KG, Tyrrell J, Rowe JB, et al. Behavioural changes in stabled horses given nontherapeutic levels of virginiamycin. Equine Vet J 1998;30:139–43.
19. Williams CA, Kronfeld DS, Staniar WB, et al. Plasma glucose and insulin responses of Thoroughbred mares fed a meal high in starch and sugar or fat and fiber. J Anim Sci 2001;79:2196–201.
20. Mahoney CR, Taylor HA, Kanarek RB, et al. Effect of breakfast composition on cognitive processes in elementary school children. Physiol Behav 2005;85: 635–45.
21. Benton D, Maconie A, Williams C. The influence of the glycaemic load of breakfast on the behaviour of children in school. Physiol Behav 2007;92:717–24.
22. Houpt KA. Ingestive behavior. Vet Clin North Am Equine Pract 1990;6:319–38.
23. Holland JL, Kronfeld DS, Meacham TN. Behavior of horses is affected by soy lecithin and corn oil in the diet. J Anim Sci 1996;74:1252–5.
24. Holland JL, Kronfeld DS, Hoffman RM, et al. Weaning stress is affected by nutrition and weaning methods. Pferdeheilkunde 1996;12:257–60.
25. Ordakowski AL, Davidson HPB, Redgate SE, et al. Characteristics of foal feeding behaviour. In: Proceedings of the WALTHAM International Symposium. Bangkok; 2003. p. 30.
26. Redgate SE, Ordakowski-Burk AL, Davidson HPB, et al. A preliminary study to investigate the effect of diet on the behaviour of weanling horses. In: Proceedings of the International Society for Applied Ethology. Helsinki, Finland; 2004. p. 154.
27. Nicol CJ, Badnell-Waters AJ, Bice R, et al. The effects of diet and weaning method on the behaviour of young horses. Appl Anim Behav Sci 2005;95:205–21.

28. Visser EK, van Reenen CG, Hopster H, et al. Quantifying aspects of young horses' temperament: consistency of behavioural variables. Appl Anim Behav Sci 2001;74:241–58.
29. Visser EK, van Reenen CG, van der Werf JTN, et al. Heart rate and heart rate variability during a novel object test and a handling test in young horses. Physiol Behav 2002;76:289–96.
30. Hothersall B, Nicol C, Kelland A, et al. Effects of diet on learning and responsive behaviour of young foals. In: Proceedings of the 4th International Equitation Science Conference. Dublin, Ireland, 2008.
31. Wilson AD, Badnell-Waters AJ, Bice R, et al. The effects of diet on blood glucose, insulin, gastrin and the serum tryptophan: large neutral amino acid ratio in foals. Vet J 2007;174:139–46.
32. Treiber KH, Boston RC, Kronfeld DS, et al. Insulin resistance and compensation in Thoroughbred weanlings adapted to high-glycemic meals. J Anim Sci 2005;83:2357–64.
33. Schloss P, Williams DC. The serotonin transporter: a primary target for antidepressant drugs. J Psychoparmacol 1998;12:115–21.
34. Schaechter JD, Wurtman RJ. Serotonin release varies with brain tryptophan levels. Brain Res 1990;532:203–10.
35. Fernstrom JD. Branched-chain amino acids and brain function. J Nutr 2005;135: 1539S–46S.
36. Markus CR, Jonkman LM, Lammers JHCM, et al. Evening intake of alpha-lactalbumin increases plasma tryptophan availability and improves morning alertness and brain measures of attention. Am J Clin Nutr 2005;81:1026–33.
37. Hoffman RM, Kronfeld DS, Cooper WS, et al. Glucose clearance in grazing mares is affected by diet, pregnancy, and lactation. J Anim Sci 2003;81:1764–71.
38. George LA, Staniar WB, Treiber KH, et al. Insulin sensitivity and glucose dynamics in foals as influenced by age and maternal diet during gestation. In: Proceedings of the Equine Science Symposium. Hunt Valley (MD); 2007. p. 5.
39. Blokland A, Lieben C, Deutz NE. Anxiogenic and depressive-like effects, but no cognitive deficits, after repeated moderate tryptophan depletion in the rat. J Psychopharmacol 2002;16:39–49.
40. Grimmett A, Sillence MN. Calmatives for the excitable horse: a review of L-tryptophan. Vet J 2005;170:24–32.
41. Malmkvist J, Christensen JW. A note on the effects of a commercial tryptophan product on horse reactivity. Appl Anim Behav Sci 2007;107:361–6.
42. Noble GK, Brockwell YM, Munn KJ, et al. Effects of a commercial dose of L-tryptophan on plasma tryptophan concentrations and behaviour in horses. Equine Vet J 2008;40:51–6.
43. Read DH, Harrington DD. Experimentally induced thiamine-deficiency in beagle dogs—clinical observations. Am J Vet Res 1981;42:984–91.
44. Medina B, Girard ID, Jacotot E, et al. Effect of a preparation of Saccharomyces cerevisiae on microbial profiles and fermentation patterns in the large intestine of horses fed a high fiber or a high starch diet. J Anim Sci 2002;80:2600–9.
45. Swyers KL, Burk AO, Harstock TG, et al. Effects of direct-fed microbial supplementation on digestibility and fermentation end-products in horses fed low- and high-starch concentrates. J Anim Sci 2008;86:2596–608.
46. Klepser TB, Klepser MB. Unsafe and potentially safe herbal therapies. Am J Health Syst Pharm 1999;56:125–38.
47. Peeters E, Driessen B, Steegmans R, et al. Effect of supplemental tryptophan, vitamin E, and a herbal product on responses by pigs to vibration. J Anim Sci 2004;82:2410–20.

48. Bhattacharya SK, Bhattacharya A, Sairam K, et al. Anxiolytic-antidepressant activity of Withania somnifera glycowithanolides: an experimental study. Phytomedicine 2000;7:463–9.
49. Davidson HPB. Herbs—a sage of all wisdom or a waste of thyme? In: Proceedings of the British Equine Veterinary Association Specialist Days on Behaviour and Nutrition. Newmarket (UK); 1999. p. 32.
50. Winskill LC, Waran NK, Young RJ. The effect of a foraging device (a modified 'Edinburgh foodball') on the behaviour of the stabled horse. Appl Anim Behav Sci 1996;48:25–35.
51. Henderson JV, Waran NK. Reducing equine stereotypies using an Equiball. Anim Welf 2001;10:73–80.
52. Goodwin D, Davidson HPB, Harris P. A note on behaviour of stabled horses with foraging devices in mangers and buckets. Appl Anim Behav Sci 2007;105: 238–43.
53. Goodwin D, Davidson HPB, Harris P. Foraging enrichment for stabled horses: effects on behaviour and selection. Equine Vet J 2002;34:686–91.
54. Goodwin D, Davidson HPB, Harris P. Sensory varieties in concentrate diets for stabled horses: effects on behaviour and selection. Appl Anim Behav Sci 2005; 90:337–49.
55. Thorne JB, Goodwin D, Kennedy MJ, et al. Foraging enrichment for individually housed horses: practicality and effects on behaviour. Appl Anim Behav Sci 2005;94:149–64.
56. Goodwin D, Davidson HPB, Harris P. Foraging enrichment for individually housed horses: practicality and effects on behaviour. Vet Rec 2007;160:548.
57. McGreevy PD, Cripps PJ, French NP, et al. Management factors associated with stereotypic and redirected behavior in the thoroughbred horse. Equine Vet J 1995;7:86–91.
58. Nicol CJ, Davidson HPB, Harris PA, et al. Study of crib-biting and gastric inflammation and ulceration in young horses. Vet Rec 2002;151:658.
59. Clegg HA, Buckley P, Friend MA, et al. The ethological and physiological characteristics of cribbing and weaving horses. Appl Anim Behav Sci 2008;109:68–76.
60. Mason G. Stereotypies—a critical review. Anim Behav 1991;41:1015–37.
61. Waters AJ, Nicol CJ, French NP. Factors influencing the development of stereotypic and redirected behaviours in young horses: findings of a four year prospective epidemiological study. Equine Vet J 2002;34:572–9.
62. Nicol CJ. Stereotypies and their relationship to management. In: Harris P, Gomarsall G, Davidson N, et al, editors. British Equine Veterinary Association Specialist Day on Behaviour and Nutrition. Harrogate: Equine Veterinary Journal; 1999. p. 11.
63. McGreevy PD, French NP, Nicol CJ. The prevalence of abnormal behaviors in dressage, eventing and endurance horses in relation to stabling. Vet Rec 1995; 137:36–7.
64. Borroni A, Canali E. Behavioural problems in Thoroughbred horses reared in Italy. In: Proceedings of the 26th International Congress on Applied Ethology. 1993. p. 43.
65. Redbo I, Redbo-Torstensson P, Odberg FO, et al. Factors affecting behavioural disturbances in race-horses. Anim Sci 1998;66:475–81.
66. Luescher U, McKeown D, Dean H. A cross-sectional study on compulsive behavior (stable vices) in horses. Equine Vet J 1998;(Suppl 27):14–8.
67. Mills DS, Alston RD, Rogers V, et al. Factors associated with the prevalence of stereotypic behaviour amongst Thoroughbred horses passing through auctioneer sales. Appl Anim Behav Sci 2002;78:115–24.

68. Normando S, Canali E, Ferrante V, et al. Behavioral problems in Italian saddle horses. J Equine Vet Sci 2002;22:117–20.
69. Ahmadinejad M, Habibi P. Abnormal behaviour of the horses in Tehran's riding clubs. Ippologia 2005;16:33–5.
70. Christie JL, Hewson CJ, Riley CB, et al. Management factors affecting stereotypies and body condition score in nonracing horses in Prince Edward Island. Can Vet J 2006;47:136–43.
71. Bachmann I, Audige L, Stauffacher M. Risk factors associated with behavioural disorders of crib-biting, weaving and box-walking in Swiss horses. Equine Vet J 2003;35:158–63.
72. Boyd L. Behavior problems of equids in zoos. Vet Clin North Am 1986;2:653–63.
73. Ninomiya S. Social leaning and stereotypy in horses. Behav Processes 2007;76: 22–3.
74. Cooper JJ, McAll N, Johnson S, et al. The short-term effects of increasing meal frequency on stereotypic behaviour of stabled horses. Appl Anim Behav Sci 2005;90:351–64.
75. Cooper JJ, McDonald L, Mills DS. The effect of increasing visual horizons on stereotypic weaving: implications for the social housing of stabled horses. Appl Anim Behav Sci 2000;69:67–83.
76. McAfee LM, Mills DS, Cooper JJ. The use of mirrors for the control of stereotypic weaving behaviour in the stabled horse. Appl Anim Behav Sci 2002;78:159–73.
77. Hillyer MH, Taylor FGR, Proudman CJ, et al. Case control study to identify risk factors for simple colonic obstruction and distension colic in horses. Equine Vet J 2002;34:455–63.
78. Archer DC, Proudman CJ, Pinchbeck GL, et al. Entrapment of the small intestine in the epiploic foramen in horses: a retrospective analysis of 71 cases recorded between 1991 and 2001. Vet Rec 2004;155:793–7.
79. Archer DC, Pinchbeck GL, French NP, et al. Risk factors for epiploic foramen entrapment colic: an international study. Equine Vet J 2008;40:224–30.
80. McGreevy P, Nicol C. Physiological and behavioral consequences associated with short-term prevention of crib-biting in horses. Physiol Behav 1998;65:15–23.
81. McGreevy PD, Webster AJF, Nicol CJ. Study of the behaviour, digestive efficiency and gut transit times of crib-biting horses. Vet Rec 2001;148:592–6.
82. Alexander F. A study of parotid salivation in the horse. J Physiol 1966;184:646–56.
83. Nicol CJ. Understanding equine stereotypies. Equine Vet J 1999;(Suppl 28):20–5.
84. Mills DS, Macleod CA. The response of crib-biting and windsucking in horses to dietary supplementation with an antacid mixture. Ippologia 2002;13:33–41.
85. Moeller BA, McCall CA, Silverman SJ, et al. Estimation of saliva production in crib-biting and normal horses. J Equine Vet Sci 2008;28:85–90.
86. Rushen J, Lawrence A, Terlouw T. The motivational basis of stereotypies. In: Lawrence AB, Rushen J, editors. Stereotypic animal behaviour: fundamentals and applications to welfare. Wallingford: CABI Publishing; 1993. p. 41–64.
87. Gillham SB, Dodman NH, Shuster L, et al. The effect of diet on cribbing behavior and plasma beta-endorphin in horses. Appl Anim Behav Sci 1994;41:147–53.
88. Pell SM, McGreevy PD. A study of cortisol and beta-endorphin levels in stereotypic and normal Thoroughbreds. Appl Anim Behav Sci 1999;64:81–90.
89. Murray MJ, Eichorn ES. Effects of intermittent feed deprivation, intermittent feed deprivation with ranitidine administration, and stall confinement with ad libitum access to hay on gastric ulceration in horses. Am J Vet Res 1996;57:1599–603.
90. Baker SJ, Gerring EL. Gastric pH monitoring in healthy, suckling pony foals. Am J Vet Res 1993;54:959–64.

91. Sanchez LC, Lester GD, Merritt AM. Effect of ranitidine on intragastric pH in clinically normal neonatal foals. J Am Vet Med Assoc 1998;212:1407–12.
92. Murray MJ. Pathophysiology of peptic disorders in foals and horses: a review. Equine Vet J 1999;(Suppl 29):14–8.
93. Nicol CJ, Badnell-Waters AJ. Suckling behaviour in domestic foals and the development of abnormal oral behaviour. Anim Behav 2005;70:21–9.

Index

Note: Page numbers of article titles are in **boldface** type.

Vet Clin Equine 25 (2009) 183–191
doi:10.1016/S0749-0739(09)00027-3

D

E

G

H

I

R

S

Printed and bound by CPI Group (UK) Ltd, Croydon, CR0 4YY
03/10/2024
01040452-0020